Praise for *Down There the Wise Woman Way*

"A comprehensive, comforting, and easy-to-read guide on pelvic health. The perfect combination of current modern treatment practices with ageless goddess wisdom."

Mary O'Dwyer, Senior Teaching Fellow, Bond University

"A one-of-a-kind book. A gentle guide to connecting with ourselves and our well-being, both emotional and physical."

Kathi Keville, *Women's Herbs, Women's Health*

"Susun Weed is one of the most important, informative, and inspirational writers of our time. Her new book, like all her others, is an essential guide to anyone seeking optimum health."

Corinna Wood, Red Moon Herbs

"A fabulous, amazing, and world-changing book. It will help us take back the night, the day, and our rightful place in the world – and in our own hearts and wombs." **Susan McLaughlin**

"Susun's newest book is intuitive, well-researched, and a fine example of integrative medicine. It bridges the gaps between natural healing and mainstream medicine, leaving nothing out."

Feather Jones, RH, AHG, herbalist, author

"Just when I thought there were too many women's health care books, one appears with a fresh perspective. This is a book of choices. Susun provides the mainstream perspective, a deeper understanding of pelvic conditions, and all the treatment options. Unlike most texts, this one is a delight to peruse. I enjoyed it cover to cover." **Sharol Tilgner**, *Herbal Medicine from the Heart*

"A crucial and empowering book. You clearly explain how my body works so I can understand and pick the best options for my health." **Maria Barresi**

"Another gifted book in the Wise Woman Series, filled with 'secrets', recipes, and wisdom. Like all of her books, its written from the heart, well researched and fully engaging. Susun brings a truth and honesty to her writings, and teachings, that is a rare gift."

Rosemary Gladstar, *Herbal Healing for Women*

"Susun brings light to all that is down there." **Pam Hyde-Nakai**

"A no-nonsense practical guide that puts the power of our health into our own hands. As with Weed's other books, this should be up there on everyone's wellness bookshelf." **Aviva Romm**, MD

"Another exciting herbal from Weed! Well-organized, comprehensive, and easy to use. Should be in every library and every home." **Gretchen Gould**, *Amazing Grease*

"Critical health information wrapped in the wisdom of our herbal traditions creates a guide useful for anyone interested in a grounded approach to an often overwhelming topic."
Bevin Clare, Tai Sophia Institute

"So clear, concise, and straight to the point, I couldn't put it down. What a gift to us all!" **Chinmayo Forro**, Alaskan midwife

"I found your work when I was in my 40's, facing a hysterectomy for fibroids, endometriosis, and cysts. Chaste tree berries made me healthy! I recommend your books to those with fertility problems, female issues, and pesky 'down there' problems."
Anonymous

"Rich in research, thought provoking, seasoned with stories and accessibe herbal remedies, this is a superbly useful reference book. Susun is a word weaver who can help you craft your own unique healing path, the Wise Woman Way."
Robin Rose Bennett, *Healing Magic: A Green Witch Guidebook to Consciouis Living*

"This long-awaited next volume in the Wise Woman Herbal Series lets us look at and laugh about what we speak of the least."
Andrea and Matthias Reisen, Healing Spirits Herbs

"Thank for delving so deeply down there, Susun. You really get to the root of things." **Doug Eliott**, *Wild Roots*

"I celebrate a new book by one of the most original herbal voices of our time. Poetic and plain-spoken. A welcome addition."
Stephen Harrod Buhner, *Lost Language of the Plants*

Down There

Sexual and Reproductive Health

The Wise Woman Way

Susun S. Weed

Other Books by Susun S. Weed

Wise Woman Herbal for the Childbearing Year
in English, French, German, Spanish, and Dutch

Healing Wise, the Big Green Herbal
in English and Japanese

Breast Cancer? Breast Health! The Wise Woman Way
in English, German, and Dutch

New Menopausal Years the Wise Woman Way
in English and Dutch

Down There

The Wise Woman Way

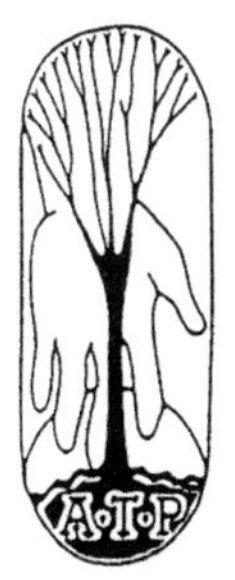

Ash Tree Publishing
PO Box 64
Woodstock NY 12498
www.AshTreePublishing.com

All information in this *Wise Woman Herbal* is based on the experiences of the author and other professionals. It is shared with the understanding that you accept responsibility for your own unique health and well-being. The results of any treatment suggested herein cannot always be anticipated and never guaranteed. The author and publisher are not responsible for any adverse effects or consequences resulting from the use of any remedies, procedures, or preparations included in this *Wise Woman Herbal.*

© 2011 Susun S. Weed

Illustrations, except as noted below, © 2011 Alan McKnight.
© 2011 for individual artists: page xx © Sophie Breillat;
page 2 © AsaRose Bond; page 28 © Derby Stewart-Arnsolen;
pages 50, 142 © Rhonda Thomas; page 66 © Tanya Pineda;
page 78 © A. Hinton; pages 84, 272, 286 © Crystalyn Abercrombie;
pages 86, 88, 89, 97, 104 © Betty Dodson; page 102 © Silvermoon;
pages 120, 302, 320 © Linda Wiebe; page 170 © Katerine Aubry;
page 206 © Kristen Kennedy; page 252 © Kate Zamarchi;
page 288 © Rose Weissman; page 318 © Livia Cavaliaro

Cover background photo and calligraphy: Alan McKnight
Cover photo of Kwan Yin statue (Moon Yin): Justine Smythe
MoonYin sculpture © 2011 Robin Noll
Cover design: Susun S. Weed

Printed and bound in the United States of America on recycled, non-chlorine-bleached paper. Green Press Initiative supporter.

Ash Tree Publishing, PO Box 64, Woodstock NY 12498
www.AshTreePublishing.com

Publisher's Cataloging-in-Publication
(Provided by Quality Books, Inc.)

Weed, Susun S.
Down there : sexual and reproductive health the wise woman way / Susun S. Weed ; illustrator, Alan McKnight.
p. cm. – (Wise woman herbal series ; 5th)
Includes bibliographical references and index.
LCCN 2010934336
ISBN-13: 978-1-888123-13-5
ISBN-10: 1-888123-13-3

1. Sexual health. 2. Reproductive health.
I. Title. II. Series: Wise woman herbal series ; 5th.

RA788.W44 2011 613.9'5
QBI10-600141

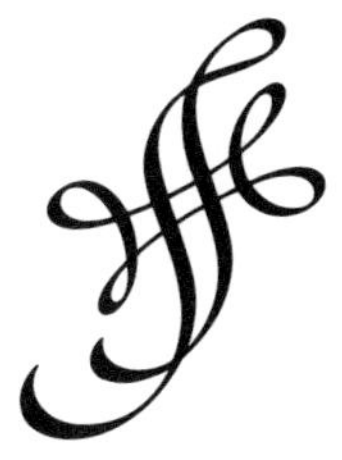

Dedicated to
my real-life guardian angels:

Keyawis Estherelke Kaplan (1940–2009)

and

Pierre Siead (born 1922)

Healers and teachers extraordinaire,
I feel your support and love always.

May it be in beauty.

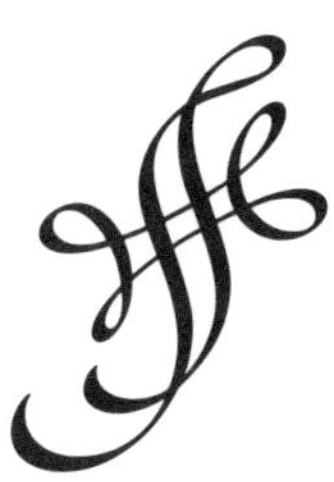

Acknowledgments

Many thanks to the many helpers and readers who help me bring the Wise Woman Tradition to life:

MoonEagle Ardnt, Colleen Belliveau, Molly Bennett, Robin Rose Bennett, Arlene Bercun, Anne BloomIsrael, Ralph Blum, Eva Castilla-Estevez, Isabel Castro, Candace Cave, Isa Coffey, Sandra Connor, Gordon Cook, Melissa Dawson, Christina C. DiEno, Betty Dodson, Ryan Drum, Doug Elliott, Sara Elisabeth, Judith Evans, Claudette Fansler, Victoria Floyd, Gena Ford, Chinmayo Forro, James Green, Michael Greenberg, Richard "RG" Guches, Holly Guzman, Teresa Harrison, Clove Haviva, Alex Heath, Teresa H., Vic Hernandez, Fern Hill, Lucretia Jones, Karen Joy, Julia Lachewitz Leh(wo)man, Lauren Lesser, Marti Long, Janice Loreta, Lisa Lyons, Michelle Lyons, Angela Macleod, Jennifer Martineau, Sasha Marts, Mary McMahon, Braida McCune, Suzy Meszoly DSH, Amy Midgley, Mary O'Dwyer, Michelle Reid, Robert Richards, Aviva Romm, Mischa Schuler, Pierre Siead, Silvermoon, Laura Slatin-Burger, David Smythe, Eleanor K. Sommer, Michelle Spence, Emily Squires, Rolan Torchco, Marge VanDorn, Sheri Winston, Dana Woodruff.

Thank you too, reader, for joining me in reweaving the Healing Cloak of the Ancients, spinning a Wise Woman web of health/wholeness/holiness into being, and reclaiming herbal medicine as people's medicine.

And a spotlight of attention, a fanfare of trumpets, a rousing round of applause, and my eternal gratitude to those who labored with me during these four years to bring *Down There* to you: Alan McKnight, for endless art. Bill McKnight and Victoria Nelson for putting the cover together. Betsy Grace Sandlin, for keeping her eye on all the details all the time and for demanding consistency. Heather Graham, for sending out manuscripts to the readers and for keeping the footnotes from driving me totally bonkers. My beloved consort Miki, for nurturing and supporting me in all ways, always. Marie Summerwood for guidance throughout. My precious daughter, Justine for keeping me focused, for creating a super website, and for doing perfect publicity. And her daughter Monica-Jean, for bringing me grandmother joy.

Contents

Part Two: Especially For Women

Part Three: Especially for Men

The Wise Woman Tradition

This book speaks from the Wise Woman in me to the Wise Woman in you. (Wo/man includes man, as you can see.) It is based on the belief that we are capable of observing our own body, heart, and mind, responding to the messages we receive, and caring for ourselves in a context of loving support and assistance. The Wise Woman Way nourishes health.

We live in the Scientific Tradition. It measures and fixes; it is covered by insurance. What is often called alternative medicine is the Heroic Tradition. It cleanses toxins from the filthy body, the dreaded colon, and the dirty liver; it runs on rules. The Wise Woman Tradition is the oldest way of healing. It nourishes the wholeness and holiness of the unique individual; it trusts the body's wisdom.

Wise Woman healing comes in cycles, adjusts to the seasons, moves in spirals, listens for harmonies, dances in rhythms and resonances with flexibile strength. Wise Woman healing focuses on nourishment: whole, healthy, holy food and rituals creating whole, healthy, holy beings.

Wise Woman herbalists (and that includes you) gather and prepare each leaf, each root, each berry with respect for its symbiotic wholeness. They seek simple, safe, local herbal remedies that have been tested in many situations and with a wide variety of people. May this book guide you.

Wise Woman healers (and that includes you) share what they know. They trust the careful experiments and the colorful experiences of generations of ordinary and extraordinary people. Herbal medicine is people's medicine. This book is my gift to you.

The Wise Woman inhabits our dreams, our visions, and our deepest memories. She speaks to us as Grandmother Growth. Her beloved consort, Grandfather Growth, accompanies her. She is the crone, She-Who-Holds-Her-Wise-Blood-Inside. She is a shaman. She is Baba Yaga. She is Kwan Yin. She is Kali. She knows the healing songs of the plants. She dances the heartbeat of the Earth. She holds out her hand to you.

Do you hear her singing? Do you feel her? Take her hand. Come.

Introduction

Aviva Romm, Midwife, MD

My mom loved bragging about my birth: She was out playing softball until four hours before she pushed me out. She told me: "Birth is normal, birth is natural. There is nothing to fear about your body. There is nothing to loathe about your body. Your body works perfectly. Trust it." Such a priceless gift from my mother.

In *Down There: Sexual and Reproductive Health the Wise Woman Way*, Susun Weed offers each one of us a similar gift. The story she weaves here, as in her previous books in the Wise Woman Herbal Series, is one of deep healing for women and men.

Down There the Wise Woman Way tells us stories about healthy cervices, healthy uteri, healthy yonis, healthy penises, healthy prostates, and healthy sex. *Down There* brings us into a healthy relationship with our bodies, and enlightens us about the places where, for too many, the sun never shines. *Down There* teaches us how to restore health when we are in distress, how to stay healthy, and how to relinquish fear and embrace pleasure. *Down There* helps us reconnect with the healing plants, and reminds us to connect our health with the health of our planet.

I know Weed's compassionate words will reach deep into your painful places and help heal them. I believe that Weed's stories can replace your stories of illness with those of healing and trust. And I am sure that the remedies gathered here will help you avoid the medical profession's ever expanding search for disease that leads to screening tests, followed by invasive tests and treatments that lead to new symptoms, new scars, new fears.

Before – and after – you go for screening, read this book. Before you follow the doctor's advice, read this book. Before you agree to a hysterectomy or prostatectomy, read this book.

I bless this addition to the Wise Woman Herbal Series. Congratulations on a fine new baby, Susun.

Aviva Romm, January 2011

Foreword

Spring is showing off: lilacs scent the breeze, late tulips shelter shy violets, bloodroot leaves unfurl, creeping phlox paints the ground, and the celandine erupts in yellow and green sprays. I'm sitting outside, renewed by floral joy and cavorting baby goats. But only for a moment, until I return to the computer, return to *Down There*, return to listening to Grandmother Growth.

There's no moon tonight. Make ready, make ready. The moon is dark tonight. Get ready, get ready. Every woman goes to the mooncave tonight.

I've been working on *Down There* since 1965, when I started collecting information from books, articles, and listening carefully to thousands of practitioners, doctors, and ordinary people talk about "down there." I met Betty Dodson. I attended Annie Sprinkle's *Sacred Sex* workshops for ten years; then taught them for another ten years. I thought about, and questioned, the accepted reasons and remedies for "down there" distresses.

Get ready. Hold my hand. Get ready, we go. The stars burn holes in the sky; no moon softens their edges. We go, we go, hold my hand, we go. We all go to the mooncave: to bleed, to share wisdom, to tell stories. We go.

In the deep memory of my womb, in the recurring stories of my ovaries, in the molten moist folds of my vulva, in my orgasms, I sought answers. I synthesized and enlivened what I had ingested. I sought the safest, simplest ways to heal the enormous energies of the pelvis, to maintain and regain continence, sexual interest and pleasure, and a host of other "down there" topics, all the while opening my heart and dreams to Grandmother Growth.

Singing, striding, together, we go. Singing we go to the mooncave. Singing, striding, climbing, we go, we go to the mooncave. Singing, singing. I would sit and sing. Help me, grandchild, sing with me. Sing the moss under my bones. Sing to me, then sit by me. We will sing the beads onto the moccasins, sing the reeds into a basket, sing the herbs into allies. We will sing mooncave songs, blood songs, birth songs, womb songs.

I get enraged by medicine that believes frightening millions of wo/men into useless – often harmful – screening tests is preventative medicine. Mammograms, colonoscopies, PSA tests, and Pap smears don't prevent anything. Do they allay fear or do they feed it? Can we be healthy when we are anxious and fearful? Fear makes me gullible; it clouds my ability to choose wisely. Instead, I wish to choose to care for myself rather than to react from fear. I want to know all the facts, so I can decide for myself what to do, helped by inner knowing, not lashed by desperation.

I'll sing you the song my grandmother's grandmother's grandmother sang when she was in this mooncave. Can you feel her in these rocks? Can you taste your ancestors in the water? Open yourself to their pleasure. Think happy thoughts. Feel good in your body.

There's sex in this book. Like Wilhelm Reich, I believe that healthy organisms need healthy orgasms for optimum health. May this book lead you to the orgasms you want; and help you to want them. May this book help you feel good in your body. May it show you how to reclaim the pleasure in your pelvis.

Feel into your body. Feel into your spirit. Lean against me. Allow your feelings to emerge. Lean against me and sing. Sing yourself to wholeness, sing yourself to joy. Let the Ancient ecstatic music move in you.

When we reconnect with the earth and with each other, we can hear each other's stories, we can hear the Wise Wo/man Within. We remember our power. We understand that our health is in our own hands, not those of the experts. We reclaim our right to decide how we heal. We value our intuition, we trust our own hearts.

Some topics I did not want to include in this book: female genital mutilation, male circumcision, and pelvic trauma. Nonetheless, I did. Other topics, such HIV and AIDs, ambiguous genitals, trans-sexuals, and gender identification issues, I have not included, though I have done my best to be aware of them and to reflect that awareness in my writing.

This book is now yours. May it empower you on your journey of health and healing. May it lessen your fear, feed your wholeness, and help you manifest a healthy, joyous, orgasm-rich life.

The moon is a silver sickle. We go, we go. We must return, return, to duty, to caring. Savor your memories, granddaughter. Remember joy. Keep your heart open to the old truths. Take my hand; let's go, let's go home.

Susun S. Weed, Laughing Rock Farm, May 2011

Six Steps of Healing

(Parentheses suggest a few of the modalities of each Step.)

Step 0: *Do Nothing* /Serenity Medicine (sleep, meditate, unplug the clock, don't look at email). A vital, invisible step. Listen to the voice of the Wise Healer Within.

Step 1: *Collect Information* /Story Medicine (low-tech diagnosis, support groups, books, dreams, divination). We want to know why. Listen to the voices of the wise healers without.

Step 2: *Engage the Energy* /Mind Medicine (prayer, homeopathy, visualization, ritual, laughter, reiki, placebos). This is the shaman's playground. It is flashy, colorful, scented, lush. Here we will it to be so, and it is as we will, with harm to none.

Step 3: *Nourish and Tonify* /Lifestyle Medicine (nourishing herbal infusions, food, movement, yoga, tai chi, walking, moxibustion, tonic herbs). We create ourselves with every choice we make.

The first four steps build health. Engage them daily.

Step 4: *Stimulate/Sedate* /Alternative Medicine (acupuncture, chiropractic, naturopathy, herbalism, hydrotherapy, massage). A good place to start when dealing with a chronic problem. Tonic herbs are safer than drugs, but overuse can lead to dependency.

Step 5: *Use Drugs* /Pharmaceutical Medicine (all prescribed and over the counter drugs, all supplements, essential oils). One of the leading causes of death in America is reactions to prescribed drugs.

Step 6: *Break and Enter* /High-tech Medicine (surgery, MRI, CAT scans, x-rays, injections, colonics, psychoactive drugs, invasive diagnostic tests). Side effects may include death and disability. Think twice about invasive screening procedures such as mamograms.

The last three steps are fast-acting, but have harmful side effects. Use them only as needed, and for as short a time as is prudent.

Using Herbs Safely

- ❖ Use one herb at a time.
- ❖ Learn about each plant from several sources.
- ❖ Avoid herbs in capsules.
- ❖ Respect the power of the plants; those strong enough to act as medicines affect the body and spirit in powerful ways.
- ❖ Remember, every plant, person, and situation is unique.

Nourishing herbs are the safest herbs; side effects are rare. Brew in water or vinegar; take in quantity, for extended periods of time. They offer high levels of protein, minerals, vitamins, and antioxidants. Nourishing herbs are safe to take with drugs. Nourishing herbs in this book include: chickweed, comfrey leaf, corn silk, dandelion leaf, hawthorn, kelp, linden, mallow, mullein, nettle, oatstraw, parsley leaf, plantain, purslane, red clover, raspberry leaf, self-heal, and slippery elm.

Tonic herbs act slowly and have cumulative effects. They are best used consistently for months or years. Tonics are safe to take with drugs. Prepare in water, vinegar, and alcohol (tinctures).

Soothing tonics are used in greater quantity: astragalus, burdock root, calendula, cleavers, echinacea, eleuthero, fenugreek seeds, goldenrod, and passionflower.

Bitter tonics aid digestion, too: buchu, dandelion root, cronewort, eleuthero, fennel seed, ginseng (American), milk thistle, motherwort, saw palmetto, tea (black and green), vitex, wild yam, and yellow dock.

Astringent tonics are often used externally: American ash, aspen, avens, barberry, bistort, black haw, coptis, cranesbill, couch grass, horsetail, oak bark, Oregon grape, shepherd's purse, tormentil, and witch hazel.

Food tonics include: turmeric, garlic, ginger, maitake, pomegranate, seaweeds, and wild mushrooms.

Stimulating/sedating herbs act quickly and have powerful effects and side-effects. They are used in the smallest effective dose and only for as long as is needed. They are problematic when combined with drugs. Daily use of stimulating/sedating herbs can undermine health. Stimulating/sedating herbs are used most often as tinctures. Stimulating/sedating herbs in this book: aloe, black cohosh, catnip, cayenne, chamomile, cinnamon, crampbark, damiana, dong quai, ginkgo, ginseng (Oriental), gold thread, guarana, juniper berries, kava kava, lavender, lemon balm, licorice, ma huang, marijuana, osha, parsley juice, parsley root, skullcap, sassafras, sarsaparilla, St. Joan's wort, sage, uva ursi, usnea, wild ginger, and yohimbe.

Potentially poisonous herbs can cause severe side-effects; they are unsafe to use with drugs. They are used in the smallest effective dose and only for as long as is needed. Potentially poisonous herbs are usually prepared as tinctures. Potentially poisonous herbs in this book: American mandrake, black walnut hulls, bloodroot, blue flag, cascara, celandine, chaparral, cotton root bark, eastern white cedar, goldenseal, horse chestnut, ivy (English), liferoot, mistletoe, myrrh, poke root, tea tree oil, thuja, and tobacco.

Notes on Homeopathic Remedies

❖ Dilutions are not given for the remedies listed in this book. Dosage range is from 10X to 1M. (Dilution is 100 times at 10x, and one million times at 1M.) In general, the greater the dilution, the stronger the remedy. Those who are very sensitive generally do better with higher dilutions. The lower dilutions are considered cruder in their actions.

❖ There is no cleansing crisis or healing crisis associated with proper use of homeopathic remedies. If your condition worsens, take an herbal remedy or seek help. *The result of taking a homeopathic remedy should be remission of symptoms.* In acute cases, this will happen quickly, often within hours. In chronic conditions, this will happen more slowly, sometimes over a few weeks.

❖ In general, one dose of the correct remedy will have the desired effect. Taking further doses is not useful. However, for chronic conditions, repetitions may be used.

❖ Homeopathic remedies work best when taken at least an hour before or after eating. Avoid all strong-tasting, strong-smelling drinks the day you take your remedy.

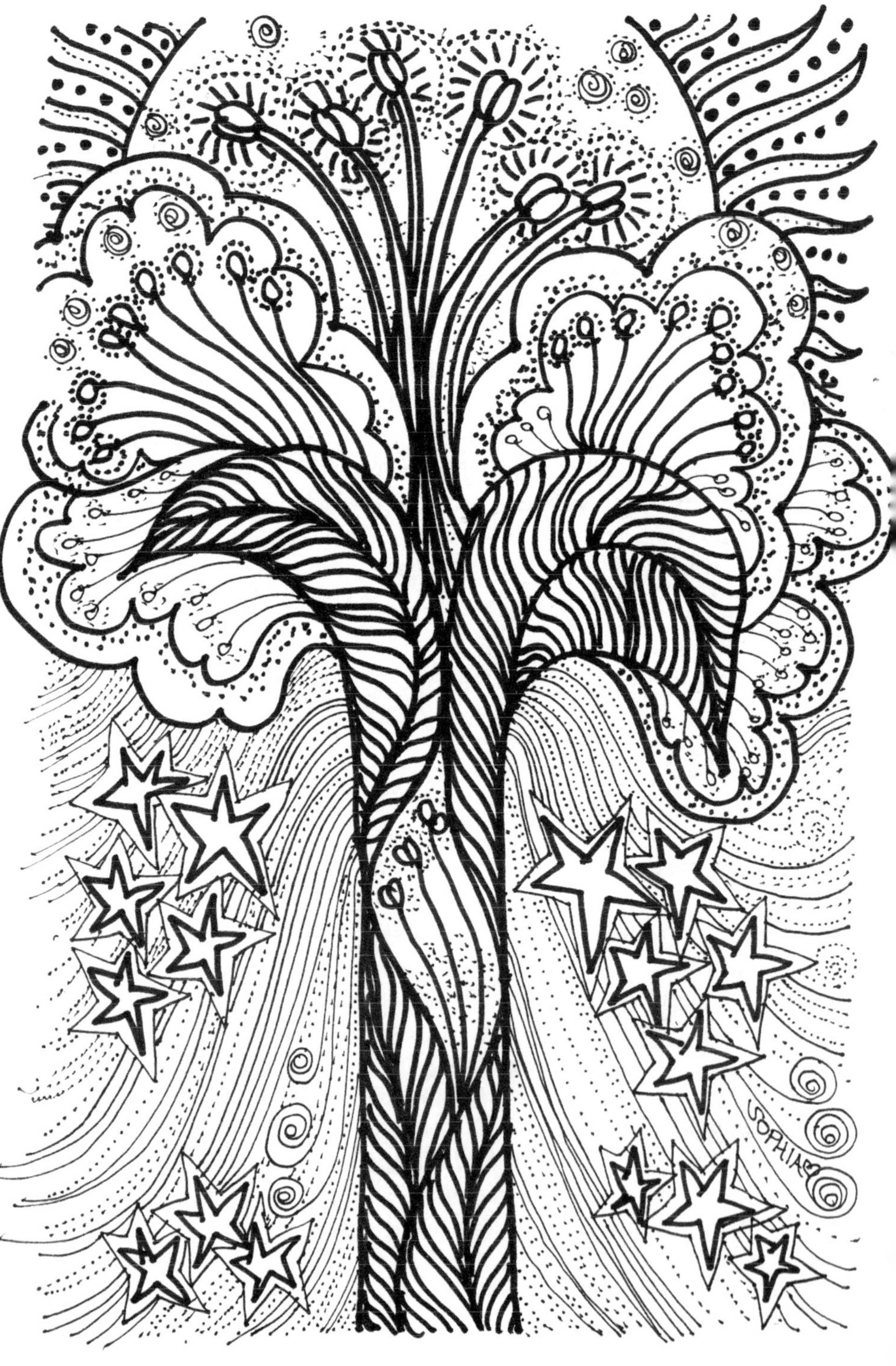
SOPHIA

Part One
For Everyone

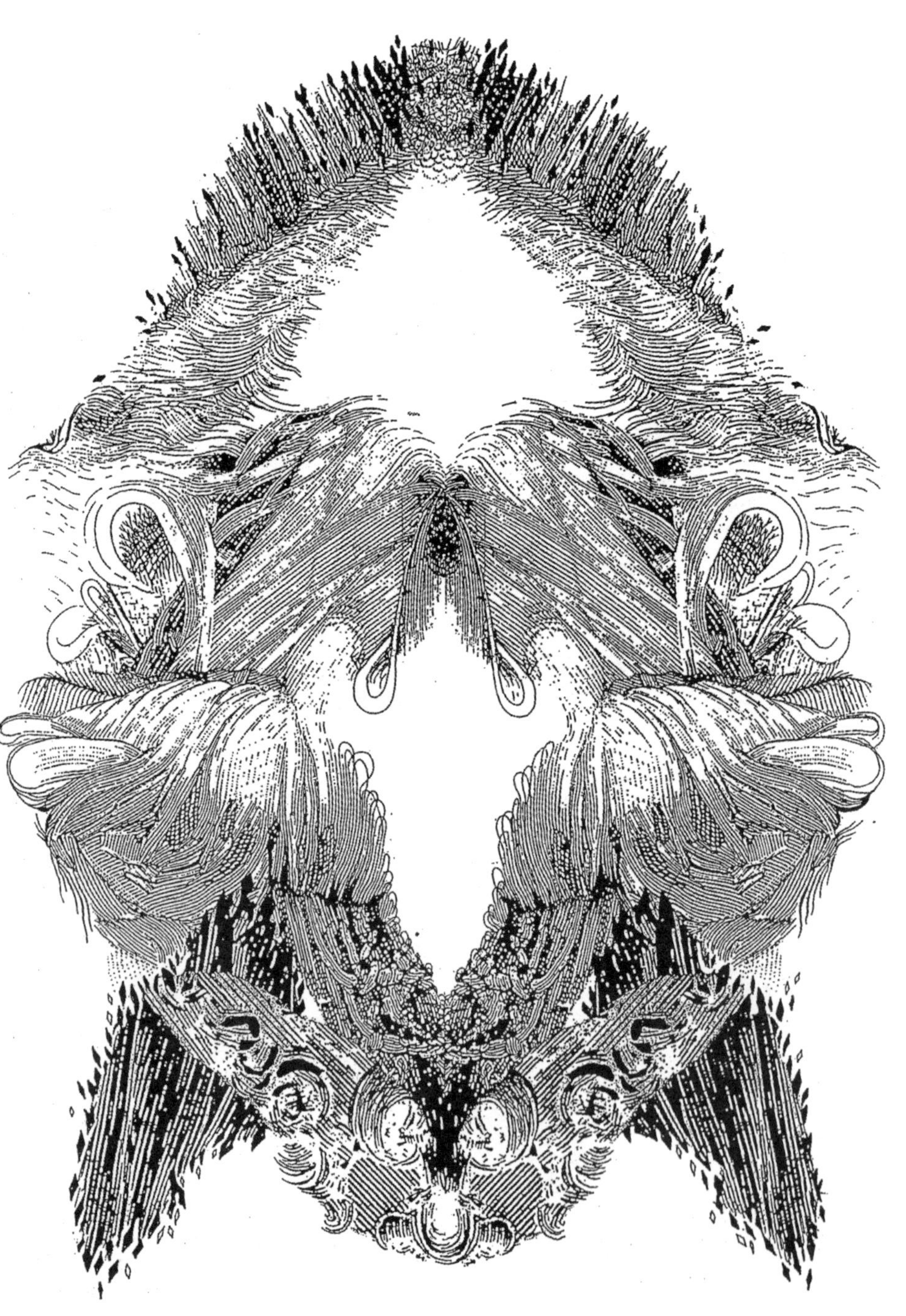

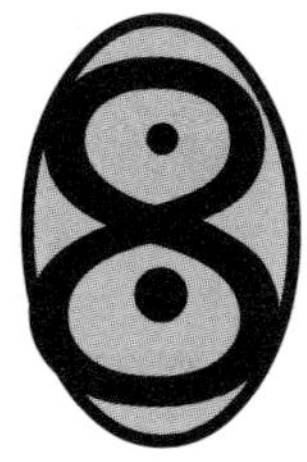

The Pelvic Floor

I am the floor. I am the ground. I am the base of your pleasure. I am the foundation of your well-being. I am the road that rises to meet you.

I am the hammock. I am the sling. I am the hands that hold. I am the cradle. I am the safety net.

I separate this from that, above from below, upright from horizontal. I hold firm. I open. I keep it all inside. I usher it out.

I am rich. I am well supplied. I have nerve endings in abundance. I throb with blood. I am a treasure. I am the setting of the jewels.

I am flexible. I stretch and bounce back. I thrive on action. Stir me. Pulse me. Use me. Ask of me. Demand of me. Keep me strong.

I am the mystical figure eight. I am infinity. I am the Mobius, the Ouroburos, the endless loop.

I am the lowest, the slowest, the most powerful. I am your first gear. I am the mover; I am the shaker.

I wrap myself around your most intimate parts. I support you in my firmness. I am your pelvic floor.

Healthy Pelvic Floor

In a healthy, well-nourished person, the tissues of the pelvic floor are well lubricated and elastic. The muscles strongly counter the downward tug of gravity. The blood vessels readily allow the engorgement of sexual arousal. The nerves freely carry signals of pleasure; and tell us, in a timely fashion, when we need to move our bowels or empty our bladder.

The pelvic floor is a continuous network of connective tissues – tendons, ligaments, muscles, and fascia – that protect the bladder, rectum, and uterus. It has two opposing functions: to keep these organs inside the body, and to provide their contents (urine, feces, babies) with a way out. In order to do both things, the pelvic floor must be tough and flexible.

There are two sets of muscles in the pelvic floor: a deep layer, the *pelvic diaphragm* (Figure 1), and a more surface layer, the *perineum* (Figure 2). Additionally, the *pelvic sidewalls* and the *accessory muscles* give pelvic support. In women, the muscular wall of the vagina helps strengthen the pelvic floor.

The healthy uterus lies parallel to the pelvic floor, tilted away from the vagina, toward the belly, causing a rounding there. A flat belly interferes with a woman's health and sexual pleasure![1] Incidentally, during sexual arousal, the uterus "stands up." After orgasm – during which it vibrates – it returns to horizontal.

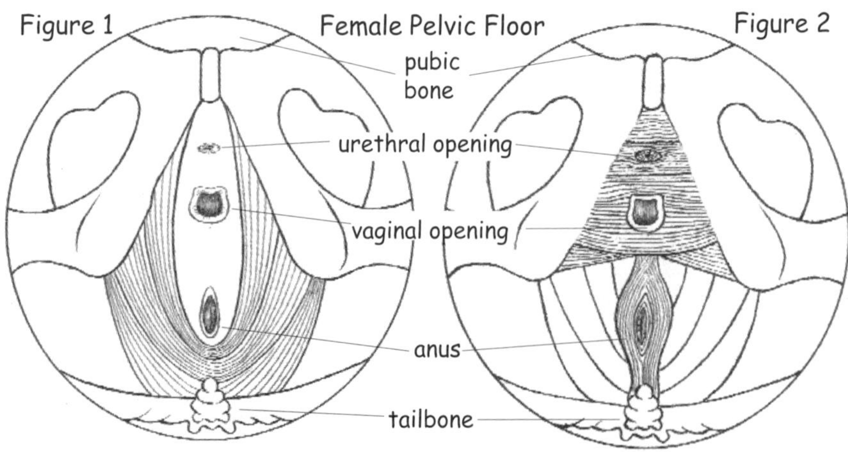

Pelvic Floor Distresses

Standing upright puts severe stress on the pelvic floor, a group of muscles which is vertical in mammals with all four feet on the ground, but horizontal in humans. Gravity and the weight of the entire abdomen and upper body press down on the muscles of our pelvic floor. Pregnancy and obesity stretch the tendons and ligaments. It is no wonder that this is a problem area for many.

Pelvic floor problems can arise from innate, functional, traumatic, or disease-related changes to the spine, pelvic bones, nerves, and blood vessels serving the pelvis. Aging, lack of exercise, and genetics are the most common causes of pelvic floor problems.

The muscles of the pelvic floor, like other muscles, grow weak if not used. Exercising them regularly helps prevent and cure **prolapse**, **incontinence** (page 34) and sexual difficulties. The special exercises for this area are called *pelvic clenches* or **Kegels**. ("How-to" on pages 10 and 14.)

Prolapses (page 6) occur when weak pelvic floor muscles allow the uterus, the bladder (**cystocele**), or the rectum (**rectocele**) to sag from their place in the pelvis down into the vagina.

Chronic pelvic pain/CPP (page 15) affects both men and women; in men it is often **chronic non-bacterial prostatitis**.

Men and women are equally likely to have **hemorrhoids** (page 19), **fistulas**, and anal **fissures** (page 24).

"The pelvic floor is important for maintaining a feeling of being carried, for the dialogue with gravity, and for our perception of the ground. [It] has an essential effect on our well-being and our vitality. . . ."[2]

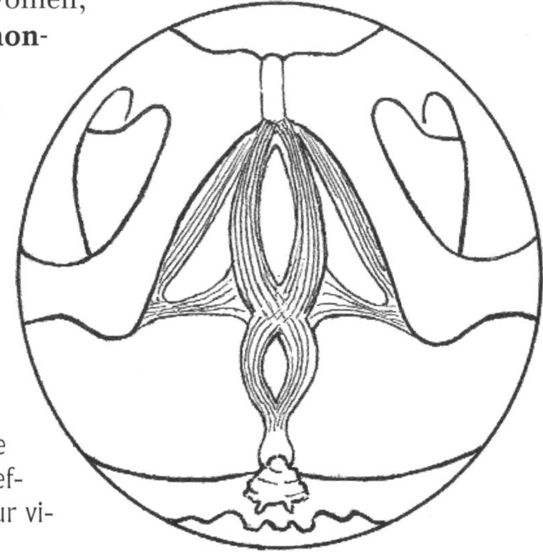

pubococcygeal (PC) muscle

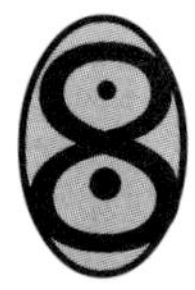

Pelvic Organ Prolapses

"I sense that you want my comfort," Grandmother Growth's voice softly echoes. "But you must stand on your own now, dear one.

"You look dejected, beaten down, despairing, sinking. Pull yourself up by your bootstraps, or pelvic floor ligaments, if you will, my child. Stop drooping and looking for sympathy. Clench your muscles. Feed your fire. Stand your ground."

"Put your heels on the ground. Let your belly come forward. Tuck your tailbone. Head up. Back straight. Be proud," growls Grandfather Growth.

"No one else can do this for you. You must find your own fierceness. Awaken your root chakra and create your own ground. Find your power. Be regal, be proud. I love you."

Step 1. *Collect Information*

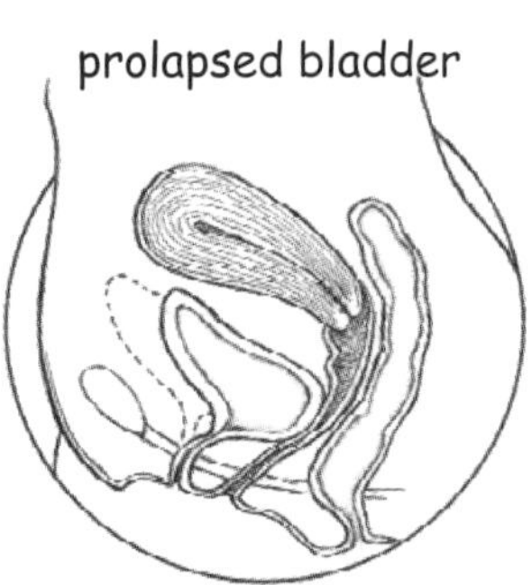

• If the uterus, bladder, urethra, or rectum prolapse (protrude) into the vagina, a variety of symptoms can be present in the belly or pelvic area: tenderness, heaviness, dull pain, difficulty urinating, difficulty defecating, leakage of urine or feces, and/or intercourse pain.

prolapsed uterus

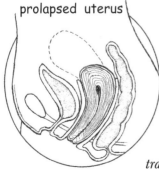

• More than ten percent of American women have some degree of prolapse. More than a quarter of a million repair surgeries are done yearly. But surgical remedies may create worse problems. There are effective, simple, safe Wise Woman ways to deal with prolapses without the risks of surgery.

• The pubococcygeal (PC) muscle (*illustrations,* pages 5 and 30) is one of the major muscles of the pelvic floor. It starts at the pubic bone, wraps around the openings of the urethra, vagina, and anus in a figure-eight and ends at the coccyx (tail) bone. The PC is responsible for the contractions of orgasm. The stronger your PC, the stronger and more prolonged your orgasms will be. The PC also helps the bladder hold urine in. If it is weak, "accidents" are likely. Pelvic floor exercises (pages 10 and 14) strengthen and tone the PC muscle.

• Bladder prolapse is usually due to a weak pelvic floor. But sometimes removing the uterus (hysterectomy) allows the bladder to fall backwards and down. When it bulges into the vagina, it is a *cystocele.* If only the urethra prolapses, it is a *urethrocele.* Both can be mildly annoying to utterly debilitating. Surgery may worsen these problems.[3]

• Prolapse of the bladder can stretch the ureters and lead to kidney problems. Protect the kidneys by drinking nettle infusion.

Step 2. *Engage the Energy*

• Prolapse is associated with helplessness and despair, as in, "I've got a sinking feeling." It may indicate a need to escape from difficulties, to sink out of sight. Instead, get in touch with your Earth-Mother-Bitch-Goddess. Affirm: "I am rising up!"

• A folk remedy from China calls for rubbing the very top of the head with a tiny bit of castor oil to counter the outflow of energy which is causing the prolapse. Energy is stored in the pelvis and organs prolapse when we use up our reserves and start to leak.

• **Homeopathic remedies** for prolapses are best taken in very high doses with the oversight of an experienced homeopath.

~ *Belladonna*: uterus leaden, falling, vagina hot and dry.
~ *Calc-carb.*: uterus chilly, flabby; constipation.
~ *Lilium*: anxiety; itchy vulva; urgent desire to pass stool.
~ *Natrum mur.*: uterus heavy, bearing down; better sitting.
~ *Nux vomica*: sharp pains, constant urge to void.
~ *Pulsatilla*: weepiness, nausea, pain in lower back and abdomen, worse with menses.
~ *Sepia*: uterus draggy, taut; sex painful; depression.

Step 3. *Nourish and Tonify*

★ A toned pelvic floor holds the organs up. The best way to tone the pelvic floor is to **exercise** it. Pioneering Dr. Kegel gave his name to the exercises he found so helpful. He believed that early morning exercises were especially important: ". . . for the patient begins the day with the perineum in a high position, whereas previously she started out with a sagging pelvic floor and considered the associated tired feeling normal."

★ To counter any kind of prolapse, the tendons and ligaments of the pelvic floor need to be strengthened, not just the muscles. My favorite herb to nourish and tonify connective tissues is **comfrey leaf infusion**, a quart or more a week, drunk hot or cold. If you are reluctant to drink comfrey, use it as a sitz bath!

• *The Family Physician*, by W. Beach, an herbal published in 1834, advises women with prolapses to use a strong decoction of **witch hazel** vaginally to tighten, tone, and pull up the pelvic organs. For strongest effect, sit in at least two quarts of witch hazel infusion and use your pelvic floor muscles to swoosh the liquid in and out of your vagina. **Oak bark** infusion may be substituted, as can **black tea** or **comfrey leaf**.

★ The "prostate herb" – **saw palmetto** – is a deep nourisher of all pelvic tissues. A dose of 10–30 drops of tincture, taken 1–3 times a day, gradually strengthens the pelvic floor, pulls prolapses up, increases beneficial hormonal responses, and counters incontinence.

★ Tincture of **black cohosh** root – a dropperful a day for 3 months – is a superb tonic to weak pelvic floor muscles and a counter to all prolapses.

Help!
Pelvic Organ Prolapse

Expect results within 3–6 months

• Commit yourself to one **orgasm** and/or one hundred **Kegels** a day.

• Experiment with **saw palmetto** or **black cohosh** tincture.

• Do an **inclined pose** daily.

• **Sitz bath** in **oak**, **comfrey leaf**, or **witch hazel** 3–6 times a week.

• Consider a **pessary** or a **sponge**.

★ Gravity can return pelvic organs to their intended places. You don't have to stand on your head, or hang in a frame, either. Even those with reflux problems can do many of these simple inversions. **Inclined poses** may seem too simple to be effective, but they have saved many women from surgery. Consistency brings the best results.

~ Lie on your back on the floor and prop your legs up against a wall, at a right angle to your body. Or sit the "wrong" way on a sofa or armchair, with your back on the seat and your legs on the back, head hanging down. Rest in this position for 15 minutes.

~ Lie on your back. Hold your knees close to your chest. Gently rock from side to side, or make circles with your hips on the floor. Continue for five minutes.

~ Kneel on a mat. Place your forearms, from elbows to hands, flat on the floor. Bend forward so your head touches the floor between your hands. Your bottom will go up. Rest there. Then slide your hands forward and your knees a little apart to push your bottom further up. Rest for a minute or two.

~ Lie on your back with your knees bent and feet close to your bottom, arms at your sides. Pull your PC muscles up and in as you raise your belly toward the ceiling. Imagine a thread pulling the tailbone up. Hold for a count of three. Release. Rest. Repeat up to ten times.

~ Lie on your back. Bend one knee. Lift the other leg up ten times. Rest. Switch legs. Rest in an easy pose.

~ Do you do yoga? Downward-facing dog, camel, plow, and shoulder stand help the pelvic floor. Rest when done.

★ Sitting upright and **cross-legged** makes the pelvic muscles do their part to keep you upright. It may be difficult at first. Per-

Dr. Kegel Says

- Before arising, contract the PC muscle five times.
- When you stand, contract the PC muscle another five times.
- Keep the PC muscle contracted as you walk to the toilet.
- Do five PC contractions every thirty minutes while awake.
- Unsure? Do a Kegel while urinating; it will block the flow.

sist! You'll not only relieve the prolapse, you'll enjoy deeper breathing, gain mental clarity, and have lots more energy. (Sitting on a chair? Pull your feet up and sit cross-legged on the seat.)

• If your **bladder** is prolapsed, it is important to empty it completely at least once a day. To achieve this, undress, kneel over a pan on the floor, lean forward onto your hands and pee into the pan.

• If your **rectum** is prolapsed, prop your feet up when you have a bowel movement. Unless you are acrobatic enough to balance on the toilet seat, use a stool the same height as the toilet.

★ **Dance!** Whether you go to a belly dance class or just groove to a beat at home, moving your pelvis strengthens your muscles.

★ **Do a Kegel exercise**: Clench the entire pelvic floor – the vagina, anal sphincter, bladder sphincter, and PC. To strengthen fast-twitch muscles that control the bladder, hold the clench for two seconds, then relax for two seconds. To strengthen the muscles involved in orgasm, hold the clench for ten seconds, then relax for ten seconds. For both: start with ten repetitions; increase to one hundred. Pelvic floor clenches can be done anywhere, anytime. Do them while waiting in a queue; do them while having intercourse; do them while washing dishes; do them now.

Pelvic Floor Clenches
Kegels

❖ Tighten and relax the pelvic floor muscles as quickly as you can, ten times. Do ten repetitions.

❖ Tighten the pelvic floor muscles and hold for a count of three, then release. Do ten repetitions.

❖ Slowly squeeze the pelvic floor muscles while counting to five – harder, *harder*, **harder**. Slowly release while counting to five. Do the whole thing ten times.

Keep the buttocks, thighs, and belly loose. To be sure you are contracting the PC, put your finger in your vagina and feel the squeeze.

Step 4. *Stimulate/Sedate*

> "After struggling with the ups and downs of pelvic floor weakness for several years, the day finally arrived when I realized I could no longer tolerate any constriction whatsoever around my torso. Tight jeans and waistbands literally squeezed my uterus out of my body . . . bras, high underwear, tights, pantyhose, and . . . skirts were no longer viable clothing options. . . ."[4]

★ While healing a prolapse, consider a **pessary**. Most are donut-shaped devices, which, inserted into the vagina, act as a "stopper" to keep the uterus and bladder from falling. A natural sea sponge may be used as a pessary as well (next page). A pessary is recommended for women who refuse surgery, women who are deemed unfit for surgery, and those who want to wait and see if surgery can be avoided. (Hopefully, this is you.)

pessary

Pessaries of linen, wool, brass, cork, or sponge have been in use for centuries. Modern medical-grade silicon ones come in several dozen sizes. It may take several tries to find the perfect size for you. If you can insert, remove, and care for a diaphragm, then you will be able to use a pessary.

Christine Kent,[5] who used a pessary for seven years while healing her prolapse, believes surgical approaches predominate because medical professionals are taught that women aren't willing or able to care for a pessary. So the current standard of care calls for a physician to place the pessary in the vagina. The patient returns each month for the pessary to be removed and cleaned.

But leaving a pessary in your vagina for that long can cause infections, open wounds (*fistula*), even cancer. "I never slept with mine in, nor did I keep it in longer than twelve hours at a time," writes Ms. Kent. Each time she removed her pessary, she washed it immediately with mild soap and warm water and put it on a clean towel to dry. Twice a week she soaked it briefly in hydrogen peroxide, using an overnight soak to remove menstrual blood.

Her pessary gave her instant relief from the pressure and drag in her belly, but it could interfere with urination, prevent voiding, or cause stress incontinence. "Sometimes my pessary was comfortable for hours on end," she says. "Other times it would be propelled out of my vagina and no way could I get it to stay in."

> "Like a brace or a crutch, the pessary is a very important helper during the process of healing prolapse naturally."[6]

• Instead of the usual pessary, try a sea sponge (page 250). It's lighter and easier to use, but just as effective.

• **Acupuncture**, by itself, or in combination with herbal or homeopathic remedies, can be helpful in correcting prolapses.

• Heavy lifting can aggravate prolapse, as can very low chairs.

★ The rhythmic contractions of **orgasm** (whether alone or with a partner) lift the pelvic organs, tone the pelvic muscles, and help reverse prolapses. Pull out the vibrator and snuggle up to your sweetie. Worried about penetration? "No problem," say the prolapsed women I've met, or whose stories I've read. No matter how weak the pelvic floor or how severe the prolapse, intercourse can be pleasurable. Prolapses are compounded by gravity; lie down, and the organs return to their proper positions.

Step 5. *Use Drugs*

> "Because it is well-known that statin use can weaken muscles, I believe it is possible that the medication may have caused my prolapse. Recently, statins have been shown to cause actual structural damage to muscles in some people."[7]

Step 6. *Break and Enter*

> "Women suffering from pelvic organ prolapse should always attempt alternative treatments before having a hysterectomy."[8]

• Despite the assurances of gynecological surgeons, women are often unhappy with the results of surgical fixes for prolapse. Pelvic floor surgeries are complicated and may lead to greater pain and weakness. A hysterectomy may change one distress for another. In any surgery, nerves are cut. In pelvic surgery, that means loss (for some women major, for others minor) of sexual sensation. Muscles are cut and sewn, adhesions form, there is often chronic stiffness, inflammation, and pain.

• Dr. Howard Kelly, one of the early founders of gynecological medicine and creator of many of the pelvic floor surgeries still in use today, proclaimed in 1900: "I do not believe pleasure in the sexual act has any particular bearing on the happiness of life."[9]

• The removal of uterus and/or ovaries is rarely justified to remedy prolapses.[10] Seek a more compassionate care giver, and go back to the earlier remedies in this chapter.

Her Story

Christine tells her whole story in *Saving the Whole Woman.*

"When my gynecologist told me I needed immediate surgery to deal with a fibroid, he asked if I was ever incontinent. 'Yes,' I admitted, 'but only occasionally.'

"'You're too young for that,' he admonished. 'Since I'm going in there anyway, I'll get rid of that problem at the same time.'

"Recovering from the surgery was 'uneventful' according to the doctor. My vomiting, extreme pain, and infections were 'normal.' But a few weeks later, my uterus was down in my vagina.

"'Prolapse' was the diagnosis. I was told by every doctor I consulted that the only cure was a hysterectomy. If my uterus was a problem, then remove it.

"But surgery had *caused* the prolapse. And left me numb down there. Sex no longer worked. My bowels were adversely affected. My entire body felt twisted. Who knew what further damage more surgery would create! I refused to lose my uterus. I sought alternatives.

"I pioneered pessary use, making it up as I went along. There were no instructions for me to follow, except the 'awesome truth' of my own body. I learned to sit cross-legged, to stand from my center, to feed myself nourishing foods, to do yoga and pelvic floor exercises, to free my breasts and belly from elastic cinches, and to reconnect with, and honor, my own power. I went to chiropractors, massage therapists, nutritionists, anyone who could offer me a piece to fit into my healing puzzle.

"It took time. It was difficult. At its worst, my uterus was boggy and heavy and protruded an inch out of my vagina. When I menstruated, the pain was excruciating. I could hardly stand, walk, or even sit up. Sometimes I bled and bled and bled. Hysterectomy lurked, beckoning me, the 'easy' way out.

It took courage, and faith in myself, as well as time, to revitalize my pelvic floor and heal my prolapse. I found my courage; I trusted myself and my body; I took the time I needed. I still have my uterus! It sits up in my pelvis, where it belongs."

Some Thoughts on Pelvic Floor Exercises

from Michelle Lyons, Pelvic Floor Specialist

There are both slow-twitch and fast-twitch muscles in the pelvic floor. Seventy percent of the total are slow twitch muscles. They are the marathoners; they maintain pelvic floor integrity most of the time. Thirty percent are fast-twitch muscles. They are the sprinters; they come into play when there are high intra-abdominal pressure events such as coughing, sneezing, or jumping.

It is important to exercise both the slow- and the fast-twitch muscles.

But it is even more important to relax all the pelvic floor muscles completely. If we do the exercises and don't relax between reps, we can develop trigger points/spasms in the pelvic floor muscles. These spasms inflame hyperactivity in the nerves associated with chronic pelvic pain, low back pain, and pain with intercourse (dyspareunia).

We want to develop a full range of motion, from all the way relaxed to maximally contracted and back to relaxed. This is what gives us control.

To relax: Breathe into your belly. Feel the belly button move out and the pelvic floor open and drop down.

To find the right muscles: Imagine trying to hold back a big stinky fart.

To contract: Breathe out and engage the muscles. Aim for a lift rather than a squeeze. Sucking your thumb helps.

Breathe! Holding your breath can weaken the muscles or send them into spasms.

Stand up tall. Poor posture puts a terrible strain on the pelvic floor muscles. Let a strong back and a strong abdomen take some of the load off the pelvic floor.

Continue your pelvic floor education with *Pelvic Power: Mind/Body Exercises* by Eric Franklin.[11]

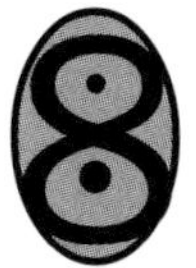

Chronic Pelvic Pain

"Put your belly on the warm sand," counsels Grandmother Growth.

"Give your pain to the Earth. Spill your guts into Her. Release your fear, your dread, your nightmares into the accepting, transformative Earth. Cry into Her. Cry out the pain of the millions of wo/men who are oppressed, raped, cut. Cry out your personal pain. Empty your belly. Trust in the process," encourages Grandfather Growth.

"And when you are done, the fire in your belly will be yours. It will blaze your path instead of burning you alive."

Step 0. *Do Nothing*

• **Relaxing** deeply and **breathing** slowly, even for fifteen minutes, is a powerful pain reliever for those with chronic pelvic pain.[12]

★ Many wo/men struggling with CPP find any **meditative practice** immediately helpful. (Hypnosis is rarely helpful.)

Step 1. *Collect Information*

"Few medical conditions are as perplexing. . . ."[13]

• At least ten million American wo/men are affected by chronic pelvic pain (CPP).[14] CPP is defined by the American College of Obstetricians and Gynecologists as any pain anywhere in the pelvis that persists for at least six months and has no apparent cause.

CPP Symptoms

- ❖ Pain radiating from pelvis to lower back, hips, thighs, buttocks
- ❖ Pain when bladder is full
- ❖ Pain on intercourse
- ❖ Pain on sitting
- ❖ Pain in the abdomen
- ❖ Menstrual-like cramps and aches
- ❖ Prostate pain

• Consider this: Men who used to have chronic non-bacterial prostatitis now have CPP. Half of all women with CPP have endometriosis.[15] For all wo/men, CPP is deeply linked to trauma.

• Down theres can become sensitized to frequently-used soaps, detergents, fabric softeners, perfumes, and spermicides, leading to itching, burning, and painful intercourse, but not CPP.[16]

• Pain during intercourse (dyspareunia) is a symptom of CPP. But prostate, bladder, and uterine infections, hormonal changes, pelvic tumors/cysts, trauma, prolapses, venereal warts, herpes outbreaks, yeast, and other STDs can also interfere with pleasure.

• Women with CPP say their pain follows the menstrual cycle, flaring up in intensity with the menstrual flow, then easing off for a few weeks. Men don't seem to have cycles with their CPP.

• The suspected origin of CPP is a bundle of nerves at the base of the spinal cord: the superior hypogastric plexus. These nerves relay pain sensations from the pelvis to the brain. When they are chronically stimulated, the signals reverse and the brain sends pain signals to the pelvic muscles. Eventually, these healthy areas respond with painful spasms called *pelvic floor tension myalgia.*

★ Structural problems abet this nerve disruption. **Yoga** relieves them all: it realigns the sacroiliac joint, strengthens the muscles of the pelvic floor and abdomen, and restores elasticity to the stretched ligaments.

• Up to two-thirds of those affected by CPP don't get a proper diagnosis.[17] Desperate for relief after years of pain, many agree to surgery, which can make the pain far worse.

Help!
Chronic Pelvic Pain

Expect results within 2–4 months

• Take 2–4 dropperfuls of **St. Joan's wort tincture** daily.

• Commit to 4–6 **acupuncture** or **massage** sessions.

• Take a course in **relaxation**.

• Drink 3–6 quarts of **nourishing herbal infusion** (page 17) weekly.

Step 2. *Engage the Energy*

• The belly is the pelvis; the pelvis is the *hara*; the hara is the center of the body. The belly is an important part of the immune system. It can remember, just like the brain. Chronic pelvic pain is a message from your center that you don't feel safe in your life/body.

★ Whether dealing with acute or chronic pain, I especially like Stephen Levine's "Meditations on Pain" in his book *Who Dies?*[18]

Step 3. *Nourish and Tonify*

• Whole-body **massage, MAM** (page 209), or electro-magnetic therapy relaxes the pelvic muscles and normalizes nerves. Weekly sessions are best until the pain is under control.

• **Nourishing herbal infusions** – a quart a week each of oatstraw, comfrey, and linden – calm nerves, ease muscle spasms, and help reduce pain from adhesions. (Make it, page 367.)

• Since all seed oils are high in omega-6 fatty acids, which are inflammatory, reducing or eliminating seed oils from the diet can bring rapid relief from inflammatory pain. Instead, use olive oil, a natural anti-inflammatory, or butter, an active pain reliever.

• A physical therapist can design an individual program to help you relieve your pain. Find one at www.womenshealthapta.org.

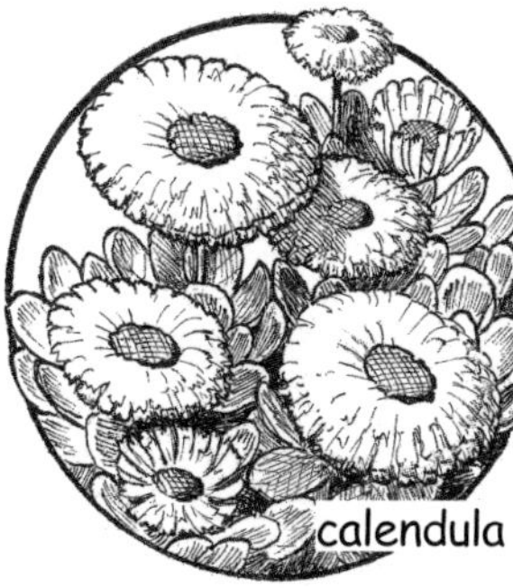

• Hot compresses (make it: page 367) of **comfrey leaf**, **castor oil**, **plantain oil**, or **calendula oil**, applied to the belly can ease pain and gently, but slowly, dissolve adhesions. Patience and persistence pay dividends. Aim for 4–7 applications a week.

calendula

Step 4. *Stimulate/Sedate*

★ **Acupuncture** successfully reverses the nerve disruption, muscle spasms, and myalgic pain of CPP. Ultrasound, electrotherapy, and biofeedback are useful for some wo/men.

• **Static magnetic field therapy**, or magnet therapy, used continuously for a month, significantly reduced chronic pelvic pain in a small double-blind study.[19,20]

★ I prefer herbal pain killers (such as **skullcap** or **passionflower** tincture and **meadowsweet** oil) and herbal muscle relaxers (such as **St. Joan's wort** tincture). Not only are they effective, they are free from side effects, and dependably non-addictive.

Step 5. *Use Drugs*

• Nonsteroidal anti-inflammatory drugs, such as **ibuprofen** or **aspirin**, ease pelvic pain. So do muscle relaxers, anti-convulsants, tricyclic antidepressants, anti-seizure meds, and opiates.

• Injections of the anesthetic **lidocaine** into tender pelvic or abdominal muscles can bring immediate, but short-term, relief. Or they can cause the pain to be expressed in other places.

• **Birth control pills** are effective therapy for some women who suffer from CPP.

Her Story

Moonflower is a homesteader with three children.

"I assumed the debilitating pain I was suddenly feeling with my period meant there was something wrong 'down there.' It took all the best diagnostic tests that modern medicine could throw at me to convince me that I did not have fibroids, cysts, endometriosis, or worse. Things I never heard of—the iliopsoas muscle and the ilioinguinal nerve—are at the root of my pain. There's no happy ending . . . yet. But acupuncture and herbs have helped a lot."

Step 6. *Break and Enter*

• Orgasm, or intravaginal/intrarectal massage, counters pelvic floor spasms fast. Do it yourself or ask for help.

• All surgical procedures, including laparoscopies, leave scar tissue (adhesions) in the soft pelvic tissues and cause nerve damage, both of which may trigger CPP. Paradoxically, surgery to remove the adhesions is recommended for wo/men with CPP.[21] This creates more scar tissue, more pain, more damage.

• CPP is responsible for 12 percent of all hysterectomies done in the USA, yet one-quarter of these women get no relief.[22]

• CPP is also responsible for 40 percent of the laparoscopic procedures done in the USA. But even when a supposed cause is found and treated, many women continue to suffer pelvic pain.[23]

• The ultimate solution for women with CPP is to **cut the nerves** in the lower back, thus preventing pelvic nerve signals from being transmitted. Strangely, this does not always work.

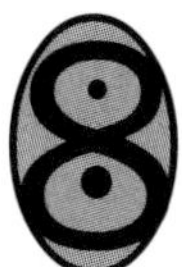

Hemorrhoids

"You are so fragile, my precious grandchild," murmurs Grandmother Growth. "But being tense and fearful will not compensate for fragility. In fact, your tension makes you more easily damaged."

"You can't keep yourself together. You've lost the will to push against obstacles. But life doesn't play fair. It doesn't stop if you give in. It keeps on moving through you, fast and furious," hisses Grandfather Growth.

"The life force, the chi, of all you ingest is absorbed through the blood vessels of your large intestine. You need vigorous veins in your pelvic floor. You want pushy veins, not loose, relaxed, laid back veins. There is a difference between being easy and being slack. Let us look for, and nourish, your flexible strength. It's becoming impossible to sit on it, isn't it?"

Their laughter spills through the twilight, sparking like fireflies.

Step 0. *Do Nothing*

"Not everyone with hemorrhoids has symptoms, and hemorrhoids should be treated only if they are bothering you."[24]

Step 1. *Collect Information*

• Hemorrhoids are inflamed and enlarged veins in the rectum and anus. Half of people over 50 have them. They may cause symptoms or not. (If they do, they are the original "pain in the ass.")

• Hemorrhoid is from Greek *hemo* (blood) and *rrhoos* (flowing, discharging). They are also called piles, from the Latin *pila*, a ball.

• Hemorrhoids may stay internal or push out of the anus. They may itch, bleed, or cause intense pelvic pressure and pain.

~ **External hemorrhoids** may fill with blood and form hard walnut-sized bluish lumps (*thrombosis*) around the anus. They are often quite painful and itchy, but generally dissipate on their own.

~ **Internal hemorrhoids** may bleed bright red blood. (Blood from colon cancer is usually dark red.) They are often painless, but may *prolapse* out of the rectum and cause pain or itching.

• What causes hemorrhoids? Pressure in the anal/abdominal area, genetics, a tense pelvic floor, a weak pelvic floor, constipation, diarrhea, pregnancy, vaginal birth, obesity, chemotherapy, radiation treatments, and sitting for long periods. About 75 percent of Americans have hemorrhoids.[25]

• It's not a hemorrhoid if you are in constant pain or bleeding persists. You may have a **fissure** or a **fistula** (page 24).

Step 2. *Engage the Energy*

• Visualize aqua light cooling and soothing the anus. Let it tighten loose tissues, ease irritation, and bring a smile to your face. If you are so inclined, imagine a hum passing through the anal blood vessels; feel the vibration bringing healing and support.

• **Homeopathic** remedies for those with hemorrhoids:

~ *Aesulus*: rectum very dry; hemorrhoids swollen, blue-purple; worse with standing.

~ *Aloe*: hemorroids like grapes; better with cold water.

~ *Ignatia*: severe rectal spasms, cutting pains, anal fissures.

~ *Hamamelis*: large, blue, sore, congested, bruised-feeling, bleeding hemorrhoids; worse in pregnancy.

~ *Nux vomica*: congested, painful; better after stool.

~ *Ratanhia*: severe pain, burning, cuts like broken glass; worse after stool or with touch.

~ *Sepia*: heaviness, prolapse, worse in pregnancy.

~ *Sulphur*: moist, large, hot, congested hemorrhoids with severe itching; worse at night, with standing.

• The homeopathic supplier Boericke & Tafel offers Alpha Hemorrhoids: a combination of horse chestnut, witch hazel, *Nux vomica*, and sulphur in a suppository to relieve pain and itching.

Step 3. *Nourish and Tonify*

★ The same things that ease constipation, ease hemorrhoids: **water**, **fiber**, **exercise**, and going to the toilet at set times.

• Ease hemorrhoids by drinking up to two quarts of herbal teas or infusions daily. **Astringents** – like black or green tea, raspberry tea, or comfrey leaf infusion – shrink hemorrhoids and counter bleeding. **Soothers** – such as linden infusion, marshmallow tea, or slippery elm mixed with honey – relieve pain. **Nettle infusion** restores youthful elasticity and tone to the anal veins.

• Aim for ten servings (25–30 grams) of **fiber**-rich foods daily: whole grains, beans, nuts, fruits, and vegetables; or supplement with soothing **flax** or **plantain seeds**/husks cooked in **oatmeal** or soaked in cold water overnight. Compared to a placebo, fiber reduced symptoms by 47 percent and bleeding by 50 percent.[26]

★ **Exercise** that moves the lower body – swimming, walking, dancing, jogging, pelvic floor clenches – helps.

• Constipated? Avoid laxatives, enemas, and colonics: they worsen hemorrhoids. A dropperful of **yellow dock** tincture moves things along without stimulation.

Step 4. *Stimulate/Sedate*

★ To ease itching quickly, apply a poultice of freshly-chewed **plantain** leaves, or **calendula** or **plantain ointment**. (Make it: page 367.)

Help!
Hemorrhoids

Expect results immediately

• Apply **witch hazel** liquid.

• Apply **plantain oil**.

• Avoid peppers, chilis, curries.

Expect results within 3–6 weeks

• Every week, sitz in a quart of **astringent** herb (like oak bark)and drink a quart of **soothing** herb (like linden).

• Take two dropperfuls of **stoneroot** tincture daily.

• Increase **fiber** and **fluids**.

• Alternating hot and cold **sitz baths** soothe pain, reduce swelling, counter itching, stop bleeding, and shrink hemorrhoids. Use plain water, or add **seaweed** or **aloe** juice. Or try alternating cold **oak bark** and hot **comfrey** sitz baths. (Make them: pages 367, 368.)

★ **Witch hazel**, a small tree native to North America, is everybody's favorite hemorrhoid remedy. You can buy witch hazel at the drug store in a bottle or in premoistened towelettes to use instead of toilet paper. Soak a cotton ball in the witch hazel, and apply to the painful area. For cooling relief, keep it in the freezer. It rapidly shrinks swelling, eases pain, counters bleeding, stops itching, soothes irritation, and encourages healing. A witch hazel bark sitz bath is even stronger. (Make it: page 368.)

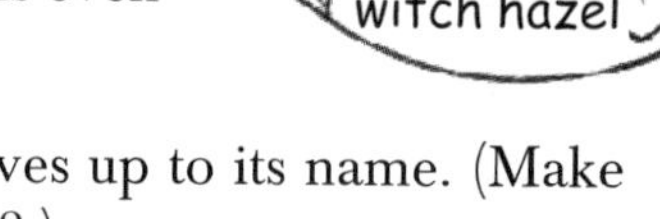

• **Sitting Pretty Salve** lives up to its name. (Make it: page 368.)

• Chilled **horse chestnut** gel shrinks hemorrhoids fast. (More: page 27.)

★ Herbalist Christopher Hobbs calls **stoneroot** "the premier hemorrhoid herb. It's miraculous."[27] He suggests two 375mg capsules of the powdered root twice a day with a full glass of water between meals. Herbalist David Winston prefers tincture of the whole fresh plant, a dropperful twice a day. Some herbalists apply tincture externally too.

• Naturopath Mark Stengler uses 200–300mg of **butcher's broom** (standardized to 9 to 11 percent ruscogenins) per day to control bleeding and pain from hemorrhoids. A daily dose of 320mg **bilberry** extract (25 percent anthocyanosides) strengthens blood vessel walls, improves circulation, and shrinks hemorrhoids.

Step 5. *Use Drugs*

• Caution: Typical topical creams like Preparation H and Anusol, anesthetic creams (names end in "-caine"), and 0.5percent hydrocortisone cream can injure skin and damage perineal and anal tissues if used for more than a week.[28] Instead, soothe with cool **yogurt**, plain **cocoa butter**, or **zinc oxide paste**.

Step 6. *Break and Enter*

> "No surgery, and especially not hemorrhoid surgery, is pain-free and without potential complications."[29]

• If there is continued bleeding, uncontrollable pain, or prolapsed hemorrhoids, and if dietary changes and herb sitz baths haven't worked, there are invasive, aggressive treaments.

~ Rubber band ligation cuts off the circulation to the hemorrhoid causing it to fall off with little or no pain,[30] though there may be bleeding or infection.[31]

~ Lancing a clot in a hemorrhoid brings fast relief.[32]

~ Lasers, electricity, or infrared energy seal off or vaporize the affected blood vessels, but there is a high recurrence rate.

~ Sclerotherapy is less expensive, less painful, and less effective than ligation. Chemicals injected into internal hemorrhoids destroy them. Side-effects include abscess formation, fecal incontinence, scarring, and infection.[33]

~ Cryosurgery freezes hemorrhoidal tissue.

~ The Keesey Technique, or *hemorrhoidolysis*, is an outpatient procedure requiring 6 to 10 sessions. An electrode conducts a current into the hemorrhoid, causing it to shrink.

~ Large, prolapsed internal hemorrhoids may need to be surgically removed. This is a *hemorrhoidectomy*. Postsurgical pain is a major problem, requiring weeks of strong medications.

~ A new outpatient procedure, PPH, or *hemorrhoidopexy*, uses a circular device to lift hemorrhoids and staple them into their original position, above the area of nerves. Hemorrhoids are pulled back into the anal canal, not removed, which minimizes fecal incontinence and stricture after surgery.[34]

> "The anal area is rich in nerves, so traditional surgery to excise . . . hemorrhoids leaves patients in considerable pain."[35]

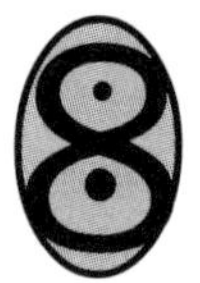

Anal Fissure, Anal Fistula

"You are being ripped in two," weeps Grandfather Growth.
"Torn asunder," thunders Grandmother Growth.
"Split from stem to stern!"
" Hooked and gutted like a fish."
"What horrible thing have you tried to consume that grappled you as it passed?" wonders Grandfather Growth.
"Have you bitten off more than you can chew? Is it eating at you from the inside?" admonishes Grandmother Growth.
"Stop sitting on it!" they yell at the top of their lungs. You vibrate.

Step 1. *Collect Information*

• An anal fissure is a tear in the lining of the anal canal that will not heal. Fissures are intensely painful and bleed profusely.

• Fissures don't heal because they trigger spasms in the underlying sphincter muscle that continually reinjure the tear.

• An anal fistula is a tear that continues through into the vagina or vulva. Because it is in contact with feces, a fistula does not heal.

Step 2. *Engage the Energy*

• Is something tearing you up inside? Are your guts in a knot? Is someone knifing you in the back? Are you in the hot seat? Do you have an itch you can't scratch? Are you getting it up the arse? Can it change?

Help!
Anal Fissure, Fistula

Expect results within 3–6 days

• Drink 2–3 quarts of **comfrey** leaf infusion a week.

• Apply **aloe vera** or horse chestnut gel; try **oak bark** sitz baths.

• Take stone root, horse chestnut (page 27), or echinacea tincture.

Step 3. *Nourish and Tonify*

★ **Comfrey leaf infusion** – internally and externally – strengthens the anal tissues, initiates rapid healing of fissures, calms fistulas, and relieves spasms. Frequent sitz baths soothe, tighten, and mend anal tissues. Frequent sips, hot with honey, strengthen the intestines throughout, helping them resist further fissures.

• Increase hydration, fiber, and exercise to counter fissures. And eat **slippery elm**. This high-fiber herb repairs, nourishes, and soothes digestive tissues. The powder can be cooked in hot cereal, or mixed with honey and slowly dissolved in the mouth.

★ Apply **aloe vera** or **horse chestnut** gel to the fissure as often as possible, or whenever there is pain.

Step 4. *Stimulate/Sedate*

★ **Oak bark sitz bath** heals anal fissures, genital inflammation, and hemorrhoids; it's antiseptic and antibacterial, too.

★ A combination of **echinacea** and **goldenseal** tinctures, applied directly to the fissure or fistula, will sting as it clears infection, tighten the tissues, and initiate rapid healing.

• This remedy from Russia gets to the root of the problem: Heat a brick in the oven until very hot. Place it in the bottom of a large metal bowl. Put some cloves of raw **garlic** on it, remove your pants, and squat over the bowl. The fumes from the smoldering garlic counter infection and prompt rapid healing.

• **Horse chestnut** (page 27) or **stoneroot** (page 22), used internally and externally, ease pain and helps initiate healing.

Her Story

Serenity channels angelic beings.

"I went to the doctor with a pain in my butt and I left bleeding and in need of surgery. I swear he split me in two when he put his finger up there to 'check things out.' They cut out a piece of my anus. It still works fine, though my BMs are thinner now."

• Plum Flower Brand Formula H is a patented Chinese herbal remedy recommended by a woman who says it keeps her fistula "under control, meaning it never gets big or discharges."

Step 5b. *Use Drugs*

• Ointments of nitroglycerin or a calcium-channel blocker are effective 50–90 percent of the time for those with anal fissures.[36] They move the pain from one end to the other though, as both (nitro more often) give many people a splitting headache.

Step 6. *Break and Enter*

• Injections of Botox (botulinum toxin) temporarily paralyze the internal anal sphincter muscle so the fissure can heal. Between 60–96 percent of patients note improvement.[37,38] Temporary leakage of gas or stool is likely. Often, only one shot is needed.

• As a last resort, for a stubborn fissure that will not heal, a piece of the sphincter muscle is removed; the spasm stops, and healing commences. This causes fecal incontinence in up to 30 percent of patients.[39]

Her Story

Lotty is a librarian in a major city.

"At first I thought it was pain from a hemorrhoid. I had a lot of pains-in-the-butt going on: an abusive boss and a difficult mother.

"The first doctor said it was a fissure. The next wanted to do invasive tests. The third was ready to wheel me into surgery. It was all very discouraging and wore me out.

"I decided my body was helping me express and understand how badly ripped up I had become. I committed to a year-long process of healing my digestive tract. I used yellow dock root, dandelion root and slippery elm powder internally. Plantain and comfrey leaf oil externally kept me pain free.

"Though at times I felt sure the fissure was getting worse, it did finally resolve after a year. I have been fissure-free and pain-free for six years now. I couldn't have done it without the loving support of my herbal and witchy friends!"

 Pelvic Floor Star: Fenugreek (*Trigonella foenum-graecum*) 

Fenugreek is an annual plant in the bean family. The nutritive and soothing qualities of the seeds have made them a pelvic floor star from the time of Dioscorides to today.

A tea of the pleasant-tasting seeds is made by steeping a tablespoonful in a pint of boiling water for no more than ten minutes. The strained liquid may be taken hot with honey, or chilled.

Frequent use of fenugreek seed tea eases irritation throughout the pelvic floor and pelvic organs. It relieves hemorrhoids and chronic pelvic pain in both men and women. It restores moisture to dry vaginal tissues and eases menstrual pain. It increases the nutrition in, and the amount of, breast milk. Fenugreek was the main ingredient in Lydia Pinkham's "Vegetable Compound."

Fenugreek seeds are rich in iron, lysine, and tryptophan.[40]

The seed oil, used externally, is said to resolve fissures quickly.[41]

 Pelvic Floor Star: Horse chestnut (*Aesculus hippocastanum*) 

Horse chestnut is a large tree found throughout the temperate regions. Its primary use is as a prepared topical gel to shrink hemorrhoids and heal anal fissures. Internal use may cause problems.

Horse chestnut is a specific against "chronic venous insufficiency."[42] Placebo-controlled trials (including one restricted to pregnant women) confirm its ability to counter inflammation and tighten veins.[43] It also relieves nocturnal leg cramps, phlebitis, rheumatism, neuralgia, and bruises, and hastens recovery after surgery.[44]

Horse chestnut contains *aescin*, which reduces the permeability of blood vessels, plus tannins and quercetin, which counter pain and swelling.[45,46] There are no side effects with "proper administration of designated therapeutic dosages."[47] A cup a day of the leaf tea, 30 drops twice a day of seed tincture, or four seed-extract caps (with 120mg aescin) a day, are considered safe dosages.

horse chestnut

Cautions: Internal use of horse chestnut can redden urine![48] It thins the blood; do not take with aspirin or coumadin.

"Susceptible patients may . . . experience irritation of the gastrointestinal tract or decrease in kidney function."[49]

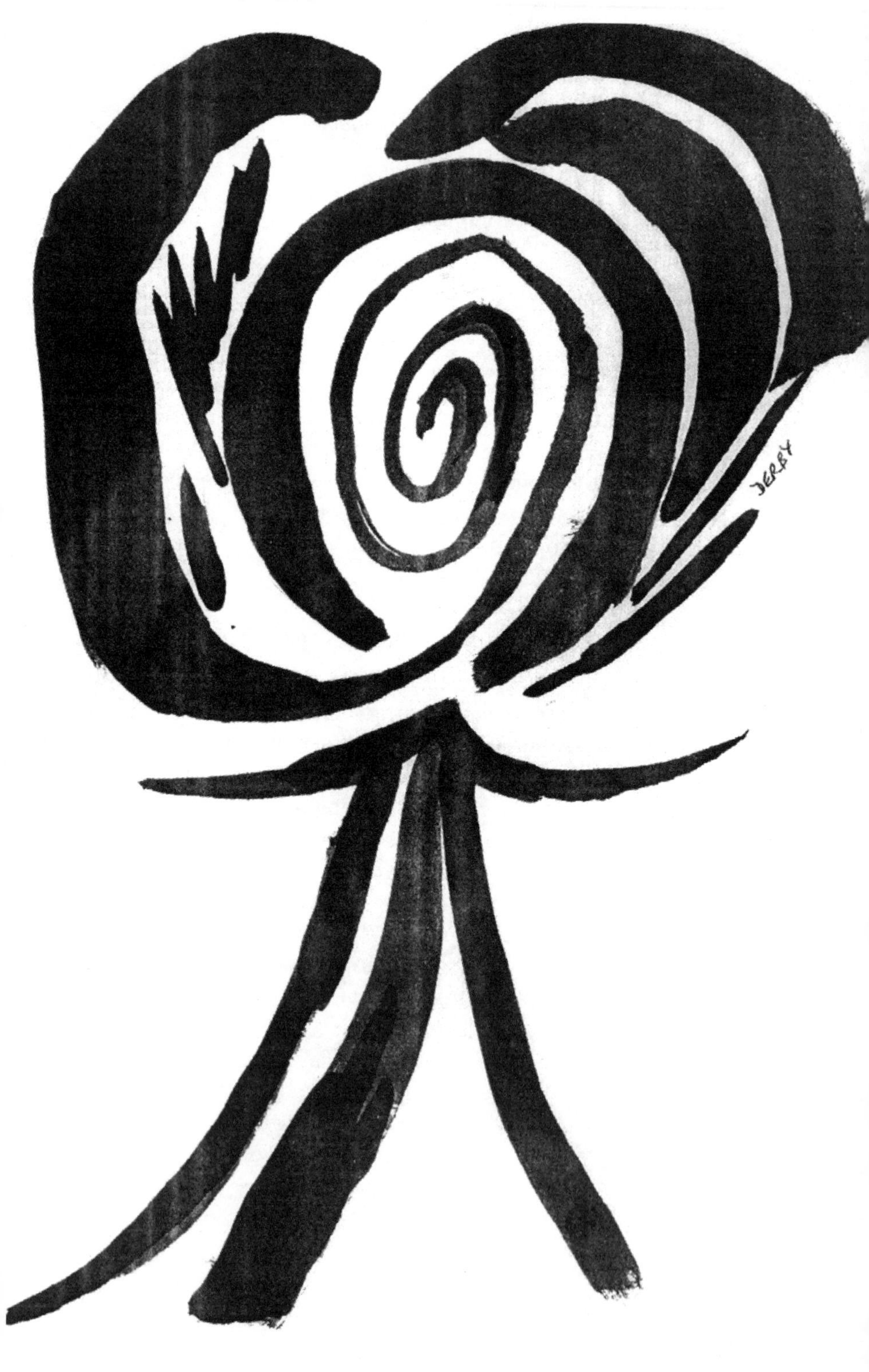

The Bladder

I am the holding tank. I am the lowest point. All flows come down to me. It all comes down to me. The blood flows 'round and 'round, and the liver decides what stays and what goes. What goes, flows to the kidneys. And when the kidneys are done with what goes 'round, it flows down to me. It all comes flowing down to me, you see.

It flows 'round and it comes down and I hold it in until it is time. Then I let it go, so it can go 'round somewhere else, back into the flow.

I am part of it all, but I am apart. I am touched by it all, but not taken. I am the container, not the contents. I offer short-term storage, no interest, no credit, just in and out, here and gone. I have no plans, no memories, no desires. Fill me. Empty me. Again. And again.

I am in the flow. I can hold it for you, but I can only hold so much.

Your rage trickles down to me. It burns me; it irritates me. Your fear of life seeps into me. It annoys me; it compresses me. Grudges precipitate and settle into me. Your suspicious nature grabs hold of me. It tears at me; it agitates me. Controlling me doesn't give you control over your life. Trust the process; surrender to the flow.

It all comes down to me. It all flows 'round and 'round, and it comes out down here. I am your bladder.

Healthy Bladder

The urinary bladder is an elastic, muscular, thin-tissued storage vessel for urine. Urine is produced by the kidneys and travels to the bladder via thin, foot-long tubes called *ureters.* The tube from the bladder to the outside is the *urethra.* An adult's bladder can hold at least 1000ml before bursting.

The bladder has an inner layer of protective, collagen-rich mucus, a middle-layer of smooth muscle (the *detrusor* – "thrust out" – *muscle*), and an outer layer of connective tissue which unites the bladder, ureters and urethra.

At the base of the bladder, smooth muscles form an internal sphincter that involuntarily releases urine. Below that, skeletal muscles – which are under conscious control – form the external urethral sphincter, giving us the choice of when to void. The average human bladder is emptied every 2–5 hours during the day.

When the bladder is about half full, stretch receptors send an impulse to the sacral spinal nerves. These send a message to the brain, causing the detrusor muscle to contract, the internal sphincter to relax, and alerting us to our need to "go." If we don't void, the urge disappears within a minute, then recurs at intervals. The tighter the stretch, the more frequent the messages to let go.

Women's bladders are constrained in size by the uterus, which lies behind it. Nonetheless, there is little difference in the capacity, or functioning, of healthy men's and women's bladders.

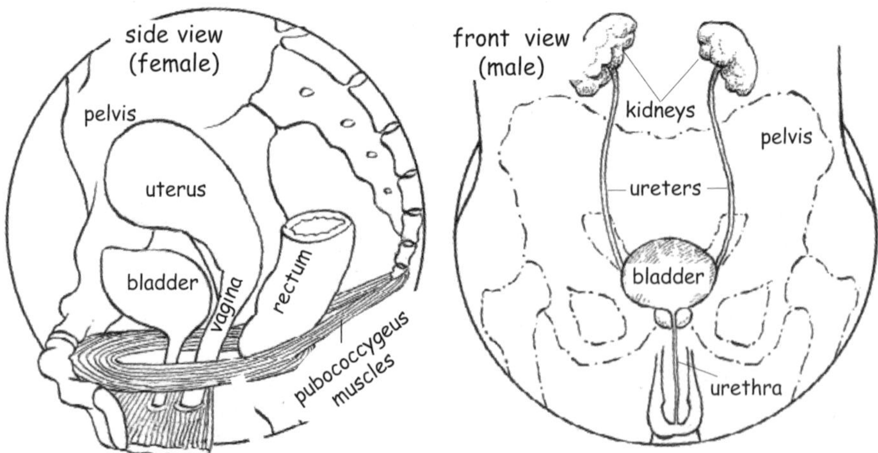

Bladder Distresses

Bladder distresses range from **retention** (can't go, page 32) to **incontinence** (can't *not* go, page 34), from mild to chronic infections/UTIs (page 59), and even to **cancer** (page 74).

If the muscles of the pelvic floor are weak, urine leaks, leading to **stress incontinence** (page 41) or **urge incontinence** (page 45). If the muscles are very lax, the bladder **prolapses** (page 6), making it difficult to empty it fully.

The bladder's proximity to hormone-rich glands – the ovaries and uterus in women, the prostate in men – gives a subtle, hormonal twist to bladder problems, especially as we age. Many women are incontinent, while men have the opposite problem: prostate swelling that causes retention.

Since her shorter urethra (4cm versus his 20cm) exposes her bladder to more bacteria, women are fifty times more likely to have **urinary tract infections** (page 59) than men. When treated promptly, with herbs or drugs, these clear quickly. If left untreated (or if the valves that keep urine from backing up into the kidneys fail to close – ureter reflux), bacteria can move into the kidneys, causing fever, chills, nausea, vomiting, back pain on one side, and even, eventually, kidney damage or kidney death.

Men's bladder distresses include prostate enlargement that squeezes the urethra, causing lower urinary tract problems (**LUTS**, page 55). Some men have a "shy" bladder (**paruresis**, page 53).

Both sexes deal with the need to urinate frequently while they ought to be sleeping (**nocturia**, page 51).

Interstitial cystitis (page 67) is an ulcerated condition of the bladder. It mimics cystitis at first. But IC gets worse, not better, and doesn't respond to treatment. IC may be related to fibromyalgia.[1]

Another problem that can cause bladder pain is urethritis, or inflammation and infection of the urethra. Bacteria – such as gonorrhea, chlamydia, *Ureaplasma urealyticum*, and *Mycoplasma genitalium* – cause this painful condition. Antibiotics – drugs or herbs (page 342) – are the treatments of choice.

Urinary Retention

"Frightened rabbits won't give birth. Frightened people hold things in their pelvises, too . . . things that hurt, that are traumatic." Grandmother Growth speaks with force, but her voice is kind.

"Your task, my spirit child, is to find a physical or mental space where you feel safe enough to let it all go, where you can let loose. Letting loose is on the right track. Shall we catch the train?"

Step 0. *Do Nothing*

• Oops, that's the problem. Seriously, though, relaxing deeply can open the valves. If it doesn't, there may be an obstruction.

Step 1. *Collect Information*

• Urinary retention is caused by: a swollen prostate gland (page 55), a phobia (page 53), trauma, surgery, or an obstruction.

★ **Obstruction is an emergency**. Catheterization can be life-saving. On the way to the hospital, take parsley root tincture.

Step 2. *Engage the Energy*

• Homeopathic *Stigmata Zea mays* is specific for relieving retained/suppressed urine.

• To trigger release: Put a warm, wet washcloth on the urethra; put your hand under warm running water; listen to water.

Step 3. *Nourish and Tonify*

★ **Dandelion**, **chickweed**, and **nettle** are three good friends who work together to increase urinary output and voiding ease. A dose is 10–20 drops of each **tincture**, repeated every ten minutes.

• The roots of **goldenrod** (*Solidago*), alone or with nettle roots, make a brew famous for relieving urinary retention.

Step 4. *Stimulate/Sedate*

• Traditional Chinese Medicine (TCM) views retention or difficulty in voiding as a *kidney yang deficiency* and *dysfunction of the Triple Burner.* The TCM formula on page 369 is complicated but effective.

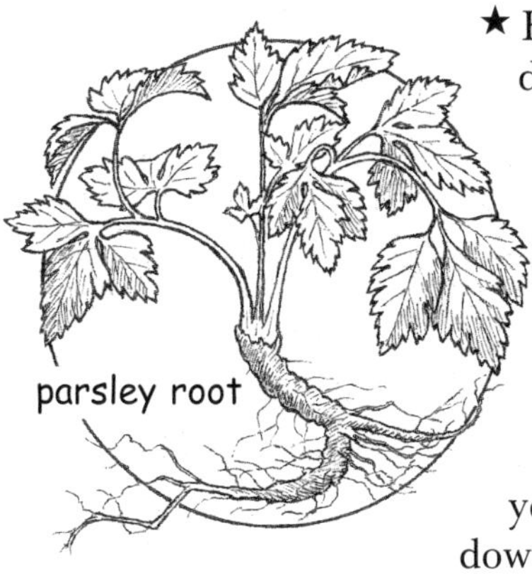

parsley root

★ Herbalists traditionally use dropperful doses, taken every 20-120 minutes, of tinctures to relieve urinary retention. Best bets: **parsley** root, **buchu** leaves, **juniper** berries, **saw palmetto** berries, or **uva ursi** leaves.

• Can't go? Run hot water over your hands or get into a hot bath or shower and squat down. Put your hand above your pubic bone; lightly push in and down, expelling the urine. Or, get on your hands and knees and let gravity help.

Step 5. *Use Drugs*

• Diuretics do work. Short-term.

Step 6. *Break and Enter*

• At least half the time, urinary retention is caused by use of a nasal decongestant or an antihistamine. Stop taking the drug and spontaneous urination returns.

• A **catheter** (a plastic tube) is passed through the urethra into the bladder to empty it when you can't. An indwelling catheter, often used after pelvic surgery, can easily cause a bladder infection. Protect yourself with cranberries (page 61).

Help!
Urinary Retention

Expect results in two hours

• Take a dropperful of dandelion or **parsley root tincture** every twenty minutes.

• Sit in a **hot bath** and relax.

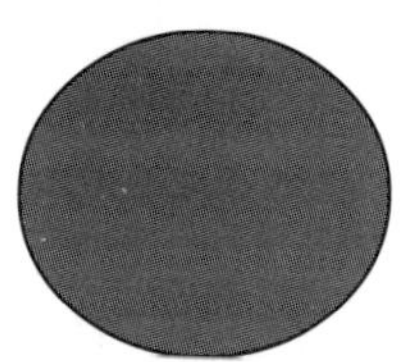

Urinary Incontinence

"Stir the heat in your pelvis or it will leak out, dear one," Grandmother Growth admonishes. "Clench your pelvic floor muscles – then release! Clench! Clench! Clench! Reclaim your power. Speak your anger instead of pissing it away. Stand tall and clench those pelvic floor muscles. Clench! Clench! Clench!

"Clench without stress, clench without tension, my precious one," Grandmother Growth soothes. "Let your pelvis be at peace.

"Clench and say 'no' out loud so your bladder doesn't have to scream it. Clench! Clench! Clench!"

Step 0. *Do Nothing*

> "To determine which type of incontinence a patient has, a doctor must perform lengthy and exhaustive tests."[2]

• You can avoid the expensive tests needed for a diagnosis of incontinence. You know if you leak and when. If not, keep a diary. For safety sake, rule out infection or bleeding with a simple, non-invasive, urine test. Then answer the questions below, and try the Wise Woman remedies gathered here. Specialists concur that at least 80 percent of those with incontinence can regain near-normal bladder control with life-style changes.[3]

 What Kind of Urinary Incontinence? 

During the last three months, if you leaked urine, was it

- When coughing, sneezing, lifting, or exercising?
  Stress incontinence, giggle incontinence (page 41).
- When you needed to go?
  Urge incontinence, overactive bladder (page 45).
- Both? *Mixed incontinence* (keep reading).

Step 1. *Collect Information*

> "There's no distinct structure around the female urethra. Age weakens all the pelvic tissues. So, as you get older, the 'gasket' doesn't work as well. It's a design flaw."[4]

• Incontinence affects 10–35 percent of women globally, including 30 million American women,[5] who spend over 17 billion dollars a years on incontinence pads and treatments.[6]

• Urinary incontinence means leakage of urine, often because of muscle weakness, but also because of muscle spasms.

~ **Stress incontinence** affects half of those who leak. Weak pelvic floor muscles can't prevent leakage when there is pressure from coughing, sneezing, laughing, exercising, or bending. Heredity, childbearing, age, and surgery can weaken muscles; herbs and pelvic floor exercises can strengthen them.

~ **Urge incontinence** (**overactive bladder**) causes a voiding urge so intense it is impossible to prevent leaks. It may be caused by muscle or nerve spasms, inflammation, chronic low-level bladder infections, an enlarged prostate, a fibroid tumor, uncontrolled diabetes, a stroke, even circulatory or neurological problems. Herbs and exercises can relax spasms, counter inflammation, eliminate infection and ease prostate swelling.

~ **Overflow incontinence** is rare. Urine leaks continually and constantly. Uncontrolled diabetes, MS, a very enlarged prostate, and prostate surgery can cause it.

~ **Functional incontinence** occurs in those who are physically unable to get to the toilet in time or who fail to get or recognize voiding signals due to Alzheimer's, dementia, MS, or paralysis. It may also result

Help!
Urinary Incontinence

Expect results in 2–4 weeks

• Do **Kegels** (page 10) or low-intensity behavioral training.

• **Avoid** soda, diet soda, coffee, alcohol, fruit/citrus juice, and high-fructose corn sweetener.

• Drink 2 cups of **nettle**, **oatstraw**, or **linden** infusion, and ½ cup cranberry juice, daily.

• Stop taking hormones (ERT, HRT, the Pill, bio-identicals).

• Ally with **dandelion root**.

from pelvic surgery or injury to pelvic nerves. Exercises and nerve-nourishing herbs such as oatstraw, passionflower, and skullcap can complement drugs.

~ **Transient incontinence** is usually triggered by a drug or infection and is relieved when the irritant is removed.

• Is incontinence linked to **age**? In men, probably. In women, probably not. Incontinence is experienced by 57 percent of post-menopausal women and 47 percent of those under fifty.[7]

• Does **childbearing** cause incontinence? No. A study comparing more than a thousand pairs of postmenopausal sisters – one who had given birth vaginally and one who had never given birth – found little difference in the incidence, type, or severity of incontinence.[8] If there was prolapse, the stage and type was similar.[9]

• **Weight** makes no significant difference to the likelihood of incontinence.[10,11] But if you are incontinent, the more you weigh, the worse it will be. Women who lost as little as three pounds had 28 percent fewer leaks; those who lost more cut their leaks by half.[12] Being **diabetic** increases incontinence risk by 70 percent.[13,14]

• If your mother or older sisters were/are incontinent, you are twice as likely to share their fate.[15] Genes predispose us to incontinence and prolapses. Caucasian women have more of those genes than African-American or Asian women.[16]

• The Women's Health Initiative found over 66 percent of 161,861 women aged 50–79 leaked in a given year. The strongest risk factors were: hysterectomy before the age of 40, first birth at age less than 20, and breast-feeding (regardless of duration).[17]

> "More money is spent on menstrual pads for incontinence than for menstruation."[18]

Step 2. *Engage the Energy*

★ **Low-intensity behavioral training** works as well as surgery, without side effects or complications, in relieving all types of incontinence.[19] Six weekly twenty-minute sessions helped reduce accidents by at least 50 percent. A third of the participants became completely dry after keeping a diary of voids and leaks, learning Kegel exercises (page 10), and training themselves to wait longer and longer between voiding.

• If your incontinence leaves you feeling ashamed, **embarrassed**, and reluctant to socialize, remember, you are not alone. A dose of 10–20 drops of calming **motherwort** tincture may make it easier for you to seek assistance and consider your options.

• **Timed urination** – voiding regularly on a schedule – helps elderly, frail, or forgetful people get to the toilet before it's too late. By slowly expanding interval length, timed urination also helps you train your bladder to hold more urine and void less often.

• **Functional magnetic stimulation** of the pelvic floor muscles, is a safe, effective treatment against stress and urge incontinence. After two twenty-minute treatments a week for eight weeks, 58 percent of women had less leakage; some were completely dry.[20]

• **Homeopathic** remedies for bladder problems cover fourteen pages in the *Homeopathic Clinical Repertory*. I have listed some here and others in the sections on stress and urge incontinence.

~ *Achillea millefolium*: chronic incontinence.
~ *Cantharis*: violent burning pain on voiding.
~ *Juniperus communis*: bladder heavy, urine scant, especially in elders. (Avoid if pregnant.)
~ *Nux vomica*: pain in the bladder, great urgency.
~ *Rhus aromatica* (or *Agrimony*): constant dribbling.
~ *Thuja* (or *Claviceps pur.*): weak bladder, great urgency.

> "The detrusor muscle is comparable to the bulbous end of the baster, reflexively contracting when nerves fire in the muscle. In order for the urinary system to function in a controlled way, the muscles must be strong, the nerves must be in good order, and the bladder itself must be in good physical condition."[21]

Step 3. *Nourish and Tonify*

• Nourish the bladder by eating more apricots, black cherries, blueberries, brown rice, beans, celery, corn, cranberries, lentils, miso, parsley, and prunes (dried plums).

★ **Seaweeds** nourish and heal the muscles, nerves, and mucosa of the kidneys, ureters, bladder, and urethra. Eating **kelps** such as wakame, kombu, alaria, and nereocystis (bull whip) cooked in soups, beans, and whole grains is more effective than taking pills.

★ Nourish and strengthen bladder muscles with 1–2 quarts of **comfrey** leaf or **nettle** leaf infusion weekly. Add a pinch of silica-rich **horsetail** for even more effect.

★ Soothe bladder mucosa with teas of **corn silk**, **plantain seed**, or **mullein**. Or use a dropperful (1–3 times a day) of tincture of **burdock** root/seed, **cleavers** herb, or **marshmallow** root.

★ **Dandelion** tea or tincture tones and tightens bladder sphincters. Regular use of 5–19 drops daily of tincture of **passionflower**, **oatstraw**, or **skullcap** strengthens the nerves of the bladder.

★ Squat, crawl, and sit cross-legged to strengthen pelvic floor muscles and counter incontinence.

★ Women who did at least forty Kegel clenches (page 10) a day for three or more months were able to control or cure stress, urge, and mixed incontinence, unlike those receiving sham treatments.[22] Women who were coached got the best results. Dr. Kegel advises five clenches on awakening while still in bed, five more when up, then five every half-hour throughout the day.

• Avoid these common bladder **irritants**: food preservatives, artificial sweeteners, flavors, and colors, coffee, alcohol, pepper, curry, black tea, tomatoes, citrus, parsley juice, and soda pop.[23]

• If incontinence makes you reluctant to be passionately **sexual** for fear you'll wet the bed, invest in a waterproof pad, please!

Out On A (Plastic) Limb

Plastic in the diet is associated with prostate cancer, PCOS,[24] and perhaps incontinence as well. Therefore I:

- Avoid microwaved food.
- Avoid food in styrofoam.
- Store leftovers in glass.
- Avoid bottled water.
- Avoid produce, meat, and fish wrapped in plastic.

• **Yellow dock** root gently aids bowel movements, freeing the pelvic floor from the pressure of constipation. The tea is too bitter for most, so tincture is preferable. A dropperful a day is the dose.

★ **Yoga**, Pilates, weight lifting, and tai chi build core strength and tone up tiny muscles in the pelvis that help you stay in control.

Step 4. *Stimulate/Sedate*

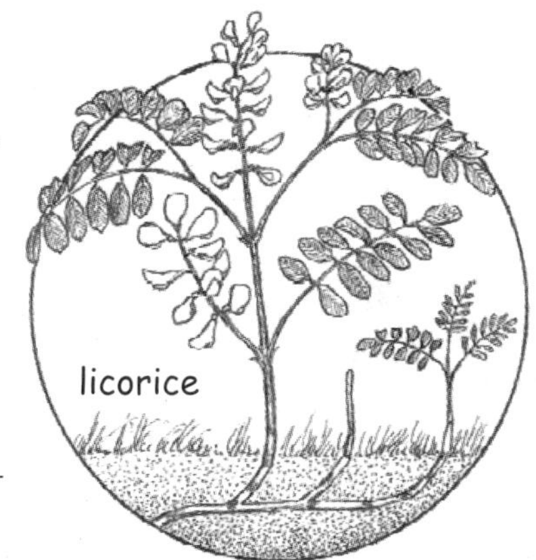

• Tinctures of **damiana** leaf, **licorice** root, **kava kava** root, **uva ursi** leaf, **black haw**, and/or **cramp bark** – in doses ranging from 1–8 dropperfuls a day – help counter incontinence. **Licorice** is a specific against "kidney insufficiency" and incontinence. Take it with dandelion to prevent electrolyte disturbances.

• Herbalist Holly Guzman, who specializes in urinary difficulties, relies on "elevator pills" to help lift and strengthen the pelvic floor. Buy them at Chinese pharmacies as *buz-hongyiqitang.* Look for *Golden Lock Pills*, too, a traditional formula against "bed wetting."

Step 5. *Use Drugs*

• A wide range of drugs – diuretics, sedatives, antidepressants, antihistamines, calcium channel blockers, and alpha-blockers – can cause or worsen incontinence.[25]

• Hormone replacement (ERT or HRT) increases the risk that a healthy woman will become incontinent, and makes the symptoms worse in women who already are.[26]

In the Women's Health Initiative study, 27,000 postmenopausal women were given either hormones or a placebo. The incidence, frequency, and severity of all types of **incontinence increased significantly in women taking ERT** or **HRT**. [27,28,29] This was true for all racial and ethnic groups,[30] and was not linked to prior incontinence. The longer the use, the greater the risk.

In HERS (Hormone and Estrogen Replacement Study), half of the women who took HRT developed incontinence, compared to a third of those who took the placebo. After only one year, the risk of weekly episodes of incontinence was three times greater among hormone users; after four years it was five time higher.[31]

• Drugs that treat incontinence can cause a rapid decline in your mental acuity. Those who take Detrol or Ditropan have a rate of **cognitive decline** that is one and a half times faster than those who did not take these drugs.[32] If you are taking medications for dementia as well, the mental decline is magnified.[33]

• Drugs always have side effects. Research carefully before use. After 3–4 months, go without to see if you still need the drug. (More information on incontinence drugs on page 49.)

Step 6. *Break and Enter*

> "In addition to being risky, surgery can cause significant discomfort — and it isn't always effective [in treating urinary incontinence]."[34]

• Mild electrical shocks, delivered in a clinic or at home with a prescription device, can relieve urge and stress incontinence.[35] The current provokes involuntary muscle contractions, which, over a period of months of daily treatments, has the same effect as Kegels: the muscles and nerves of the bladder are strengthened.

• FDA-approved **Urgent PCNe uromodulation** looks like acupuncture, but isn't. A needle is inserted near the ankle to stimulate a bladder-controlling nerve that goes up the leg to the pelvis. Twelve thirty-minute sessions reduced leakage by at least half for most participants.[36]

Odor-Free

Chlorophyll (taken orally) reduces/eliminates urine odors.[37] One of the richest sources of chlorophyll (yes, even more than wheat grass), is **nettle infusion**. Chlorophyll pills work, too.

Stress Incontinence

Step 0. *Do Nothing*

• Limiting fluids, especially before exercise, can help.

Step 1. *Collect Information*

• Repeated childbearing can weaken pelvic muscles. And some birthing situations make it more likely.

~ Women who receive an epidural, or who deliver by C-section, are twice as likely to have stress incontinence as they age.[38]

~ Women who tuck their chin and hold their breath during the peak of a labor contraction (coached pushing) give birth more quickly, but increase their risk of stress incontinence.[39]

• Stress incontinence is common after prostate surgery.

Step 2. *Engage the Energy*

• **Homeopathic** remedies for those with stress incontinence:

~ *Belladonna*: leakage starts after childbirth or surgery.
~ *Causticum*: unaware of leaks on coughing, walking, sneezing.
~ *Ferrum*: tickling sensation in bladder/urethra, better at night.
~ *Nux vomica*: leaks laughing, coughing, sneezing; great urge.
~ *Pulsatilla*: leakage worse for sitting, walking.
~ *Sepia*: bearing down sensation with leakage, also at night.

Step 3. *Nourish and Tonify*

★ Nothing is as **effective** at countering incontinence as pelvic floor exercises (page 10). Dr. Kegel called stress incontinence "pelvic fatigue syndrome." Any wo/man bothered by incontinence, prolapse, or a desire for stronger orgasms will benefit.

• To nourish the bladder, drink two or more quarts of **comfrey leaf** infusion a week. Adding more **fat** to the diet helps, too.

★ Make the effort to **stay active**. Exercise strengthens the muscles of the back, belly, and thighs, making the pelvic floor stronger, and incontinence less likely. Many women give up sports because jumping, tensing their thighs or buttocks, or lifting weight causes leakage. Protect yourself with a liner, a pad, or protective underwear. Or fight back with a tampon.

Women who wear a **tampon** while exercising stay significantly drier.[41] (It holds the pelvic floor up.) A rubber pessary or a **sea sponge** tampon (page 250) does it too, and can be reused many times. Or try a plug. Really! There are tiny urethral plugs that stopper the urethra to prevent leaks.

Step 4. *Stimulate/Sedate*

• There are four primary nonsurgical medical remedies currently in use to treat stress incontinence: pessaries, electricity, estrogen, and physical therapy. An NIH-sponsored summary of over 96 clinical trials found: Pessaries and plugs do decrease leakage, but don't cure. Electrical stimulation has no effect. Oral estrogen makes incontinence worse. Physical therapies – **Kegels** and bladder-retraining – **produce the most consistently beneficial results**, helping more than half of the women using them.[40]

Step 5. *Use Drugs*

• Actually, *don't* use drugs. Prescription drugs are not effective in relieving stress incontinence, with the possible exception of duloxetine – an antidepressant which blocks re-uptake of serotonin and norepinephrine in the spinal cord, thus stimulating the nerve that contracts the urethral sphincter.

• Pseudoephedrine activates the autonomic nervous system and causes the urethra to tighten, but only in about 10 percent of those who take it; and it raises blood pressure.[42]

• Topical vaginal **estrogen cream** may relieve your stress incontinence, especially if menopause aggravated it.

> "Everyone who is incontinent has weak pelvic floor muscles. Those with stress incontinence deny the problem, pay little attention to bladder signals, and are surprised when a slight physical exertion forces urine out. The urge patient, on the other hand, is preoccupied with bladder signals . . . and rushes to the toilet at the first signals. . . [and] the brain learns to stop inhibiting the reflexive contractions of the bladder. . . ."[43]

Step 6. *Break and Enter*

★ A new surgical option may revolutionize the treatment of stress incontinence. Under local anesthesia, muscle cells are cut from the biceps. They are grown for six weeks, or until there are 60 million of them. Injected into the muscle that controls the flow of urine, they proliferate and rebuild the sphincter, restoring full bladder control in 90 percent of the women within 24 hours.[44,45] Ferdinand Frauscher, MD, of Innsbruck, co-developer of the technique says: "The whole procedure . . . takes just 10–15 minutes. It reverses the effects of aging. . . ."[46] Most women (80 percent) retained complete bladder control for a year afterward. Long-term data are not yet available.

> "Getting help when surgery is needed can be challenging, because female reproduction and urology are separate medical specialities. Urologists know little more than the basics about female reproductive organs . . . few doctors in either specialty know much about treating middle-aged and older women."[47]

• Surgery to resolve incontinence is neither easy nor always successful. If you do decide to go for it, a *urogynecologist* – someone who specializes in female urinary problems – is preferred.

• **Collagen** injections, used to bulk up weakened bladder muscles, have to be repeated every six months, can cause allergic reactions, and generally provide only partial relief.

• **Trans-vaginal radio frequencies** – applied by means of a thin probe inserted into the vagina during a twenty-minute, local anesthesia, outpatient, surgical procedure – heat up and break down pelvic floor muscles and the urethra. The resulting scar tissue gives firmer, surer control. Three-quarters of women who have the procedure, called Renessa, were continent or improved at the one year follow-up.[48,49] No long-term studies are available.

• **Weight loss**, even a little, even as a result of bariatric surgery, reduces the severity of both urinary and fecal incontinence.[50]

• Think having a C-section instead of a vaginal birth will protect you against later incontinence? It won't.[51,52]

• A **hysterectomy** may help – but only if you are already incontinent. In a study of 1200 women, 89 percent of those with severe, and 62 percent of those with moderate incontinence experienced improvement after a hysterectomy. However, 17 percent of those with mild or no prior incontinence experienced leakage in the year after surgery.[53] Middle-aged women with hysterectomies had a 60 percent higher risk of incontinence later in life.[54]

> "For women who aren't satisfied with partial relief, surgery is the treatment most likely to succeed."[55]

• Surgical corrections for incontinence used to be limited to the Burch (49 percent cure rate) or the fascial sling (66 percent cure rate).[56] These are now obsolete. A minimally invasive procedure, the midurethral sling (65–90 percent cure rate), places a narrow strip of plastic mesh under the urethera. It takes 15–30 minutes under local anesthesia. About 10 percent of women have an adverse reaction to the polypropylene mesh.[57] Bladder perforation occurs in 6 percent of retropubic slings (TVT).[58] Transobturator slings (TOT) avoid the bladder but cut into the vagina.

> ". . . no woman should have to live with stress incontinence, as long as a qualified surgeon performs the procedure."[59]

The FDA has received over 1,000 reports of adverse events following pelvic reconstructive (urinary sling) surgery with synthetic mesh-based materials. They issued a **Public Health Notification.** Signs of complications include: yellow discharge, chronic vaginal infection, persistent bleeding, paniful intercourse, and (yikes!) protrusions of mesh through the vaginal wall.

Urge Incontinence
Overactive Bladder

"My dearest," Grandmother Growth says with a wink, "your power is in your belly. When you pee too much, you piss away your strength. When you fear the life force that lives inside you, you can't retain it, you lose it.

"Gather yourself up. Take yourself in hand. Hold yourself with a firm grip. Bear up. Pull yourself up, not by your bootstraps, but by your pelvic floor. Sweet child, contain yourself by opening yourself to life. Allow life to pulse and vibrate in every cell. You can do it. You can."

Step 0. *Do Nothing*

• Spare yourself the health risks of invasive tests. The majority of cases of urge incontinence are idiopathic, that is, they have no known cause. Try some of these simple, safe, effective remedies.

Step 1. *Collect Information*

• About 34 million Americans have an urgent and frequent need to urinate more than ten times in 24 hours.[60] Most are older than 40, and one-third to one-half are men.

• The "urge" in urgent bladder comes on so quickly and so powerfully that there isn't time to get to a toilet, even if you are standing right next to one! For some, even the thought or sight of a toilet causes leakage.

Help!
Overactive Bladder

Expect results in two weeks

• Use a **visualization** daily.

• Do your **Kegels** every day.

• Keep a voiding **diary**; retrain your bladder; use **biofeedback**.

• Drink a quart or more **comfrey leaf** infusion each week.

• Diagnostic tests rarely reveal a reason for urge incontinence, and they may be harmful. If you don't have an enlarged prostate, a bladder infection, vaginal yeast overgrowth, interstitial cystitis, fibromyalgia, or multiple sclerosis, then your incontinence is caused by **abnormal nerve signals** to the bladder that initiate spastic muscle contractions, uncontrollable urges, and urine leaks.

• A **bladder diary** lists the times of day you urinate (including leaks), the amount of urine you void, what you drink and eat and when, and medicines you took. Over a period of a week or two, patterns emerge that can help you retrain your bladder.

> "About 30 percent of women [with overactive bladders] get better simply by understanding what's happening and thinking about it."[61]

Step 2. *Engage the Energy*

★ A powerful **visualization** coupled with a physical trigger can put you in control of your bladder, fast. Choose an image, visualize it repeatedly, then use it to help prevent leaks and urgency. Visualizing for even two minutes a day controls incontinence faster than drugs. Use the physical trigger while you visualize, and eventually it, alone, will be enough to control your urge.

Sit alone in a tranquil environment (a bathtub is fine); close your eyes and imagine vividly. Use all your senses: see the scene, taste it, smell it, feel its texture, listen to it. As in a dream, you can create whatever you want. Allow yourself time to create your visualization and make it real; don't try to do it all at once. Create your own visualization or try one of these:

~ Visualize the nerve messages flowing between the bladder and brain as a stream. Build dams and locks along the stream to slow it down. Squeeze your fist in a slow rhythm.

~ Visualize the bladder nerve pathway as a road. Imagine the cars and trucks on the road. Then visualize toll booths at intervals, starting at the bladder and working your way up to the brain. Gently bite your lower lip.

~ Visualize a large strong hand gently but firmly pushing up between your legs, strengthening your pelvic floor, lessening the voiding urge, and giving you warm comfort. Smile.

• **Homeopathic remedies** for those with urge incontinence:
- ~ *Arnica montana*: constant urging, bladder feels full and sore.
- ~ *Cantharis*: intolerable urgency, burning leakage.
- ~ *Nitric acid*: painless incontinence; urine smelly, like a horse.
- ~ *Ph-ac.*: milky, watery, profuse urine gushes out.
- ~ *Rhus tox.*: urine dark, scanty; worse at night or when sitting.
- ~ *Sulphur*: sudden, intense, uncontrollable urges.

★ **Biofeedback** using electrical or pressure-sensing devices can increase awareness of the bladder, thereby foiling urge incontinence. Biofeedback is so well-studied, and so effective in relieving incontinence, that Medicare covers the cost.

Step 3. *Nourish and Tonify*

★ **Retrain your bladder**. Counter the urge by gradually lengthening the time between visits to the toilet. With practice, your nerves will signal less frequently.

• Food additives such as potassium sorbate, aspartame, and food colorings aggravate urge incontinence.[62]

★ Including at least 25 grams of real **fiber** from whole grains, beans, and nuts in the daily diet may significantly ease overactivity in the bladder and help end urge incontinence.

• **Caffeine** makes the bladder contract. No wonder women who take in 300mg of caffeine a day (3 cups of coffee) are 70 percent more likely to have an overactive bladder.[62A]

Step 4. *Stimulate/Sedate*

★ For **men** with overactive bladders, herbalist Terry Willard uses a tea of equal parts **parsley** leaf, **corn silk**, and **dandelion** leaf to reduce urine acidity and ease bladder irritability. When needed, he adds wild yam root to soothe and valerian to calm.[63]

★ **Saw palmetto berries**, in tincture or tea, relax the smooth muscle in the bladder neck and help reduce overactivity.

• Herbal nurse Martha Libster uses **ma huang** to reduce swelling and relax the spastic muscles of overactive bladders.[64]

• Heat and inflammation underlie an overactive bladder. Herbalists in India counter this with cooling, soothing **infusions** of **marshmallow** root, **plantain** leaf, or **mullein** leaf. **Linden** or **comfrey** infusions do the same.

• If your problem is severe, add 1–4 tablespoons of powdered **turmeric** to your daily quart of infusion.[65]

• If you can't get the knack of doing pelvic floor clenches (Kegels), don't despair. Engage a pelvic floor physical therapist to act as a personal trainer for you and your bladder.

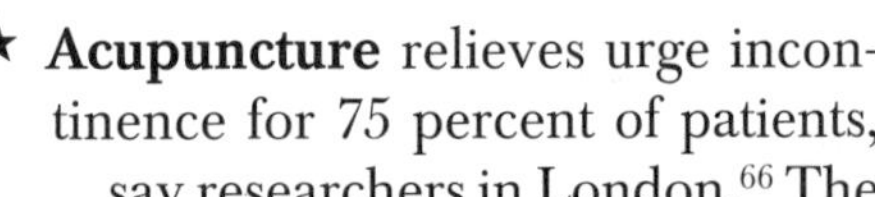

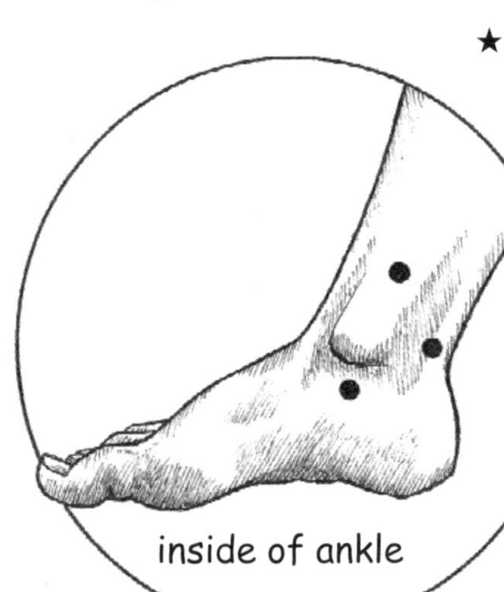

★ **Acupuncture** relieves urge incontinence for 75 percent of patients, say researchers in London.[66] The Oregon Department of Health agrees. As few as four weekly treatments increased bladder capacity, reduced urgency and frequency, and improved the quality of life just as well as drug or behavioral therapies.[67] Do it yourself: Press hard for 2–3 minutes on each indicated spot (illustrated, left), which will be tender, on both ankles, daily for three months.

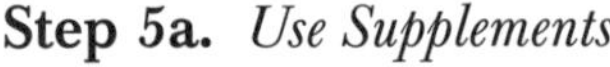

Step 5a. *Use Supplements*

• An herbal extract containing hops and uva ursi with alpha-tocopherol acetate (vitamin E) eased bladder irritability/pain and lessened urinary incontinence in 772 of 915 patients.[68]

• **Magnesium** deficiency triggers muscle spasms and urge incontinence.[69] Supplements of 200–600mg daily may help. Or up your magnesium level with infusion of oatstraw or nettle.

• Vegans and vegetarians with overactive bladders probably lack **vitamin B_{12}** – a critical nutrient found only in animal foods. Vitamin B_{12} deficiency causes uncontrollable bladder spasms.[70] The cure is a healthier diet; eat eggs, fish, organic dairy, and meat. Vitamin B_{12} cannot be absorbed from oral supplements. Want a test? Have your methylmalonic acid level checked; it's a better indicator of deficiency than tests for vitamin B_{12} itself.[71]

Step 5b. *Use Drugs*

★ "Water pills" and tranquilizers can aggravate an overactive bladder. Herbal diuretics – like **corn silk**, **burdock** root, or **dandelion** – don't. Neither do herbal tranquilizers like **St. Joan's wort**, **passionflower**, or **motherwort** tincture, 1–4 dropperfuls daily.

• For a current list of drugs that cause incontinence and bladder woes, check www.worstpills.org.

• Antimuscarinic, anticholinergic, and antispasmodic drugs – such as Ditropan, Detrol, and Sanctura – relax the bladder's detrusor muscle and extend the time between urge and voiding. Drugs are "better than nothing, but their effect is minimal (a reducction of one urination a day compared to placebo)."[72] The "side effects may be nearly as troublesome as the incontinence itself."[73] And dangerous: increased blood pressure and heart rate, arrhythmias, inhibited secretion of stomach acid, saliva, and sweat, dry mouth, constipation, worsening of glaucoma, confusion, impaired attention, and memory problems.[74]

★ Although topical vaginal estrogen cream can calm an overactive bladder, low **estrogen** doesn't cause incontinence. In fact, postmenopausal women who take oral estrogen have more incontinence and worse urinary symptoms than those who don't.[75]

• Tofranil (imipramine), an antidepressant, in conjunction with an antimuscarinic can tighten the urinary sphincter and relax spasming bladder muscles. There are side effects.

• Gelnique is an antispasmodic drug applied topically to calm an overactive bladder. After twelve weeks of use, 27 percent of women had complete relief of symptoms.[76]

Step 6. *Break and Enter*

• Two last resorts, both invasive, experimental, and costly:

~ Botox, delivered to the bladder lining via catheter, blocks nerve impulses that trigger overactive bladder.

~ Surgical implantation of a *sacral neuromodulator* relaxes spasming bladder muscles.

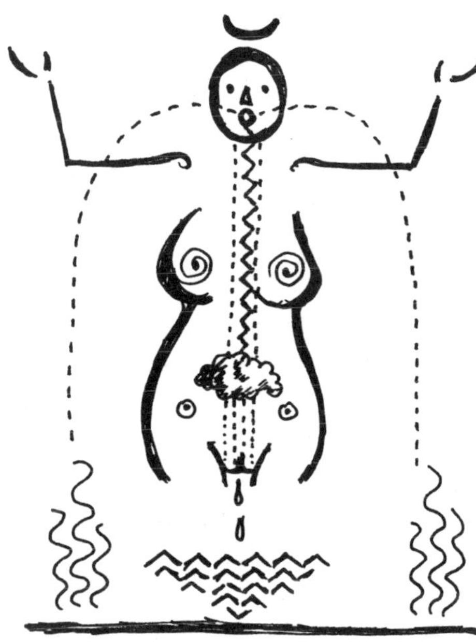

Her Story

Randi is a well-educated African-American woman who has had Parkinson's for more than twenty years.

"Over the past five years, my bladder has become more and more overactive. The primary medicine I use to deal with my Parkinson's is the Ayurvedic remedy, *mucuna pruriens.* It has to be taken in water, and that aggravated the situation. Eventually, I started taking oxybutin; but it became less effective over time, and it made my bowels so sluggish that I fell into the habit of using colonic irrigation (high enema) every month!

"Then I read Susun's article on comfrey. I got the summary of the comfrey research from the Henry Doubleday Research Institute here in the UK. They refuted the claims that comfrey could not be ingested. I started to take comfrey tea.

"The results were fast and dramatic. No more urinary urgency! Then I noticed my constipation, or rather, I didn't notice it. It was gone, too.

"By sheer coincidence, earlier this year I bought a *Symphytum uplandica* to plant in my herbaceous garden. It is so easy to grow! I dry it and make my tea; for the first time in a long time, I feel like I have some control over my health. Parkinson's isn't easy to live with, but my bladder and bowel problems were the straw that broke this camel's back. Thanks to comfrey, neither of them bother me now."

Nocturia

"When we lived wild, fire kept us safe," muses Grandmother Growth. "When we lived wild, night creatures were kept away by the steady glow of fire. When we lived wild, we kept alert all night long, listening for predators, keeping the fire going.

"You are no longer wild, my beloved. You don't need to feed the fire, but your body remembers and wakes you up at night. Honor your part in protecting the young when this happens; smile. And remind your bladder that you are not alone, not solely responsible for the fire.

"Yes, you are allowed to rest my dear, to take a break from eternal vigilance. Spiral down into deep dreams. Rest. Trust. Rest."

Step 1. *Collect Information*

• Nocturia – waking to urinate more than twice a night – is common during menopause and as we age. The real risk is that you'll fall on the way to the bathroom in the dark. Women with nocturia are 26 percent more likely to fall, and 34 percent more likely to break a bone.[77] Protect yourself. Keep a chamber pot by your bed. Remove scatter rugs. Keep a flashlight handy. (Nightlights disturb deep sleep.)

Help! Nocturia

Expect results in two weeks

• Are your medications to blame? If so, change them.

• Drink **nettle infusion** or **cranberry juice** daily.

• Drink less in the evening and more during the day.

• As we age, a natural shift in the timing of urination occurs. Instead of being most active during the day, the urinary system gets into gear at night, alas.

• Hypertension, diabetes, stroke, kidney disease, and bladder tumors also cause nocturia, as does prostate enlargement. (LUTS, page 55; BPH, page 329.)

Step 2. *Engage the Energy*

• Homeopathic remedies for those with nocturia include: *Apis*, *Argentum nitricum*, *Arnica montana*, *Arsenicum*, *Belladonna*, *Benzoicum acidum*, *Causticum*, *Equis hyemale*, *Ferrum metalicum*, *Graphites*, *Kalium nitricum*, *Kreosotum*, *Lac caninum*, *Magnesium phosph.*, *Natrum muriaticum*, *Nitricum*, *Pulsatilla*, *Rhus tox.*, *Sepia*, *Silicea terra*, and *Sulphur*.

Step 3. *Nourish and Tonify*

★ My favorite herbal remedy for menopausal women with nocturia is **nettle infusion**. It rebuilds healthy adrenal function, deepens sleep, and resets the bladder clock. The initial response to drinking nettle infusion is more frequent urination, but this rarely continues for more than a few days, after which frequency and urge normalize.

★ **Quercetin** is a strong antioxidant. It is the preferred helper for men with nocturia because it decreases urinary and pelvic inflammation and inhibits cell damage in the kidneys, too. Find quercetin in oak bark, nettles, cranberries, and blueberries.

Step 4. *Stimulate/Sedate*

• Limiting fluid intake to a little **water only** in the four hours before bed helps. Volunteers who reduced fluid intake by 25 percent had 34 percent less urgency, a 23 percent reduction in daytime frequency, and a 7 percent decrease in nocturia.[78]

Step 5. *Use Drugs*

• Diuretic blood pressure medications can worsen nocturia. Instead, try 1–2 dropperfuls of **hawthorn** tincture twice a day.

• Desmopressin acetate, DDAVP, a prescription hormonal nasal spray, blocks the urge to urinate. Elders who use it before bed can shift the timing of their urination toward daytime.[79] It is harsh on the heart and kidneys, though, and can imbalance electrolytes.

• Except for doxazosin, no drugs make a significant difference for men whose enlarged prostates wake them repeatedly.[80]

Paruresis/Shy Bladder

Step 0. *Do Nothing*

• That's what most of those with a shy bladder do: nothing. They can't urinate. They don't talk about it. They don't seek treatment. And in the worst case scenarios, they don't leave home.

Step 1. *Collect Information*

• About 20 million Americans and 2 million Canadians, most of them men, deal with shy bladder; for 10 percent of them, paruresis is incapacitating.[81]

• Shy bladder is a *phobia.* There is no physical cause for it.

• The thought that someone else may be watching, listening, or aware of one's urination produces excruciating embarrassment and extreme anxiety in those with bashful bladder. This anxiety causes the smooth muscles of the urethra to clamp down, making it impossible to void, no matter how strong the desire or effort. In mild cases, voiding in public is impossible. In the worst cases, urination is so blocked that catheterization is needed to release it.

• Holding urine in the bladder for long periods can weaken the elasticity of the bladder and increase the risk of infection.

Step 2. *Engage the Energy*

• Psychoactive substances such as **peyote**, **mescalin**, **psilocybin**, and **LSD-25** are the shaman's choice for helping those with phobias. Consider this true story: "As the effects of the plant began to come on, reality shifted, and I felt terror. I was sure that everyone was not only watching me, but reading my mind as well. My guide laughed: 'They are only concerned with themselves. Set aside your big ego and your wish to be the center of attention. You are just another human, invisible to others. Laugh at your fear; send it away.' And I did."[82]

• Don't have access to psychoactive plants? **Visualize**. Or try **graduated exposure therapy**, the only accepted orthodox treatment for those with paruresis.[83]

• **Emotional Freedom Technique** is a free-of-charge, self-guided, long-established, easy, powerful cure for all phobias. It includes humming, tapping, and repeating a mantra of self-love.

• Social phobias do run in families. Often, **the first step in healing paruresis is to share with others.**

• Those with paruresis may also have panic attacks, claustrophobia, obsessive-compulsive problems, and a deep fear of germs.

• The "tremendous levels of frustration and despair" experienced by paruretics is not relieved by psychoanalysis.[84]

Step 3. *Nourish and Tonify*

• **Corn silk tea**, or the liquid from canned corn, soothes and heals overstretched bladder tissues.

• Be kind to your nerves with **oatstraw infusion**. Regular use of 2–4 cups a day will rebuild the nervous system, so you can handle more stress with less anxiety.

Step 4. *Stimulate/Sedate*

• Keep a bottle of anxiety-relieving **motherwort tincture** in your pocket. A dose of 1–2 dropperfuls, taken on the way to the toilet, relaxes mind and muscles. A dropperful under the tongue stops rapid heartbeat, eases heavy breathing, and counters panic.

Step 5b. *Use Drugs*

• More than half the men answering a recent survey said they were unable to produce a urine sample on demand for a drug test, especially if they were under surveillance.[85]

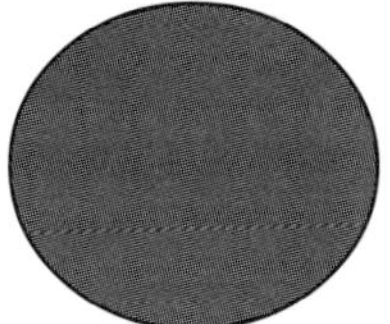

LUTS
(His) Lower Urinary Tract Symptoms

Step 1. *Collect Information*

• LUTS can be caused by benign enlargement of the prostate (page 329), prostatitis (page 338), or cancer (page 351).

• The most common LUTS are:
 ~ Frequent urination at night (nocturia, page 51)
 ~ A weak, inconstant, start-and-stop flow of urine
 ~ Difficulty initiating urination, delays of up to a minute
 ~ Intense urgency, often with little result
 ~ Straining to urinate
 ~ Dribbling and leaking after urination
 ~ Being unable to empty the bladder completely

Step 2. *Engage the Energy*

• **Homeopathic remedies** for men with LUTS:
 ~ *Clematis*: dribbling, stops/starts, last bit burns severely.
 ~ *Ignatia*: frequent urgency but unable to pass urine.
 ~ *Kreostum*: involuntary, hurried urination; as if a lump is pressing down on the bladder.
 ~ *Sepia*: feeble, slow, thick urine, cutting pain beforehand.
 ~ *Serenoa serrulata*: dribbling.
 ~ *Sulphur*: ineffectual, painful efforts to urinate.

Step 3. *Nourish and Tonify*

• For freedom from LUTS, eat **pumpkin seeds** daily.

★ Trinovin, a standardized extract of red clover, reduces LUTS. Drinking 1–2 quarts of **red clover infusion** a week will too, and at a fraction of the cost.

Step 4. *Stimulate/Sedate*

• **Horsetail** herb **tea** eases the prostate, soothes the urinary tract, improves sphincter function, and tones bladder muscles. Dose is 1–2 cups daily.

horsetail

★ **Saw palmetto** is the herb of choice for men with LUTS. Regular use of the **tincture** (not capsules) improves the strength of urine flow, decreases dribbling, eliminates residual urine, and counters nocturia. A dose of 2–4 dropperfuls twice a day works quickly.

• If LUTS is particularly severe, German herbalist Rudolf Fritz Weiss suggests 1–2 tablespoonfuls of ground pumpkin seeds twice a day plus a dropperful of tinctures of saw palmetto and echinacea.[86]

★ Pygeum (page 337) and **nettle root** (page 334) seem particularly helpful for men dealing with LUTS. In a placebo-controlled study, men taking these herbs for one month reported significant increases in urine flow, substantial reduction in residual urine, and fewer trips to the bathroom at night.[87]

★ A twenty-minute soak in **hot water** (105° F) eases pain fast.

• To help force urine out, press a finger behind the scrotum and pull up to the base of the penis.

"It's not just a convenience problem. It wrecks your entire life."[88]

Help!
LUTS

Expect results in 2–4 weeks

• **Relax** in a **hot bath**.

• Take a dropperful each of **saw palmetto** and **St. Joan's wort** tinctures twice a day.

• Limit use of antihistamines, decongestants, diuretics; alcohol, coffee, tea, soda; acidic foods.

Step 5a. *Use Supplements*

★ Dr. Carlton Fredericks says copper-zinc superoxide dismutase, injected by a veterinarian is "remarkably helpful."[89] He also suggests 1000mg **vitamin C** twice a day; but men who take even 250mg a day are 83 percent more likely to have LUTS than those who don't.[90,90A]

Step 5b. *Use Drugs*

• When the prostate is enlarged, it doesn't just swell, it creates new muscle tissue. **Alpha blockers** help muscles relax, relieving urinary symptoms within a week for three-quarters of those with prostate swelling. Side effects include sudden drop in blood pressure on standing, fatigue, and retrograde ejaculation (semen goes into the bladder instead of out). Generics have more noticeable side-effects than Flomax (tamsulosin) or Uroxatral (alfuzosin). Instead: Use dropperfuls of St. Joan's wort tincture to relax muscles.

• Men who also take Proscar (side effects: page 335) are 67 percent less likely to need surgery than men who take no drugs.[91]

Step 6. *Break and Enter*

★ If you **cannot urinate**, sit in hot water. Take a dropperful of parsley root tincture. If you still can't go, get to the nearest emergency room for catheterization. Refuse further surgery.

• To relieve LUTS symptoms, the urinary channel can be widened surgically with laser heat (TURP), radio-frequency waves, or needles (TUNA).

~ In transurethral resection of the prostate (TURP), a small laser is threaded through the urethra and used to destroy the offending tissues. General anesthesia is required, and 3–5 days in the hospital. The success rate is quite high – about 95 percent – with fewer than 10 percent needing a second procedure. Incontinence and erectile difficulties are rare (about 6 percent).[93] The major drawback is infertility. Orgasm is pleasurable, but scarring sends semen retrograde, into the bladder instead of out. A study of 400,000 men who chose TURP found that – within five years – they were more likely to require additional prostate surgery than men who had refused surgery and they were more likely to die than those who chose the more severe prostatectomy surgery.[92]

~ Transurethral needle ablation (TUNA) is done in a doctor's office with a local anesthetic. A small scope is passed through the urethra and into the prostate where radio waves or microwaves destroy the troublesome tissues. TUNA is especially effective at improving urine-flow rates, with a success rate of 70 percent.

☆ Bladder Star: Comfrey *(Symphytum uplandica x)* ☆

An herb that can improve muscle tone in the bladder, ease irritation in the bladder lining and ureters, heal all surfaces, counter inflammation, and create resilient health throughout the urinary system is a true bladder star. That's comfrey – *Symphytum.*

The *allantoin* in comfrey is a superb healer of mucus surfaces, such as those lining the bladder and ureters. Comfrey gives almost immediate relief to those with **interstitial cystitis** and works to counter **urge incontinence** and **overactive bladders**. Comfrey's anti-inflammatory action relieves **urethritis** and **prostate swelling**, too. The astringent tannins in comfrey help tone and tighten the bladder and pelvic floor muscles, countering **stress incontinence**. Comfrey also relaxes the detrusor muscle.

The lavish amounts of minerals, vitamins, and protein found in comfrey allow the body to engage in any repairs that are needed and may counter **bladder cancer**.

A **sitz bath** of the leaves or roots works well for anyone reluctant to consume comfrey. But, for best results, **comfrey leaf infusion,** a cup or two a day, gets my vote.

I feel safe drinking comfrey leaf infusion made from commercial bulk comfrey, and have been doing so, at the rate of at least two quarts a week, for more than twenty-five years. For decades, Lois Johnson MD has done blood work on all her clients taking comfrey, and has never seen any elevation of liver enzymes.[94]

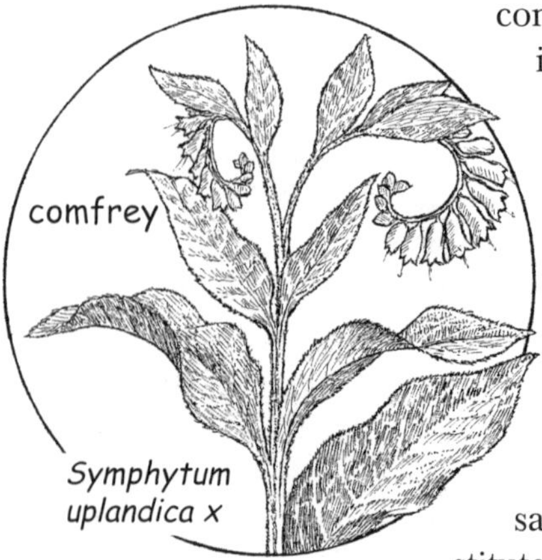

comfrey

Symphytum uplandica x

I am convinced that the majority of the comfrey leaf for sale in the United States is *uplandica*, despite labels claiming it is *officinalis.* Common garden comfrey is *Symphytum uplandica x* – "Russian comfrey" or "blue comfrey" – a tall plant with blue-purple flowers. *Symphytum officinalis*, a small plant with yellow flowers, is rarely grown or used.

Still hesitant? Christopher Hobbs, third-generation herbalist, says broadleaf plantain is a great substitute for comfrey leaf.

Urinary Tract Infections/Cystitis

"Fire in your belly is good, my child," Grandmother Growth assures you. "It fuels your creative potential, gets you going, and heats up your desire to manifest. But fire in your bladder is not. When heat goes in, but doesn't come out, it can scorch you.

"You are overheating, my dear. You are all steamed up and under far too much pressure. You have taken in more than you can process, concentrated what needs to be diffused, held onto what needs to be emptied.

"Look inside and ask yourself what is raging? What are you 'pissed off' about? What makes you burn with shame? Shake with fear? What needs to be eliminated from your life?

"Take a deep breath. Take gentle care of yourself. I love you."

Step 0. *Do Nothing*

• Nothing. It's one of the classic symptoms of a bladder infection: You feel like you really, really, really have to go, right now, even though you just went, or just tried to, but *nothing* happens!

• The fewer sexual partners one has, the less likely one is to get cystitis.[95]

Help!
UTIs

Expect results in 3–4 hours

• Drink lots of lemon-water or **cranberry juice**.

• Take a dropperful of uva ursi, echinacea, or **yarrow tincture** hourly.

• Sit in a **hot bath** and relax.

Step 1. *Collect Information*

• Urinary tract infections – UTIs or cystitis – are the most common form of bacterial infection. One third of all women will have one by the age of 24.[96] Virtually every woman will have at least one acute UTI during a lifetime; many have chronic cystitis. (Men can, but rarely do, get urinary tract infections.)

> "Bacteria irritate the wall of the bladder. [Cystitis is] the bladder's equivalent of a bad sunburn."[97]

• UTIs are usually caused by *E. coli* (*Escherichia coli*), a common fecal bacteria which accounts for 82–85 percent of infections. Other bacteria that cause UTIs include: *Staphylococcus saprophyticus* (4–8%), group B streptococci (6–8%), proteus (3%) and klebsiella (3%).[98] Chlamydia and trichomona organisms can also cause cystitis.[99]

• Bacteria get to the bladder mostly from the anal area (wipe carefully) and intercourse, but also from diaphragms, spermicides, catheters, surgery, and trauma. Wearing a bloody menstrual pad for hours can allow *E. coli* to proliferate, crawl up the urethra and start an infection. Diabetic women get more UTIs.[100]

• Bacteria that do make it to the bladder are usually flushed out with urination. But about half of *E. coli* have a special hairy tip – called a *P fimbria* – that helps them cling to the bladder wall.[101]

★ Untreated bladder infections increase the risk of incontinence and can damage the kidneys. **Take action** at the first hint of a UTI.

• Symptoms of cystitis include frequent, intense urges to urinate, often with little result or with burning pain, and bloody, cloudy, or strong-smelling urine. Low-grade chronic bladder infection symptoms are subtle: depression, fatigue, and low energy.

• Should you take antibiotics for a non-symptomatic bladder infection? Just say "No!" Sexually-active women often have bacteria in the urine – especially after spermicide or diaphragm use.

★ Three or more UTIs a year is a chronic problem. Persistent, chronic bladder infections are a symptom of bladder cancer. If your UTI goes on for more than three months, seek help.

Step 2. *Engage the Energy*

• **Homeopathic** remedies for those with bladder infections:
  ~ *Apis*: stinging, hot pain when urinating.
  ~ *Cantharis*: scalding, bloody urine; constant urge.
  ~ *Sarsaparilla*: pain at end of urination, dribbling.
  ~ *Staphysagria*: UTI caused by intercourse or anger.

• Energy healers say to put yellow-brown zirconium or green nephrite gemstones on your bladder or suck on them before sleep.

Step 3. *Nourish and Tonify*

★ **Cranberries** (*Vaccinium macrocarpon, V. oxycoccus*) prevent and counter UTIs. Daily use of cranberry juice or pills reduced by half the rate of infection in Canadian women who had two or more UTIs a year.[102] Finnish women reduced UTIs 50 percent by drinking 2 ounces of cranberry juice daily.[103] It works for "elderly" women, too.[104] Daily consumption prevents infections.[105]

How? Substances in cranberries – proanthocyanidins, fructose, quinolinic acid, glycoproteins, d-mannose, and tannins – work synergistically to make life hard for *E. coli* and infectious bacteria.

Proanthocyanidins bind to the P fimbria and prevent them from attaching to the bladder, thus short-circuiting the infection. An especially slippery fructose keeps bacteria without a P fimbria off balance, too.[106] Quinolinic acid – converted by the liver into hippuric acid, known to counter infection – protects the kidneys.

Reach for cranberries to prevent, rather than eliminate, UTIs. A dose of 500mg of cranberry extract is as effective as 100mg trimethoprim in preventing infections.[107] If it's too late for that, mix cranberry juice half and half with strong hibiscus tea.

Any cranberry, in any form, even canned, works.[108] Raw cranberries are the least effective; cooked berries much, much better. Cranberry pills are expensive, but best for those with acid reflux problems. Juice with high fructose corn syrup or artificial sweeteners are to be avoided. I favor pure, unsweetened cranberry juice concentrate. Sououououuur!

Expand Your Horizons

All berries in the Vaccinium genus are effective against cystitis. Instead of cranberries, try **blueberries** (*Vaccinium corymbosum*), bilberries (*V. myrtillus*), or cowberries (*Va. vitis-idaea*).

★ **Marshmallow** roots, leaves, and flowers, when infused in water, contain a nourishing mucilage that soothes irritation, eases pain, stops inflammation, increases macrophage activity, and helps rebuild the bladder's lining, so future infections are less likely. (Make it: page 367.)

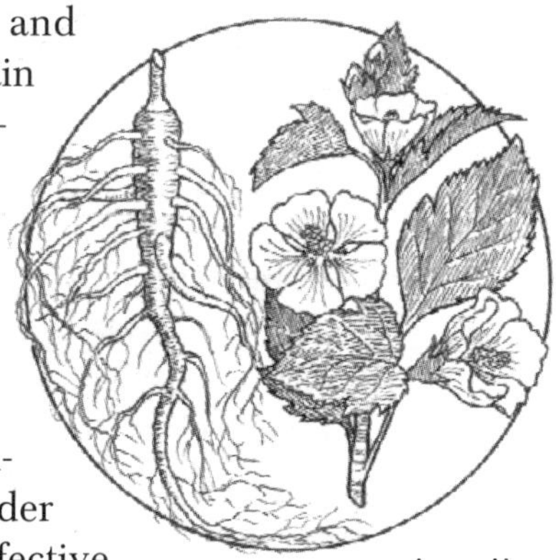

marshmallow

★ **Hibiscus**, a relative of marshmallow, kills the bacteria that cause bladder infections. A tea of the flowers is as effective as the antibiotic chloramphenicol.[109] Hibiscus works well with cranberry as a preventative, especially for women who have eight or more UTIs a year. Ingesting hibiscus tea daily can reduce occurrence of infection by 77 percent.[110]

• Herbalist Rosemary Gladstar's **Bladder Helper Tea** (page 369) was created for women with chronic cystitis. A cup a day is a preventative; to counter a UTI, it is drunk in quantity.[111]

• **Chamomile** tea (*Matricaria*) tastes good, soothes the bladder, and has been shown to kill cystitis-causing bacteria.

• Special peptides found in the urinary tract are the body's first line of defense against bacterial infections.[112] To make more of these peptides, eat **more protein** and drink more nettle infusion.

• **Watermelon** increases urination, and that keeps bacteria from lurking in the bladder. But the flesh is sugary (feeds bacteria) and acidic (can irritate bladder lining). So eat the **seeds** instead.

Step 4. *Stimulate/Sedate*

★ If you feel a bladder infection building, **flush bacteria out** by drinking – water, cranberry juice, herb tea, black or green tea, or nettle infusion. Your goal is to drink enough to provoke urination hourly. Bacteria reproduce quickly. *E. coli* in the bladder can double every twenty minutes. Flush them out! When enough bacteria accumulate, they link together and form a tough film which thwarts attempts to dislodge them. Don't delay. Drink more now!

• Be prepared! Have the herbs you'll need on hand before you need them, so you can help your bladder at the first twinge of discomfort.

★ Add a tablespoon of dried **horsetail** herb to any herbal tea, or use it alone, to help halt a bladder infection.

★ **Avoid hot, spicy foods** – curries, salsas, chile peppers, and hot peppers of all kinds. They irritate the bladder.

• Urologist Dr. Larrian Gillespie says **chiropractic** adjustments help women with chronic cystitis by relieving nerve pressure which then allows the bladder to empty completely. Residual urine in the bladder is a setup for infection.[113]

★ Sitting in **hot water** eases bladder pain fast. For extra relief, add a handful of **fresh pine** or **cedar** needles.

• **Don't wash** down there with soap. Women who wash their vulva are four times more likely to get a bladder infection.

★ **Yarrow** goes right to work killing bacteria in the bladder. A dropperful of tincture taken hourly, or frequent sips of a strong tea, will bring fast relief. Yarrow is a bladder star (page 77).

★ In my experience, **echinacea** root tincture, alone or in combination with **yarrow** tincture, is more reliable in clearing both acute and chronic bladder infections than antibiotics. I use a dose of 2–4 dropperfuls of echinacea, every 1–2 hours for acute UTIs. Add 10–20 drops yarrow if you wish. As symptoms abate, or in chronic conditions, a dose every 4 hours will do. I continue until all symptoms cease. (See: "Instead of Antibiotics," page 342.)

Simply Prevent UTIs

- Eat a quart of **yogurt** a week.
- Drink/eat **cranberries** and **hibiscus**.
- Stay **well-hydrated**.
- Wipe from front to back, or blot.
- Avoid douches, sprays, panty liners.
- Really empty your bladder, always.
- Pee right after intercourse.
- No spermicides, no diaphragms. (Regular use increases risk by 400%.)[114]

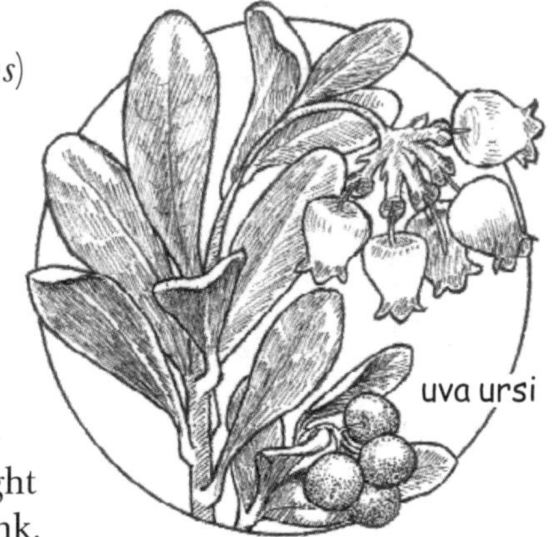

★ **Uva ursi** (*Arctostaphylos*) strengthens the bladder while eliminating acute and chronic infections. Dropperful doses of the tincture taken 3–6 times a day work well, but I prefer the reliable action of the infusion. To make it: Put one ounce uva ursi leaf in a quart/liter jar. Fill with boiling water. Steep, tightly covered, for eight hours or overnight. Strain and drink.

• **Reflexology** and **accupressure** help defeat chronic cystitis.

• My favorite herbs for those with bladder infections:
~ **Buchu** relieves urgency and strengthens the system.
~ **Cleavers**' astringency tones, tightens, and moves fluid.
~ **Corn silk** is intensely soothing and healing.
~ **Echinacea** clears infection fast.
~ **Horsetail** counters spasms and strengthens the bladder.
~ **Juniper berries** disinfect the entire urinary system.
~ **Marshmallow root** is a sweet soother.
~ **Roses** and rose hips are pain relieving and soothing.
~ **Uva ursi** rids the bladder of bacteria; tonifies, too.
~ **Yarrow** keeps you clear and keeps you going.

Use them as simples, or mix up a tea that suits you; tinctures work too. A dose is usually a cup of tea, or a dropperful of tincture, taken several times a day. And check out **Bladder Buddy Tea** and **Bladder Blast** (both on page 369).

• **Coffee** drinkers increase their risk of bladder infections by 20 percent, but not their risk of bladder cancer.[115]

Step 5a. *Use Supplements*

• Vitamin C (500mg of **ascorbic acid**), taken every few hours, can knock infections out, alone or with antibiotics. Expect to pee a lot while doing this. Your bowels may loosen as well. This is a cure; it is not a preventative. **Caution**: Ascorbic acid can aggravate, may even precipitate, interstitial cystitis and vulvodynia.

Step 5b. *Use Drugs*

A single dose of antibiotic is enough to quench most UTIs.[116,117]

• Antibiotics are notorious for giving women vaginal yeast infections. Take probiotics or yogurt during and after treatment.

• Over-the-counter, nonprescription drugs – such as Pyridium – ease the painful symptoms of cystitis, but don't kill the bacteria, which are free to move into the kidneys and cause grave damage.

• Postmenopausal women with recurrent bladder infections may find symptomatic relief with vaginal **estrogen cream**.

• **Bactrim**, a combination of two **antibiotics** – 80mg trimethoprim and 400mg sulfamethoxazole – taken for three days is the current standard of care for those with UTI.[118,119] Side effects are slight. A small dose, taken daily or only after intercourse, is used to prevent UTIs. (Cranberries are as effective and safer.)

• **Avoid** Cipro (ciprofloxacin), Tequin (gatifloxacin), Levaquin (levofloxacin), Floxin (ofloxacin), and Noroxin (norfloxacin). All are expensive, interfere with pregnancy, and cause nausea.[120,121] Or try a single large dose rather than the regular three days' worth.

Nitrofurantoins are safer during early pregnancy, but must be taken for seven days (instead of three) and are more nauseating.[122] Trimethoprims (Proloprim or Trimpex) have worse side effects – as does Monurol (fosfomycin).

• In the future, will UTIs be a thing of the past? If the **vaccine** Urovac is successful, the answer could be yes. A full-strength suppository followed by three booster suppositories more than halved infections in a group of women with chronic UTIs.[123]

Serious Symptoms

Bacteria that cause bladder infections can damage the kidneys.

Seek immediate help if these symptoms accompany a UTI.

- Blood in the urine
- Pain in the back or side
- Fever
- Nausea or vomiting

Step 6. *Break and Enter*

• If a short course of antibiotics does not clear your UTI, if you have more than three infections a year, or if your doctor suspects cancer or kidney disease, s/he may wish to do invasive diagnostic procedures. First, try the remedies in Steps 3 and 4. **Ultrasound** may be the safest test. **Cystoscopy** can irritate the urethra. The dyes used in **intravenous pyelograms** can cause severe allergic reactions. Both pyelograms and **CT scans** use x-rays, which are cancer-inducing, especially to the ovaries (and testes).

• One in four hospital patients will have a **urinary catheter**. Catheter-induced UTIs account for 40 percent of all hospital-acquired infections,[124] many of which are antibiotic resistant.[125] Protect yourself: Take yarrow or echinacea tincture 4–8 times a day, and drink or eat *Vaccinium* berries daily (page 61).

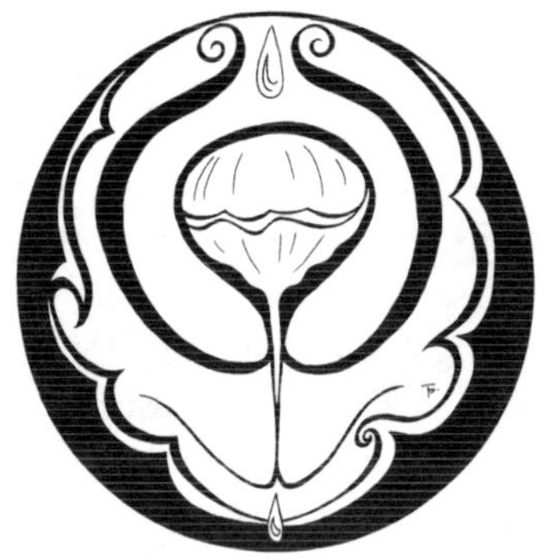

Her Story

Sarah is retired and volunteers at a local food bank.

"I got my first bladder infection at the age of two, just after my sister was born. I was "pissed off" that I wasn't the only child anymore. Despite lots of drugs and endless doctor visits, my bladder infections kept getting worse and worse. I remember lying on a gurney in a hospital hall while the doctors argued about whether my appendix was infected or not; they couldn't believe my excruciating pain was from a 'mere' bladder infection.

"Finally, as a young adult, I 'discovered' uva ursi. The first time I used it to counter a bladder infection — drinking two cups daily for a week — was pretty much the last time I had any pain in my bladder. That was sixty years ago."

Interstitial Cystitis

"Did you really think you could swallow all your feelings, my dearest, my own? Of course you want to be nice, to accommodate, to smooth the way. But look at what it has done to you. You have worn yourself out. Like an old shirt, you are threadbare. The lining of your bladder is punched full of tiny holes, and they are bleeding.

"Crying will not help now. This is the time to take your own safety seriously. It is time to stand up for yourself. Soothing will help a little, and I offer you comfort. But there is so much more to do."

Step 0. *Do Nothing*

• De-stressing decreases the pain of interstitial cystitis (IC) by up to 50 percent. Meditate. Take a nap. Soak in a hot bath. Take it easy. Breathe deeply. Do nothing.

Is It Interstitial Cystitis?

If you answer yes to two or more, you may have IC.

❖ I've had a bladder infection that lasted longer than 3 months.

❖ I've gotten a negative culture when I thought I had a bladder infection.*

❖ My bladder infections resist all treatments.

❖ My symptoms occur daily.

❖ I'm reluctant to leave home for fear I won't make it to the toilet in time.

❖ My pelvic pain interferes with my sex life.

❖ I have endometriosis, vulvodynia, fibromyalgia, chronic fatigue, and/or irritable bowel syndrome (IBS).

* About one-third of such women do have an infection.

Step 1. *Collect Information*

> "It [interstitial cystitis] was thought to be a rare, postmenopausal condition, but we found the average age of onset to be 40."[126]

• Approximately one million Americans, 90 percent of them women, suffer from IC, an ulcerated condition of the bladder lining.

• Interstitial cystitis causes burning pain on urination, a need to urinate several times an hour, and severe pain "down there." These are also symptoms of UTIs, STDs, kidney disease, bladder cancer, and some neurological disorders. Some urologists, since there is no definitive test for IC, "don't believe in it." Others have "never heard of it." When all other problems are ruled out, IC is the diagnosis. For most women, a correct diagnosis takes 4–7 years.[127]

• IC is "a chronic inflammatory condition of the bladder wall." But the pain may originate in the muscles or nerves. Interstitial cystitis may coexist with vulvodynia (page 93) and/or fibromyalgia, causing pain that is extremely difficult to pin down, and even harder to treat.

Step 2. *Engage the Energy*

★ **Biofeedback** teaches you how to turn off your pain response.

• Is IC connected to paranoia or grudges? Oriental healers connect bladder pain to a "withholding" attitude. Affirmations for women with IC: "I am safe right here and right now." "I give my grudges to Universal law." "I am free and at ease."

• Cranial-sacral treatments relieve IC pain for some.

Help! Interstitial Cystitis

Expect results in 2-4 months

• Take an **anti-inflammatory herb** daily.

• Look at your diet (page 72).

• Do 100 **Kegels** a day.

• Stop taking vitamin pills.

Step 3. *Nourish and Tonify*

★ **Soothing herbal infusions** – of mallow, comfrey, or linden – ease pain, counter inflammation, and heal the little ulcerations of IC. Use them as sitz baths several times a week and/or drink 1–2 cups a day. (Make it: page 367.) Persistence brings big changes.

• To soothe and heal inflamed bladders fast try: Hot **slippery elm tea** with honey or **flax** seeds soaked in cold water overnight and consumed, or ground and cooked in with oatmeal.

• What you eat affects your bladder.[128] Those with IC will want to **avoid** or limit artificial sweeteners, food preservatives, tofu, carbonated drinks, coffee, tea, chocolate, alcohol, vitamin C/ascorbic acid (added to many foods), and multivitamins. (More, page 72.)

• **Enjoy** bladder-soothing foods like rice, barley, winter squash, yams, carrots, green beans, and peas often.

• **Yoga**, progressive muscle relaxation, and bladder retraining are techniques that have helped those with IC.

★ **Pelvic floor lifts**/Kegels (page 10) strengthen bladder muscles, increase lymphatic circulation, restore blood flow, tonify the bladder wall, reduce pain, and diminish symptoms.

Step 4. *Stimulate/Sedate*

★ The urine of those with IC shows high concentrations of inflammatory substances. **Anti-inflammatory herbs** are allies:

~ **Black cohosh** root tincture, 10–15 drops taken 2–3 times a day, when pain is sharp, stabbing, or icy.

~ **Licorice** root tincture, 20 drops taken 2–3 times a day; deglycerized is less likely to raise blood pressure.

~ **Oak bark** tea, freely, when everything else has failed.

~ **Osha** root tincture, 3–5 drops as needed, when the belly feels heavy and full.

~ **Poke** root tincture, 1–2 drops a day, when pain is cyclical, deep, and congested.

~ **St. Joan's wort** tincture, 20–30 drops as needed, when pain is electric-like.

Help Now!
Interstitial Cystitis

Expect results in 30 minutes

• Drink a teaspoonful of **baking soda** dissolved in water.

• Drink **slippery elm** as a tea or mix powder with honey and eat.

★ **Ginger compresses** on the abdomen can increase blood flow to the bladder, strengthen the muscles that help with bladder control, and encourage release of pain-blocking hormones. Steep an ounce of fresh, grated ginger (or a tablespoon of powdered ginger) in a quart of boiling water. Soak a cotton cloth in it and apply over the pubic bone; repeat as desired.

• **Hops** eases bladder irritation, nervousness, and pain that prevents sleep. The tea sipped, or tincture taken 10–15 drops at a time, is antispasmodic, sedative, relaxing, and antibacterial.

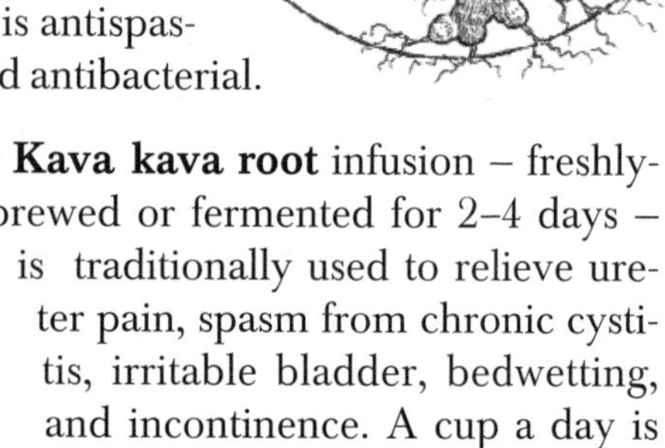

• **Kava kava root** infusion – freshly-brewed or fermented for 2–4 days – is traditionally used to relieve ureter pain, spasm from chronic cystitis, irritable bladder, bedwetting, and incontinence. A cup a day is an effective dose.

Step 5a. *Use Supplements*

★ Taking 500mg of **L-arginine** three times a day reduces IC symptoms by raising levels of coenzyme nitric oxide synthase, often low in those with IC.[129] This can initiate an outbreak of genital herpes, however.

• **Chondroitin sulfate**, **sodium hyaluronate**, and **glucosamine sulfate** repair ulcerations and heal the bladder wall.[130]

Step 5b. *Use Drugs*

"Drug therapy had the best-reported outcomes. . . ."[131]

• **Elmiron** (pentosan polysulfate sodium) is the only FDA-approved oral medication for IC. Over half the women using it had improvement; 30 percent reported no change; 4 percent deteriorated.[132] Long-term use is required. Like **slippery elm,** it repairs defects in the bladder lining, replenishes the protective mucus surfaces, and forms a protective coating.

• **Prelief**, an over-the-counter medication (calcium glycerophosphate) that neutralizes food acids, benefits 60 percent of those who take it; 36 percent say it has no effect.[133]

• Those who have allergies in addition to IC often have elevated amounts of histamine-releasing mast cells in their bladder wall. Reduce them with **hydroxyzine hydrochloride** (Atarax), quercetin supplements, or a cold water infusion of mallow roots.

Her Story

Kay is now postmenopausal. Her story starts in 1970.[134]

"My bladder infection was hardly cause for alarm. Little did I know that I was embarking upon a course of pain, repeated treatments, and frustration that would last for three decades.

"Three urologists all said my urethra was too narrow ('urethral stenosis') and I'd have UTIs repeatedly unless I had it dilated. It never occurred to me to ask how other patients had fared with this treatment before agreeing to it. I believed them.

"Over the next five years, I had ten dilatations, each followed by instillation of silver nitrate into my bladder and a course of antibiotics. After the first dilation, I experienced 'urgency and frequency' for six months. After the tenth dilation, it was chronic. I felt like I had to urinate, urgently, every second. Painful gas and bloating also became chronic, along with overwhelming fatigue. I feared the treatment had been a terrible mistake.

"Known for over a century — and now called 'interstitial cystitis,' or 'painful bladder syndrome' — my problem is still not medically validated, and is considered 'incurable.'

"In 1981, a urologist advised me to give up dairy, wheat, sugar, and about 130 other foods. My bladder pain was reduced only slightly, but the fatigue, gas and bloating were resolved.

"Over the next twenty years I saw at least thirty specialists. Finally, in 2003, I found one who limited my diet to six foods, asked me to take L-lysine, and treated me for 'small intestinal bacterial overgrowth.' Today I take no drugs and am pain-free at last."

• Other drugs used by those with IC include: Neurontin (gabapentin), to relieve nerve pain (as St. Joan's wort tincture does); Bicitra (sodium citrate), an alkalinizing agent; and Urised, an anesthetic, antiseptic, bladder relaxant (as is yarrow tincture).

❖ Chronic Cystitis & IC ❖

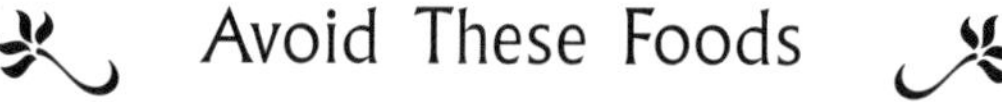

Avoid These Foods

- ❖ All spicy foods
- ❖ Ascorbic acid (vitamin C), in juices, preserves, multi-vitamins, health foods
- ❖ Fruits: apple, apricot, banana, cantaloupe, cranberry, grapes, raisins, grapefruit, guava, lemon, orange, peach, pineapple, plum, prunes, rhubarb, strawberry, watermelon
- ❖ Meat/fish: anchovies, pickled herring, caviar, chicken liver, cold cuts, corned beef, pork
- ❖ Dairy: cheese, sour cream, yogurt
- ❖ Beans: fava beans, lentils, lima beans, all nuts, soy sauce
- ❖ Drinks: coffee, tea, alcohol, carbonated drinks
- ❖ And: aspartame, avocado, aloe vera, chocolate, ginger, onion, mayonnaise, pickles, rye, saccharine, tomato, vinegar

Include These Healthy Foods

- ❖ Whole grains: brown rice, corn, quinoa, kasha, spelt, millet, whole wheat (pasta, bread, crackers, cookies)
- ❖ Seeds: sunflower, pumpkin, sesame (tahini and gomasio)
- ❖ Fruits (*cooked*): blackberry, black currant, blueberry, cherry, gooseberry, kiwi, lychee, pomegranate, raspberry
- ❖ Vegetables (*cooked only*): cabbage family plants, eggplant, leafy greens, summer squash, winter squash, potato, sweet potato, root vegetables, peas, seaweed, mushrooms
- ❖ Meat: turkey, chicken, venison, all fish, goat cheese
- ❖ Drinks (*not in plastic*): nourishing herbal infusions, goat milk, full-fat organic milk, filtered tap water
- ❖ Fats: olive oil, organic butter, pumpkin seed oil, coconut oil, roasted sesame oil

Step 6. *Break and Enter*

> "Most [of the 1,300] respondents said that the surgeries — hydrodistention, bladder instillation, urethral dilatation — either worsened or had no effect on their symptoms."[135]

• **Cystoscopy** is an invasive diagnostic procedure. It can irritate the bladder and worsen IC symptoms. You may wish to refuse it. Under local anesthesia, a tiny scope is threaded into the bladder through a tube placed in the urethra. This allows the interior of the bladder to be checked for small Hummer's ulcers or tiny bleeding sores (glomerulations) that are characteristic of IC.

• A **potassium sensitivity test** (PST) can identify 70–90 percent of IC cases. However, it will irritate the bladder and can cause a worsening of IC symptoms.[136] Do you really need it?

• BCG (*Bacillus Calmette-Guéin*, a weak tuberculosis bacterium), hyaluronic acid, or DMSO (dimethyl sulfoxide) **instilled directly into the bladder** help relieve pain. **BCG** reduces pain and frequency in more than half of patients.[137] **Hyaluronic acid** heals defects in the lining of the bladder. The pungent garlicky smell of **DMSO** leaks from the patient's pores for days after a treatment.

• **InterStim** is implanted in the abdomen to send mild electrical pulses to the sacral nerve. This dampens abnormal signals and can provide "significant improvement in IC patients previously unresponsive to other therapies."[138]

Her Story

Robin is a single, hardworking, young professional.

"I was never formally diagnosed with IC, but I had all the symptoms: burning urination, urethral pain, bladder spasms. The pain was horrible.

"I created a food diary, logging everything I ate and noting symptoms. For six months I ate only foods that "agreed" with me. I eliminated the usual irritants, plus a few personal ones, such as avocado, that set my bladder on fire. I put pumpkin seed oil on everything.

"Marshmallow root tea gave me tremendous relief. The only thing that eased the burning in my bladder faster was a few sips of baking soda in water . . . magic! It's been four years since I had any pain."

• TENS (transcutaneous electrical nerve stimulation) delivers electric pulses – via implanted wires or devices inserted into the vagina or rectum – which increase blood flow to the bladder.

• Some IC sufferers are in so much pain that they have their bladder removed. But suprapubic and pelvic pain often persist after surgery. Even cutting the sacral nerve is not guaranteed to eliminate pain. Try the Wise Woman ways gathered here, instead.

Bladder Cancer

"What is cancer?" asks Grandmother Growth, her dark eyes serious. "Is it 'stuck' energy? No, it is moving energy. It is dangerous because it is movable. If cancer stayed where it started, very few would die of it.

"Envision the cancer in your bladder. What can slow it down? You need strong medicines now. Lean on me a while. Let us sing a song."

Step 1. *Collect Information*

• Bladder cancer is the fourth most common (and the eighth most deadly) cancer among American men, and the tenth most common cancer among women, with approximately 60,000 new cases and 13,000 deaths per year.[139]

• Most bladder cancers are "pussycats," not "tigers." At least 80 percent of bladder cancers are "chronic and slow-growing."[140]

•Who is likeliest to be diagnosed? A **white** (twice as likely as black) **man** (twice as likely as a woman) who is **sixty** or older, lives in the north or northeast (40 percent more likely than in the south), smokes tobacco (doubles risk), rarely drinks water, and has a parent, grandparent, or sibling with bladder cancer.[141]

• About half of men's bladder cancers, and a third of women's, are from **tobacco** use (but not secondhand smoke).[142] About one-quarter are due to ingestion of solvents and aromatic amines – either from occupational exposure or from contaminated ground water – found in paint, chemicals, rubber, textiles, leather goods, machine shops, beauty salons, and printing plants.[143,144]

• Blood in the urine is the most common symptom of bladder cancer, occurring 70 percent of the time. Don't look for red – unless you ate beets – but a rusty color. Other symptoms include pain on urination, difficulty in starting or stopping the flow, *increasing* urgency, and an *increasingly* frequent need to void.

• Most urinary bladder cancers are limited to the inner lining.

Step 2. *Engage the Energy*

• Take an imaginary journey into your bladder. Call your helpers, guardians, and guides. Put their hands on the lining of your bladder, from the inside, and allow the energy of health to pour through you and vibrate in every cell.

Step 3. *Nourish and Tonify*

• **Red clover** infusion, medicinal **mushrooms**, **burdock**, and **kelp** nourish and enliven the immune system and kill cancer cells.

• Two servings a day of **yogurt** lowers risk of bladder cancer by 40 percent (45 percent for women; 36 percent for men).[145]

Step 4. *Stimulate/Sedate*

• Herbs strong enough to kill cancer are poisonous if misused.

~ **Celandine** root tincture is an Old World remedy for all bladder and liver problems. A dose is 5–10 drops, 1–2 times a day.

~ **Poke** root tincture kicks the immune system into high gear. Start with one drop a day! Work up to 10–15 drops a day.

~ **Mistletoe** injections are a mode of complementary cancer care favored in Germany and elsewhere in Europe.

~ **Chaparral** herb tincture is the desert's cure for anything nasty. Start with 1–2 drops 1–3 times a day and increase as needed.

• Does keeping well **hydrated** and emptying the bladder frequently lessen the risks of bladder cancer? One study did find men who drank six or more cups of water a day halved their risk of bladder cancer vs. men who drank a cup of water or less daily.

Step 5. *Use Drugs*

• Compared with similar cancer-free individuals, those with bladder cancer were three times as likely to have used **permanent hair dyes** at least once a month for fifteen years or more.[146] Even using them once a month for a year doubles risk.[147] Hair dressers and barbers have five times the risk after ten years on the job.[148] Semipermanent dyes (such as henna) appear to be safe.[149]

Step 6. *Break and Enter*

> "Treatment [of bladder cancer] is all over the lot — from mild to mutilating. . . . [We found those] treated least aggressively survived just as long. . . . Initial high-intensity treatments failed to prevent the need for more interventions in later years."[150]

• Diagnosis of bladder cancer is made through cystoscopy and urine cytology, which looks for nuclear matrix proteins (NMP) from the cancer.[151, 152] NMP is useless for screening.[153]

• Simple bladder cancer is scraped away under local anesthesia on an outpatient basis. Healing is usually complete in two weeks. Most of the time (70 percent), simple bladder cancer will recur, so regular follow-up monitoring is a must.[154]

• Follow-up monitoring, 3–4 times a year, by cystoscopy and NMP will find 99 percent of all recurrent bladder cancers.[155]

• Radiation and chemotherapy instead of surgery? This cures only 40 percent of the time, and requires regular follow-up tests.[156]

• If the bladder must be removed (*cystectomy*), it can be replaced with a lab-grown bladder, or a piece of your own intestine.

• Since there are only eight thousand cystectomies done in America each year, it is vital to seek out a university medical center or a large hospital for the best outcome.

☆ Bladder Star: Yarrow (*Achillea millefolium*) 

Yarrow flower (tea or tincture) counters urinary infections, relieves pain, restores tone to the bladder, counters incontinence, eases urinary tract spasms, and aids those with bladder cancer.

Yarrow not only destroys infective bacteria in the bladder, it strengthens the bladder wall, so repeat infections are less likely, and it doesn't promote vaginal yeast, as antibiotics do.

Expect relief from pain in minutes, lessening of fever in hours, and complete remission of bladder infections in a couple of days when using a dropperful of the tincture of the fresh flowering herb hourly or taking frequent sips of strong yarrow tea.

To kill *all* the bacteria in your bladder, it is important to take yarrow tincture 4–6 times a day for 7–10 days. For double insurance, take a dropperful of uva ursi tincture 2–3 times a day, too.

To tonify the bladder, counter incontinence, and heal IC ulcers, the dose is up to a dropperful of tincture or a cup of tea daily.

Blood in your urine? Reach for the yarrow!

Yarrow is not recommended during pregnancy.

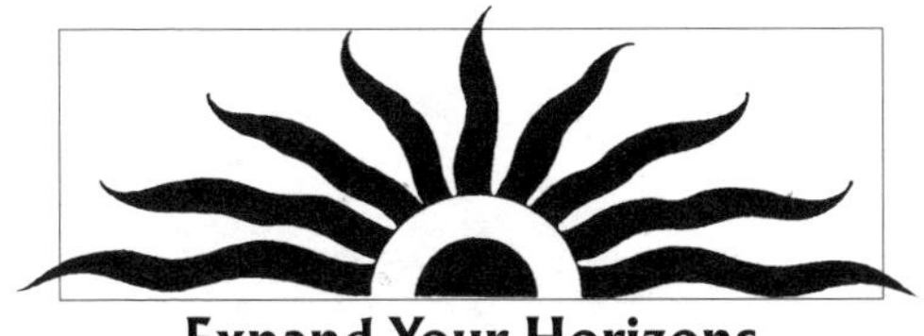

Expand Your Horizons

Many *Asteraceae* family plants – such as yarrow, echinacea, and chamomile – strengthen and heal the bladder. So do:

- Oxeye daisy (*Crysanthemum leucanthemum*) flowers
- Spanish needles (*Bidens* species) flowers
- Pearly everlasting (*Anaphalis margaritacea*) flowers
- Goldenrod (*Solidago* species) flowers or roots
- Black-eyed Susan (*Rudbeckia hirta*) roots

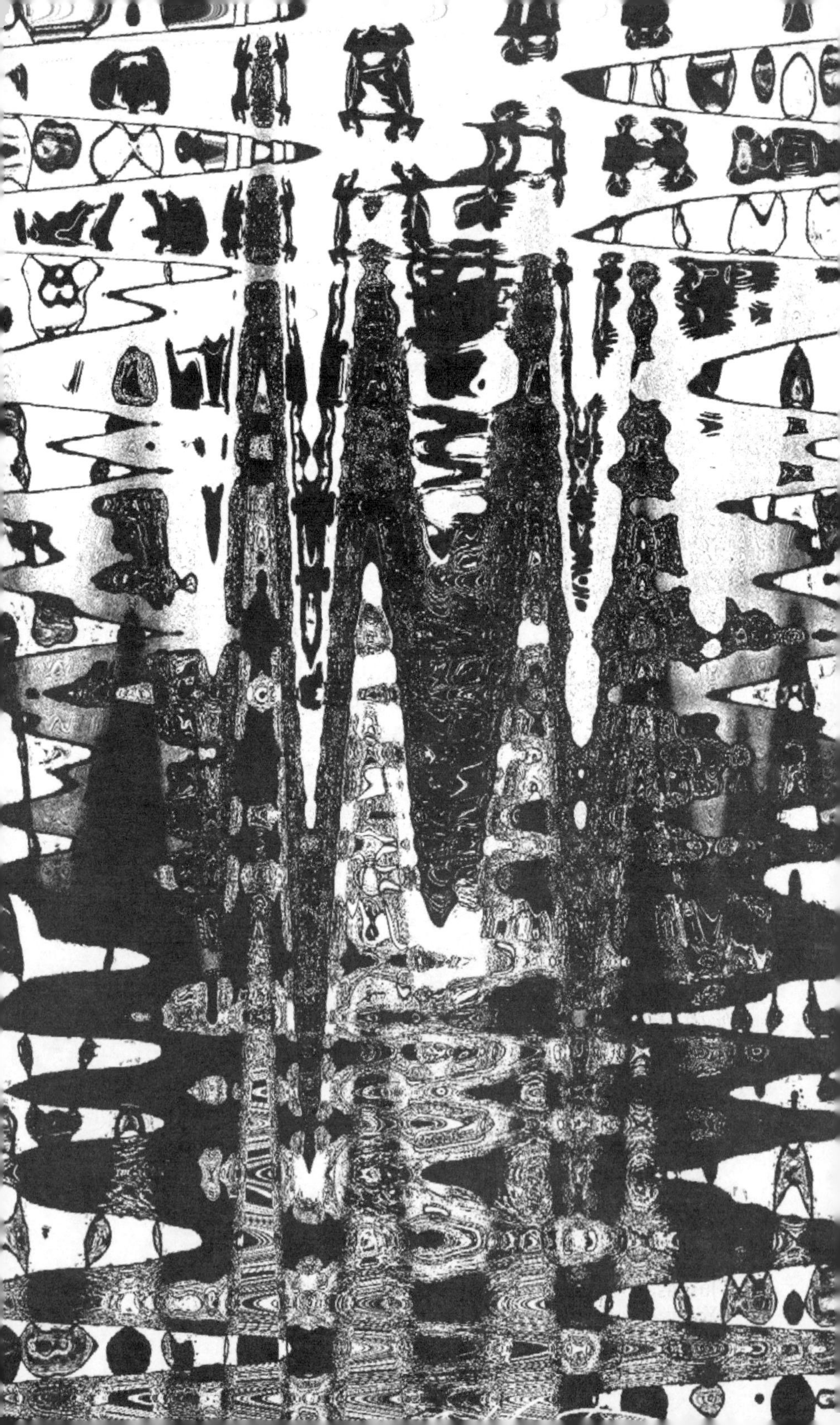

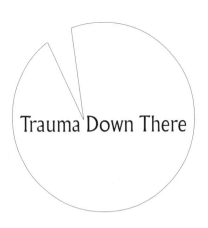

Trauma Down There

Grandmother and Grandfather Growth stand on either side of you. Their smiles curl the corners of their mouths; there is sadness in their eyes. They each take one of your hands. You feel like a small child as you walk with them. Sunlight slants through the trees in golden streams; there is the faint sound of a small waterfall. The ground rises up to meet your feet; it is yielding, soft, springy. Why are tears coursing down your cheeks?

"We cry with you." The words vibrate in your heart and you wince. "It is hard to feel the joy of life when you have been hurt, especially by those who ought to care for you. But we do not cry for your injuries, precious one, grievous though they are. We cry because you cling to your pain. Dear grandchild, pain is inevitable. It is not your fault. It is part of life. You are not to blame. You did not call this upon yourself. There is no guilt in being abused. Your shame is a slap in the face to yourself.

"Let shame and blame, guilt and suffering flow out your feet and into the transformative Earth. She knows all and cherishes all. Give the brutality, the viciousness, the betrayal, the horror, the rage, the wounding to Her. Trust Her ability to change it into food and medicine, shelter and beauty. You have nothing to lose but your burden. Put it down and open your heart. You live in love; let it in."

Step 0. *Do Nothing*

> "All the violence, fear, and suffering
> That exist in the world
> Come from grasping at 'self.'
> What use is this great evil monster to you?
> If you do not let go of the 'self,'
> There will never be an end to your suffering.
> Just as, if you do not let go of a flame with your hand,
> You can't stop it from burning your hand."[1]

• This section is for all of us, men and women. It is for those who have been impacted by trauma, and it is for those whose compassion reminds them that anyone can be the next target. It is drawn from my own experiences and from a few of the many excellent teachings on the paths to recovery of Self after abuse.

There is no one right way to heal from trauma.

Step 1. *Collect Information*

> "My definition of trauma grew to include any sort of stimuli that could send a person hurtling away from his or her body."[2]

• Where to begin? How to condense? Sexual trauma is so formative to our sense of Self that it needs more than a chapter, more than a book, more than a library. Healing may take a lifetime.

• By "trauma" I mean an assault, whether physical or mental, chosen or forced, blatant or hidden.

Primary traumatic events for women include rape, incest, pelvic surgery, clitorectomy, vaginal surgery, pregnancy and birth (whether vaginal or by C-section), sterilization (having your tubes tied), abortion, and exposure to cultural/religious views of women as worthless, evil, and the cause of all sin.

For men, primary traumatic events include circumcision, prostate surgery, war, sterilization, bullies, inappropriate advances/actions from male or female caretakers when young, and rape.

And all of us are traumatized by exposure to cultural/religious views of the body as filthy, and down there as dirty and shameful.

• By my definition, virtually every woman alive, and a significant number of men, deals – in body, mind, emotion, and spirit – with the effects of "down there" trauma. If not directly in one's own life, then indirectly, in the lives of family, friends, and countless others, both living and dead.[3]

• One out of three American women will be violently sexually assaulted in her lifetime.[4,5] One in four women and one in six men in the USA experiences sexual violence before the age of eighteen.[6] Most rapists – 99 percent – are men; 91 percent of those raped are women.[7] Nearly half of all rapes (43 percent) are gang rapes.[8] Men can stop this; organizations to help you on page 401.

• Some of the consequences of trauma include panic attacks, poor focus, weak boundaries, depersonalization, poor grounding, loss of self-esteem, hypervigilance, sleep disturbances, flashbacks (intrusive memories), suicidal thoughts, post-traumatic stress disorder, depression, apathy, paranoia, loss of appetite, low libido, CPP, dyspareunia, painful menses, and mental/muscular pains.

• Those who have experienced abuse often feel a strange mix of feelings: anxiety, embarrassment, guilt, humiliation, rage, shame, terror, isolation, abandonment, violence, and vulnerability. All your feelings are real and important; a safe space and a wise guide can help you "depathologize" your emotional stew so it can nourish you instead of poisoning your life.

• Trauma causes problems "down there." And pre-existing down there problems are aggravated by trauma.

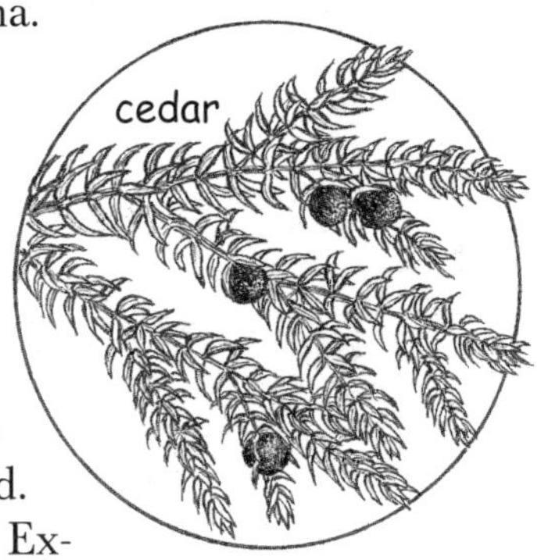

cedar

Step 2. *Engage the Energy*

• Indulge your need for **security** and **safety**. Not with locks and alarms, but with mindfulness meditation.[9,10] Or by burning cedar, sagebrush, or sweet grass. Inhale. See the fear and rage moving away with the smoke. Exhale. Expand. Inhale. Send your roots into the ground. Exhale. Let go. Inhale. Feel protected. Exhale. Smile.

★ Gang-rape survivor Linda Jean McNabb[11] felt broken until the *Course in Miracles* awakened her "indestructible being." Once she remembered that no action can harm the **indestructible soul**, she forgave herself for what happened and got on with her life.

★ Energy healing and symbolic reorganization speed recovery from trauma. Shaman Sandra Ingerman uses **soul retrieval**.[12] Shaman Anya Keifer uses this **visualization**: "Look left and inhale images of your trauma. Then look right and exhale them. Sit up straight. Breathe; keep turning your head left and right until the images fade. Then hold your breath, turn your head sharply left and right to shatter the experience into pieces. Center your head. Breathe out." **Recapitulation** (page 199) is another useful tool.

- Homeopathic remedies for healing after trauma include
  - ~ *Aconite*: extreme fear, anxiety, panic, as if near death.
  - ~ *Arnica*: tissue damage, psychic shock, stoic responses.
  - ~ *Staphysagria*: feels violated, especially after surgery.
  - ~ *Stramonium*: panic, nightmares, fears dark, being alone.

Step 3. *Nourish and Tonify*

• Healing from trauma requires the coordinated efforts of our senses, our brains, our eternal spirits, and our social network. *Open your eyes. Allow yourself to be seen.* It is not enough to know the steps of healing, one must feel them as well. *Express your anger: directly and through art or acting.* Tell your story. *Create a sanctuary where you can cry and rage, drift and dream.* Healer Karla McLaren says real forgiveness requires true anger, true despair, and true fear.

• To reset the nervous/endocrine systems and end distress, try **oatstraw infusion**, lemon balm tea, and a diet rich in **animal fats**.

★ Relieve post-traumatic stress disorder and flashbacks fast with **Traumatic Incident Reduction**.[13]

Her Story

Eva Maria is single, unemployed, and in her mid-thirties.

"I was conceived during a rape. I feel anger at my mother that she betrayed me, that she didn't abort me. She is my rapist. I envision my fetal self trapped in her belly, clawing my way out of her. I hate my mother and can never forgive her. This is the biggest tragedy in my life: that I cannot love my mother and so I cannot love myself.

"I know it is horrid, but when a human who has not known rape from conception is violated, I smile a sad smile and whisper: 'Now you know what I've known from the beginning. Now you know my pain.'

"My emotional pain — unlike physical pain — is not seen or acknowledged by others. It manifests in self-harm. Cutting myself helps me reconnect with my body. It releases endorphins in my brain that create an addictive high. When I need to cut myself I have an uncontrollable tingling in the back of my throat, like suffering from intense thirst; there is no way to resist. The pain of not hurting myself becomes greater than the pain of doing it. I have never felt in control of self-harm. It is a scary, threatening, uncontrollable ride.

"There is no healing for me. My essence is a wound. How can I deconstruct myself from the trauma when it created me?"

Step 4. *Stimulate/Sedate*

> "... healing [trauma} ... is always totally original, deeply emotive, and achingly beautiful. [There are] no shortcuts, no magic techniques, and no road map — it is a soul-making process...."[14]

★ **Motherwort** tincture stops panic attacks fast. Carry a bottle in your pocket or purse; a dropperful in some liquid will restore sanity in seconds. And do remember to breathe.

• **Passionflower** tincture or tea, taken first thing in the morning, can calm hypervigilance and ease sleep disturbances. Start with a dropperful; cut back if you feel too sleepy; increase if needed.

Her Story

Hanna is in her twenties; she was violently raped last year.

"Trauma recovery is so crazy. On one hand, I am supposed to tell my story and feel the repressed feelings. On the other hand, I am not supposed to get suicidal or homicidal. When I get into my feelings, they overwhelm me. The intensity of my anger and my grief have put me in the psych ward a few times already. I really think I might kill someone.

"Life itself seems 'unsafe' to me now. I am so broken down by this. I am constantly on edge. New research says somatic therapies are best because the body's cells hold the memories. Should I change my therapist? Recovering is more difficult than enduring the rape. I just want it to be all over."

Step 5. *Use Drugs*

> "...there is a certain blessing to be given to the substances and behaviors that have helped us survive our unrelieved suffering."[15]

• Many who are traumatized turn to alcohol and drugs. Others engage in risky behaviors. Go back to Steps 2 and 3.

Step 6. *Break and Enter*

• Some respond to sexual trauma (especially in childhood) by cutting themselves as adults. Some seek institutionalization. Let your wounds "become not endless tragedies, but **portals through which we can discover our true power and resilience**."[16]

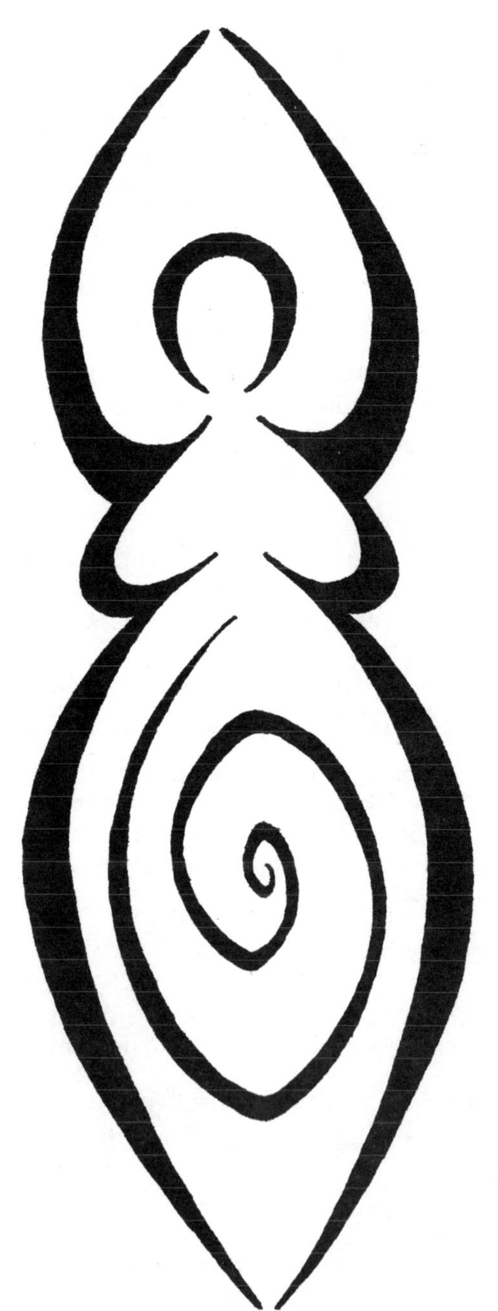

Part Two

Especially for Women

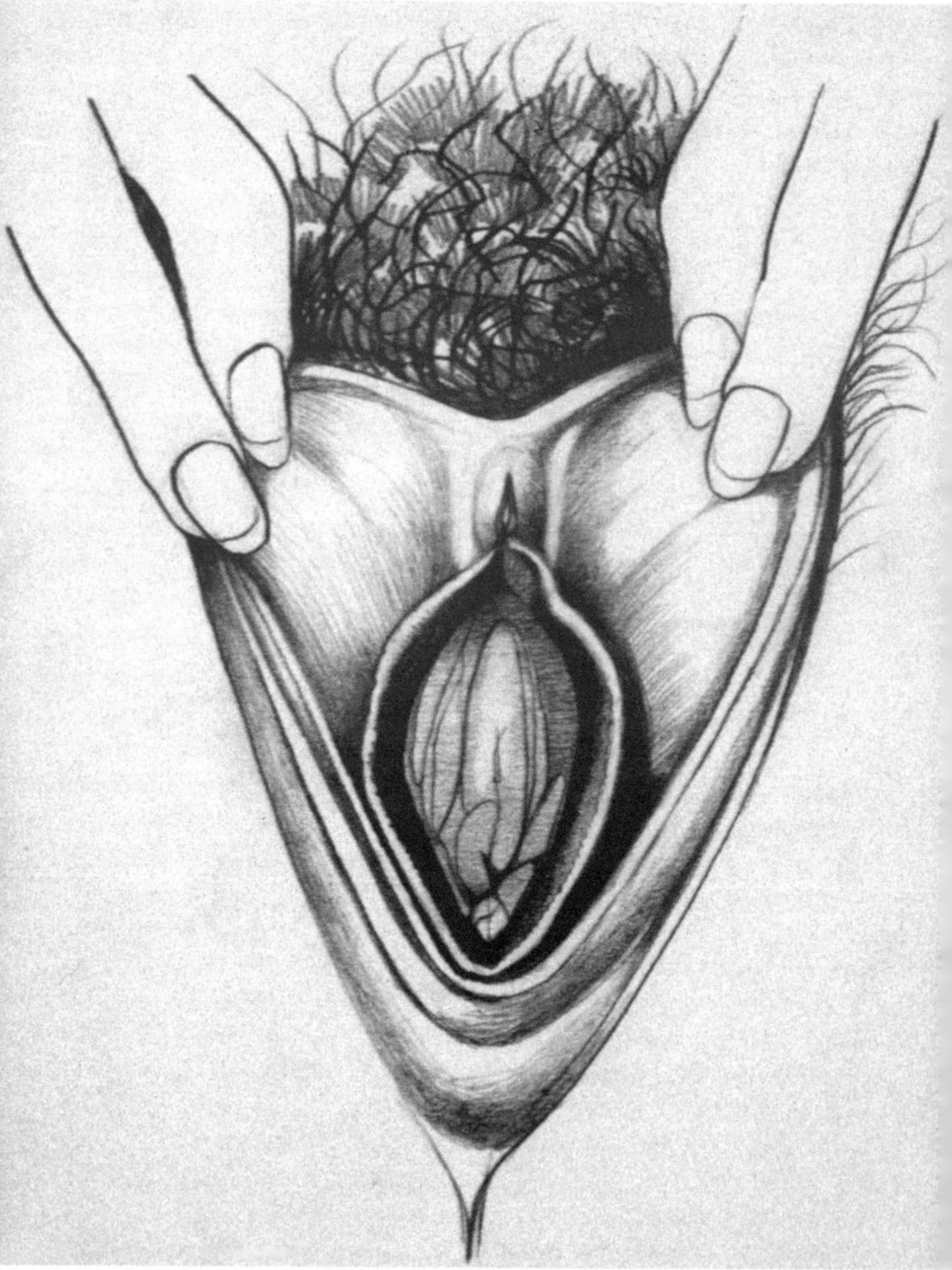

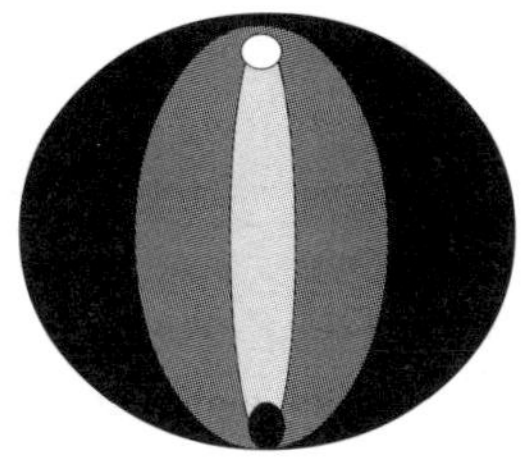

The Vulva

We are the protectors, the first guardians of your inner treasures. We enfold, we surround, we wrap your creative power, delicately and securely. Proudly we show ourselves, fiercely we protect.

We look ethereal – flowing and floating, waving and weaving – and so beautiful in our gowns of mauve and pink, pearl and coral. Like the blush of dawn, we blush. Like the glow of health, we glow. Like the dusky sky of evening, we are dusky. We are satiny. We are silken. We are velvety. We are smooth and strong. We are taffeta. We are suede. We are closely woven and tough.

We are the ones who open and close the outer gates. We are the muses who sing to those who journey within. We are the ones who kiss those who venture out.

We dance protection. We sparkle with joy. You call us lips, and like your lips, we have our moods. We mirror the health of that which we enclose. When you feel abraded by life, we hurt. When you spread us without tender care, we cry. When you cannot reject that which harms you, we scream in agony.

We will not be neglected. We will pin up our dresses and flash our red petticoats. We will scream. We will rage. We will burn with an unquenchable fire. We will wake you in the night. We will be heard. We will be respected. We will always, and ever, be here to remind you of your own worth, your own power, your own beauty.

We are the lips of your vagina and the mound of your pleasure. We are your vulva.

Healthy Vulva

The vulva, Latin for "covering," includes all the external female parts, including the *mons veneris* (Mound of Venus), the clitoris, and the lips that surround the vagina (singular: *labium*; plural: *labia*). The vulvar area contains millions of nerve endings and plays a major role in sexual response and pleasure.

There are two sets of vulval lips: one thicker, one thinner. The thicker lips lie outside the thinner ones. Previously, the thicker, outer lips were referred to as the *labia major* (big lips), and the thinner inner lips were called the *labia minor* (little lips). However, the inner lips are often longer and larger than the outer lips, so those terms are erroneous and in the process of bring replaced.

The size and the shape of the labia vary (sometimes a lot) from one side to the other on most women, and from one woman to another as well. Like snowflakes, all labia are unique.

The labia, like the lips of the mouth, are colorful, plump and moist when healthy. The entire vulva is protected by a waxy film that shields it from urine, bacteria, and vaginal secretions.

Beautiful drawings, sculptures, and art celebrating vulvas can be found in the works of Betty Dodson (below),[1] Tee Corrine,[2] Max Dashu,[3] Judy Chicago,[4] and Morgan Hastings.[5]

"Many historians find feminine symbolism in religious architecture: two sets of doorways, inner and outer (the labia); a central hallway (the vagina) leading to an altar (the uterus)."[6]

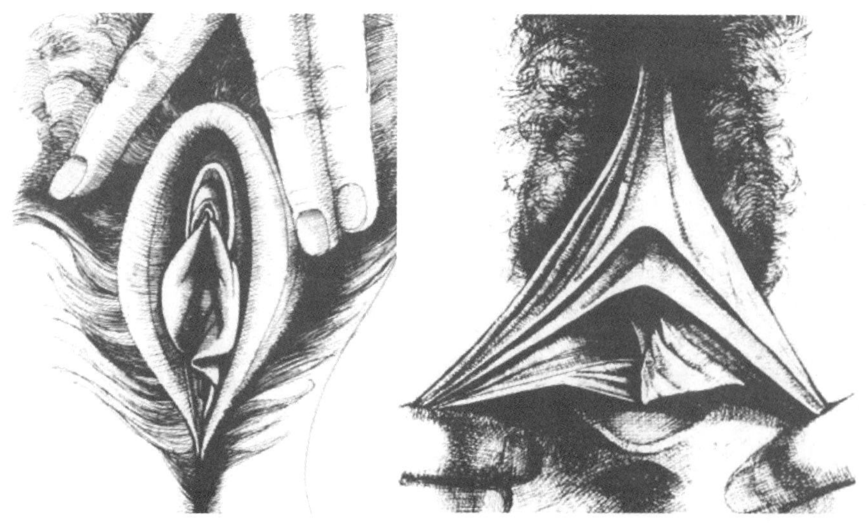

Vulvar Distresses

The vulva responds to physical and mental stressors. It can be an "early warning system" that stress is becoming too intense. The vulva can be extremely sensitive; the causes of disturbance to its health can be difficult to diagnose.

Most commonly, the vulva is irritated by **infections** such as herpes (page 160), genital warts (page 176), and yeast overgrowth (page 146). Infections cause alkaline vaginal discharges which irritate the vulva, leaving it lumpy, bumpy, itchy, burning, upset, and, in extreme cases, disfigured. The vulva may become painfully irritated by **parasites** such as trichomonas (page 150), lice, or scabies (both on page 91).

A minor vulvar problem, but one that can cause considerable discomfort and itching, is **varicosities** in the labia (page 90).

If vulvar pain does not respond to antibiotic, antiparasitic, and anti-yeast medications, and **cancer** (page 101) is ruled out, the diagnosis is **vulvodynia** (page 93). This "mysterious" condition was "relatively common a hundred years ago."[7] It disappeared for fifty years, and now seems to be making a comeback.

Occasionally, environmental irritants (such as laundry soaps, dyes and flame retardants) or skin diseases – such as **lichen scleroses** or **hyperkeratosis** – cause vulvar problems.

"Women want so much to know . . . what they look like. We must be brave enough to look, and that is a challenge for many. Give yourself permission to look at, touch, and love your vulva."[8]

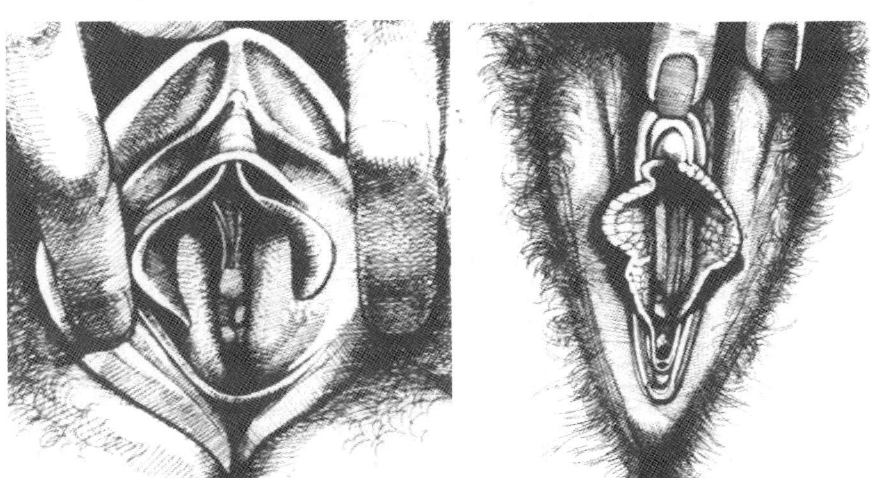

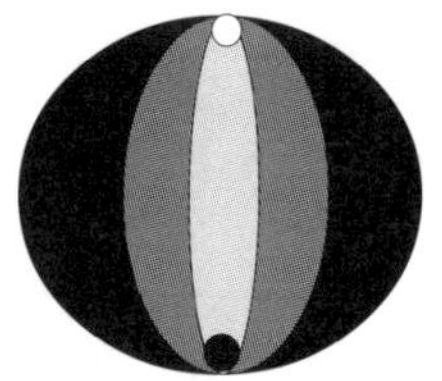

Minor Vulvar Distresses

Grandmother Growth beckons. Your bare feet step carefully through the emerging reeds, bringing you to her side.

"Squat here, just in the water, granddaughter," she urges, her eyes atwinkle. "Move slowly. Hunker down over the water. The sun is at just the right angle to make a mirror of it.

"Turn a little. There! Look! Look up between your legs. Look upon your vulva. Now, softly, quietly, put your hand there. Feel what you have seen. Take your time. Let your eyes close. Open your inner ears. Listen closely. Pay attention."

Vulvar Varicosities

• Veins return blood to the lungs and heart. Since they must work against gravity, it is no surprise that sometimes they fail. When a vein relaxes, it droops, causing a varicosity (in the anus, a hemorrhoid; *see* page 19). Some vulvar varicosities are visible; some aren't. Some bleed, others itch, and some are painless.

• A varicose vein in the vulva can interfere with sitting and sex. **Touch** your vulva. Skin on skin eases pain and nourishes the nerves. Gentle **massage** also helps heal vulvar varicosities.

• Herbal salves (such as **Sitting Pretty**, page 369), sitz baths (next page), and fumigations (below) are quite effective in reducing and eliminating vulvar viscosities. **Pelvic inversions** (page 9), done regularly, ease pain and counter swelling.

★ Chinese herbalists treat vulvar problems with **fumigation**. How to: Herbal roots such as dong quai, astragalus, plantain, and peony are boiled in water until it darkens. To fumigate: Place the steaming hot pan of herbs/water on the floor, squat over it or sit on the edge of a chair with open legs, and let the vapor steaming up from the pan condense on the vulva. The liquid may be saved, reheated, and reused for further fumigations, or as a sitz bath.

• **Sitz baths** (page 368) of soothing herbs like linden, mallow, or comfrey, or of astringent herbs like yarrow or oak bark, are allies who heal and ease vulvar pain. For fast, fast relief, apply **cold witch hazel** directly or as a compress (page 367). Ahhhh.

Pubic Lice, "Crabs"

If you have lice – soft-bodied, bloodsucking parasites – in your pubic hair, they will make your vulva itchy and red. Lice that live on pubic hair are called crabs. They travel easily from one warm body to another; sex is not required for transmission.

To get rid of lice without chemicals, suffocate them with generous applications of oil. Thick oils like castor oil or coconut oil work best. Many herbalists add a drop of essential oil to poison the lice. I don't. Essential oils can irritate, aggravate, and burn the vulva; in rare cases, they can precipitate vulvodynia. **I avoid essential oils.**

Don't sleep with anyone if you have crabs. Instead, spend your time doing laundry. Wash all your underwear, pants, and sheets with bleach. Dry them in the sun to eradicate the lice eggs. Vacuum your bed, your bedroom, your bathroom. "Hysterical hygiene" is safer than harsh poisons – and often more effective.

Scabies

Scabies is a contagious microscopic mite that burrows under the skin and causes an agonizing itch – the seven-year itch. Scabies can be caught from a person, a damp towel, or a dirty sheet. They enter the webbing between the fingers or toes, and spread to the armpits, groin, and vulva. The itch is particularly intense at night; sufferers injure themselves scratching in their sleep.

A hot, hot bath with green soap (available at drugstores) every day for ten days, followed by the lavish application of Bag Balm (a sulphur-based ointment) plus "hysterical hygiene" in bath and bedroom is usually enough to kill scabies. I avoid essential oils.

What Do You Call That?

What do *you* call *your* vulva? How do you address your vagina? My granddaughter calls it "yoni." Others say: powerbundle, fancy bit, dignity, coochi snorcher, "down under" cuz I'm from Australia, va-gha-gha, pussy (it's warm and fuzzy, and purrs when I'm happy), quim, fannyboo, snatch, honey pot, nappy dugout, nishi, poonani, hey-nonny-no, joy box, tottita, mimi, power box, pink credit card, and cunt, in honor of the goddess Cunti/Kunda/Kali.

Inga Muscio believes that the word "cunt" unites all women. She acknowledges that it is the "ultimate one-syllable covert verbal weapon any streetwise six-year-old or passing motorist can use against a women." Nonetheless, she claims it as a word of power. I do too. This venerable name – kund, cund, kunt, to use alternative spellings – is the root of "kundalini" and many English words such as "country," "cunning," "ken," and "kin."

My dear friend Mary Rose, a serious student of anatomy, finds it curious, and so do I, that many uniquely females features of the body are named after the men who "discovered" them.

~ Egg tubes are "Fallopian tubes" because Gabriele Fallopio, a sixteenth century Italian anatomist, named them.

~ Vulvovaginal glands are "Bartholin's glands" because Caspar Bartholin, eighteenth century Dutch anatomist, named them.

~ The urethral sponge, or *corpus spongiosum* erectile tissue was named the "G-spot" by our contempory Dr. Ernst Gräfenburg.

~ The suspensory ligaments, thin bands of connective tissue that support the breasts internally are "Cooper's ligaments."

~ The areolar glands, which encircle our nipples and protect them during breast-feeding, are known as "Montgomery's glands."

~ Pelvic floor lifts are commonly called "Kegels." Yogis call them *mula bandha*. Feminists call them "pelvic clenches."

~ The recto-uterine pouch, the area behind the uterus and in front of the rectum, is referred to as the "Pouch of Douglas."

"Why not use the simple anatomical terms?" Mary Rose asks. In the few instances where they are cumbersome, women ought to be in charge of the names, she contends. She urges all of us to reclaim our lives by reclaiming the naming of our body parts, one word at a time. "*Rosa cava*" (rose's cave) is her name for the recto-uterine pouch.

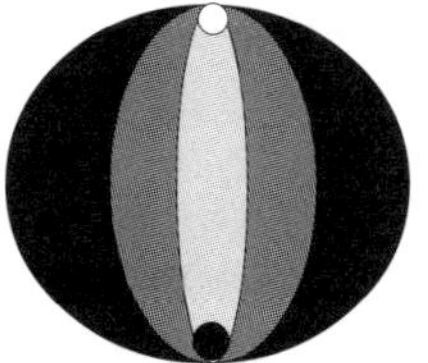

Vulvodynia

"There is pain at your root, dear daughter," Grandmother Growth says, as a tear finds its way through the wrinkles of her cheek. "Roots hold us firm. They transmit the energy of the Earth to us, filling us with strength and power, giving us the courage to protect ourselves and all we love. Our roots connect us to our Ancestors, and to all who will follow us.

"What disturbs your root, dearest? What burns your base? What shakes your belief in your own power? What deprives you of your strength? What prevents you from actively protecting what you love? Be gentle with yourself. Protect yourself. Soothe the deep and hidden parts of yourself. Do not cut away the offending tissues, sweet daughter.

"When you hurt down there, when your vulva burns with pain, when any touch to your genitals causes you to cry out and shudder, when you cannot sleep, when you weep with frustration, then – pay attention granddaughter – then you must return to your roots or lose them. Listen to the Ancient Ones within. Sit on the Earth. Remember, we love you."

Step 0. *Do Nothing*

• If you hurt down there, avoid potential irritants. No douching. No "feminine hygiene" products. No soap down there. No essential oils in your bath. *Go naked down there* – or wear loose cotton undies (the leg elastic can be an irritant) washed in hypoallergenic soap. **Avoid fabric softeners**. Use cotton menstrual pads, not tampons. No tight pants. Get out of your bathing suit as soon as possible; better yet, swim nude. Approach bicycling and horseback riding with caution, if at all. Avoid chlorine.

• Don't drink chlorinated water, and stay out of chlorinated swimming pools and hot tubs. A filter that removes chlorine from your drinking water is a lot less expensive than bottled water, and much healthier for you and the planet. You inhale chlorine gas from hot water, so a filter for the shower is critical.

Step 1. *Collect Information*

• A fifth (16–20 percent) of American women aged 18–64 have had one or more episodes of vulvar pain lasting at least three months.[10,11,12] The University of Michigan Health System says 28 percent of women will experience vulvar pain at some point in their lives.[13] About six million women have chronic vulvar pain.[14]

• For fifty years, modern medicine misdiagnosed and mistreated women with pain down there. They were labeled hysteric or frigid, given ineffective medications, and subjected to questionable surgeries. Many of them – driven by intense pain – were willing to believe or try anything in pursuit of relief.

As the twentieth century ended, however, vulvar pain was accepted as real and named: *vulvodynia* (VVD). It's also known as vulvar vestibulitis, vulvar pain syndrome, burning vulva syndrome, focal vulvitis, vestibular adenitis, and vestibulitis.

• Women with VVD have burning, stabbing, shooting, stinging pains in their vulva, vagina, urethra, and/or rectum. Pain may be constant, caused by *any* contact, or only during intercourse. It can be so excruciating – "like a fire that won't go out" – that it prevents normal activities like walking, driving, sitting, and sex.

• What causes VVD? Perhaps injury to, or irritation of, nerves serving the vulva – from surgery, a deep-seated infection, or cellular memory of previous trauma. But muscle spasms, a genetic defect, and even hormone disturbances, especially in postmenopausal women, may also be to blame.

• Massage therapist Candace Cave says: "Spasm of the *adductor magnus* muscle, which attaches to the pelvis right at the groin, may be diagnosed as vulvar pain. The symptoms are so similar."

• Thirty percent of young women with VVD have a genetic defect that increases response to inflammation. Any irritation of the vulva (or bowel, bladder, or surrounding muscles) causes *cytokines* (immune factors, such as interleukin-1) to be produced. These women cannot turn them off as others can, and thus suffer chronic inflammation and pain.[15] Herbal anti-inflammatories (page 69) can break this cycle.

• Women with vulvar pain frequently have endometriosis, fibromyalgia, irritable bowel syndrome, and/or interstitial cystitis too. They may be hyper-aware of pelvic sensations. Try the "Meditation for a Secure Vagina" on page 125 to help calm sensitivity.

Step 2. *Engage the Energy*

• Are you itching for a change? Are you burning to break free?

• Dr. Laurie Steelsmith notes that "pent up frustration, resentment, and anger" contribute to vulvar pain. Christiane Northrup, MD, believes: "A woman sets the stage . . . for chronic vulvar problems when she *lacks the courage to change* [or to reach out for help in changing] the negative aspects of unhealthy relationships."[16]

★ There are many **homeopathic remedies** for vulvar pain and inflammation.[17] Lower dilutions (10x–30c) treat acute pain, while higher dilutions (200c and up) treat chronic pain.

~ *Aconite*: superficial inflammation, soreness.
~ *Apis*: severe itching, burning, pain.
~ *Cimicifuga racemosa*: pain radiates from the back to the vulva; soreness; painful menstruation.
~ *Eryngium campestre*: with bladder involvement.
~ *Hamamelis*: with prolapse, fullness.
~ *Ignatia*: vulva, feet, and hands chilled, icy.
~ *Piper cubeba*: irritation and burning pain.
~ *Pulsatilla*: pain brings nervousness, depression.
~ *Rhus tox.*: burning pain, itching, irritation after urination; pruritis, erythematous and erysipelatous lesions.

• **Biofeedback** teaches you how to use your mind to ease your vulvar pain. It is AMA approved, and covered by most insurers.

Step 3. *Nourish and Tonify*

★ A healthy diet and daily consumption of a quart of nourishing herbal infusion – red clover, oatstraw, chickweed, or linden, one at a time, in rotation – will ease pain and supply you with all the nutrients you need to heal your vulva, including lavish amounts B vitamins, vitamin E, magnesium, and calcium.

~ **Red clover infusion** supplies minerals and phytoestrogens to strengthen the vulva, easing swelling and inflammation. It has been used for hundreds of years as a specific against vulvar pain.[18]

~ **Oatstraw infusion** nourishes the nerves, making them less sensitive. It soothes emotions, and restores hormones, too.

~ **Chickweed infusion** nourishes vulvar tissues, cools burning tissues from the inside out, and helps eliminate infections.

~ **Linden infusion** is anti-inflammatory. It soothes and heals the vulva, the vagina, and all the blood vessels serving them.

★ **Yogurt** and quercetin-rich **oak bark tincture**, taken orally and applied directly, relieve vulvar pain fast. Plain yogurt also improves digestion and immunity, both of which integrative practitioners believe are critical to reversing VVD.

• Since vulvodynia can be triggered by chemicals, **eat** mostly **organic** foods; avoid preservatives, chemicals such as phosphoric acid (in carbonated drinks), artificial sweeteners, food dyes, preservatives, soy protein isolate (in energy bars and Bragg's aminos) and nitrates (in preserved meats).[19]

• It is possible that food acids, especially **oxalic acid,** can trigger inflammation and vulvar pain. Many women with VVD have high levels of oxalic acid in their urine. Does it come from food or is it overproduced by their bodies? About 15 percent of women with VVD and interstitial cystitis benefit from eliminating/reducing oxalic acid in their diets.[20] (See page 97, "Oxalic Acid in Foods.") Results vary; dietary change can do nothing or they can be a miracle.

• Low-acid diets can be quite nourishing, although many greens, fruits and vegetables are high in plant acids and must be avoided. Vegetarians will be adversely affected by a low-acid diet.[21] Instead of such a diet, they may wish to take **calcium citrate**.

Help!
Vulvar Pain

Expect results in two weeks

• Take one dose of one **homeopathic** remedy, once.

• Take off your underwear.

• Drink two or more cups of **linden infusion** a day.

• Eat fruit cooked; no juice, no raw.

• Eat a quart of yogurt a week.

Oxalic Acid in Foods[22,23]

(mg per 100 grams)

Enjoy! Eat all you want of these. Lowest in oxalic acid (0–1mg per 100 grams): beef, natural beer, Brussels sprouts, butter, boiled cabbage, cooked broccoli, cheese, chicken, eggs, hamburger, lime juice, mangos, melons, nectarines, potatoes, rice, white wine (all 0mg); fish (0–5mg); store milk (.1mg); cauliflower, cooked turnip, cucumber, lemon juice, oatmeal, pasta, pineapple, canned peas (all 1mg).

Eat with caution. Mid-range in oxalic acid (2–10mg per 100 grams): raw tomatoes, mushrooms, Guinness stout, lettuce, onions, radishes, beets, pears, carrots, sardines, corn, asparagus, cranberry juice, strawberries.

Limit or avoid these foods. High-range in oxalic acid: kale (13), blueberries (15), green peppers (16), okra (12), blackberries (18), eggplant (18), green beans (15–20), rutabaga (19), celery (20), summer squash (22), Concord grapes (25), dandelion greens (25), escarole (31), coffee (33), Ovaltine (35), grits (41), raspberries (53), sweet potato (56), tea/black, green, white, iced (75–85), gooseberries (88), leeks (89).

Totally avoid these foods. Highest in oxalic acid: cooked rhubarb (860), cooked spinach (750), Swiss chard (645), cocoa powder (623), frozen spinach (600), poke greens (479), boiled beets (675), pickled beets (500), black pepper (419), beet greens, lamb's quarters, sheep sorrel, Essiac, pecans (202), wheat germ (269), soy crackers (207), tofu, peanuts/peanut butter (187), okra (146), plain chocolate bar (117), parsley (100).

Greens, raw or cooked, are high in food acids. Avoid these **high-oxalic greens** if you have VVD or IC: beet greens, chard, lamb's quarters, poke greens, sheep sorrel, spinach. Approach these mid-range greens with caution: collards, dandelion, escarole, kale, mustard greens, nettle, watercress.

Note: **To neutralize these acids, take calcium citrate.**

"I endured a succession of treatments — all unsuccessful — including electrocautery, antibacterial, antifungal, and antiviral medications, removal of my vestibular glands, and six treatments with laser surgery followed by two operations that involved cutting away the tissue in the painful area."[9]

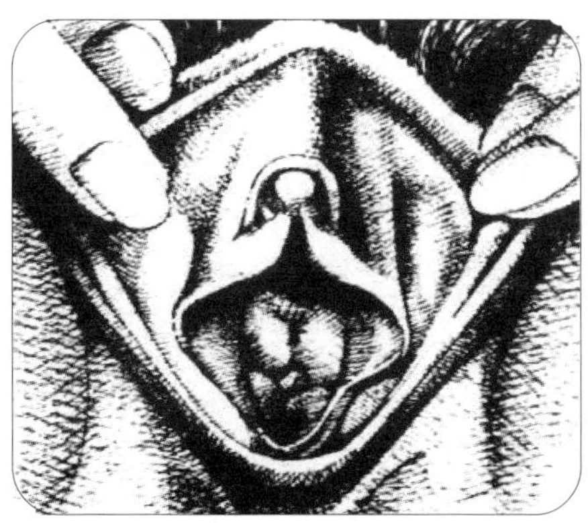

"The more women try to clean, disinfect, or perfume their vulva, the more problems they have."[24]

Step 4. *Stimulate/Sedate*

★ Herbalists and homeopaths agree that **St. Joan's wort** is the best remedy when there is nerve pain. Herbalists use the infused oil topically plus tincture internally (a dropperful 2–12 times a day, depending on the severity of the pain). St. J's relieves pain quickly – often within a few days, restores healthy nerve functioning, and helps destroy any hidden viral infections, including herpes. Homeopaths use high dilution doses of *Hypericum perforatum* to change the energy and break the cycle of chronic pain.

★ **Oat sitz baths** soothe the vulva and normalize nerves. Simmer a handful of oatmeal in a gallon/4 liters of water for thirty minutes, then strain and add liquid to a hot, hip-level bath and soak your pain away. Or buy Aveeno, powdered oatmeal, at your drugstore, dissolve some in warm water and sitz in that.

★ A **yarrow sitz bath** numbs sensitive nerves and soothes irritated tissues. Pain relief can last for hours. Make it: page 368.

• Chinese herbalists believe vulvar pain comes from "static blood and cold deficiency." To warm and move the blood, they use **dong quai**, **wild yam**, and/or **astragalus** tinctures, 1–3 dropperful doses daily. Or a cup a day, taken in sips, of **wild ginger tea**.

★ **Comfrey sitz baths** ease pain immediately. Midwives worldwide have told me how healing comfrey is to the vulvar area. Its allantoin creates strong, stretchy skin that loves life and laughs away pain, irritation, and sensitivity. Make it: page 368.

More Help!
Vulvar Pain

If you still have pain after 2 weeks, do the prior remedies, plus these.

• Take a dropperful of **St. Joan's wort tincture**, 1–12 times a day.

• Cut down on, or even eliminate, **oxalic acid** in your diet; or take **calcium citrate** with meals.

• Take a **sitz bath** 2–3 times a week for 6–8 weeks with **oak bark**, **chamomile** flowers, **comfrey** leaf, or **yarrow** flowers.

• Keep a spray bottle of water, witch hazel lotion, yarrow tincture, or oak bark infusion by the toilet and spray your vulva after urinating. Then pat dry with a very soft cloth. No rubbing, no wiping. Ahhh . . .

• To relieve pain, try sitting on a **donut pillow** or try **electromyography** with physical therapy.

★ **Self-heal**, also known as heal-all, is a common, weedy, virtually-scentless mint which grows in cities, lawns, and the edges of woodland trails. Herbalist Dr. James Duke recommends it for its high levels of antioxidants. Those who believe that a viral infection is at the root of vulvar pain rely on self-heal's antiviral properties. The dose of tincture of the fresh flowering plant is 1–3 dropperfuls daily. Self-heal may be used safely for months or years.

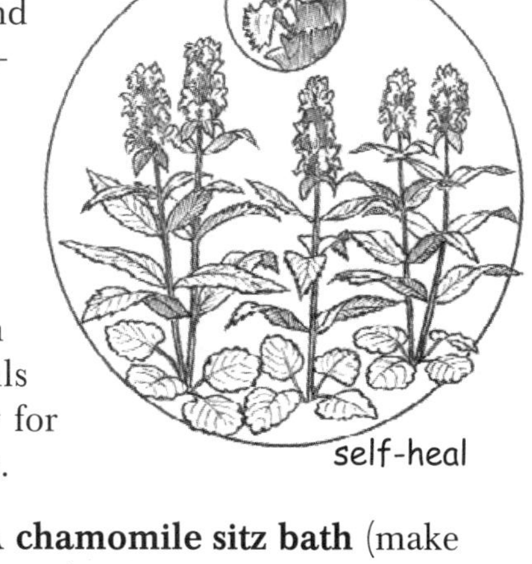
self-heal

★ A **chamomile sitz bath** (make it: page 368) relaxes painful muscles, counters spasms, kills bacteria, aids in healing, and offers powerful anti-inflammatory benefits for both immediate and long-lasting relief. **Chamomile** oil/ointment (make it, page 367) counters inflammation as well as hydrocortisone, and better than nonsteroidal anti-inflammatories like 5% bufexamac or 0.75% fluocortin butyl ester.[25]

chamomile

Step 5a. *Use Supplements*

• **Calcium citrate**, 200mg taken four times a day plus a low-acid diet (page 97), eases vulvar pain even for women who've given up. This is not a cure. Pain returns if you stop taking the calcium ciitrate or eat high-acid foods. For fewest side effects, start with one dose a day, taken on an empty stomach, immediately upon waking. Do this for three days.[20] Then add a tablet before dinner for three days, then one more at lunch, and finally one at breakfast, for a total of four doses a day.

★ A daily dropperful of **yellow dock** root tincture counters calcium citrate's tendency to constipate.

Step 5b. *Use Drugs*

★ Topical drugs deliver more vulvar relief, with fewer side effects, than oral medicines. Women with VVD swear by **estrogen creams** and **topical anesthetics** (like lidocaine).

• VVD women who took 250mg of N-acetyl glucosamine twice a day for four months, reported significant remission of pain.

• There are no specific drugs designed to treat VVD. However, some women and practitioners find these helpful:[27]

~ Antihistamines, to relieve swelling
~ Muscle relaxants, such as Flexeril, to ease pain
~ Anticonvulsant, anti-epilectic drugs, such as Neurontin
~ Interferon
~ Tricyclic antidepressants, such as Elavil or Prozac, in very, very small doses, to reduce neurotransmitter sensitivity

• High acid drugs and supplements – such as aspirin and ascorbic acid (vitamin C) – can trigger vulvar pain. Regular use of immune-suppressing drugs, birth control pills, and/or antibiotics may trigger vulvar pain.[28]

Step 6. *Break and Enter*

> "I was told that the [vulvar] biopsy [to rule out cancer] would be 'very minimally painful.' This is a flagrant misrepresentation. The injection of the anesthetic brought short term relief, but by the time I got dressed again I was in agony. The recovery was excruciating; it was almost three weeks before I could drive. The only good thing was that the acute pain was so severe that I couldn't feel the vulvar burning. The procedure caused me severe psychological pain as well."[29]

• If muscle spasms are causing your vulvar pain, electrical stimulation of the pelvic floor can help loosen them. Be sure you have tried other remedies first.

• In extremity, some women have the offending vulvar nerves surgically removed. This is completely successful only 37 percent of the time, although 87 percent of women do report some improvement or lessening of symptoms. Twice-weekly **acupuncture** sessions are an excellent alternative to surgery.

• Vestibulitis is vulvar pain centered in the vestibule, which is the entrance to the vagina. Surgical removal of the sensitized tissues is helpful for at least 76 percent of women.[30] **Avoid laser** vaporization of the tissues; it thins the tissues, leaving them less elastic and more sensitive to pain,[31] and healing is slow.

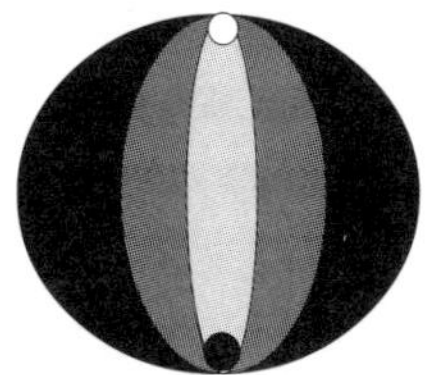

Vulvar Cancer

• Although rare, cancer of the vulva does occur; there are about 3,200 new cases diagnosed annually in the USA.[32] Nearly 800 American women a year die of vulvar cancer.

• *To reduce risk of all types of cancer:*
  - ~ Eat miso and tamari daily.
  - ~ Drink red clover infusion or eat burdock root regularly.
  - ~ Eat four servings of cabbage-family plants a week.
  - ~ Enjoy lavish amounts of onions and garlic in food.
  - ~ Meditate instead of smoking tobacco.
  - ~ Rest and sleep deeply.

• If you are dancing with vulvar cancer, the remedies suggested for other cancers (pages 75, 200, 244, and 284) can assist you.

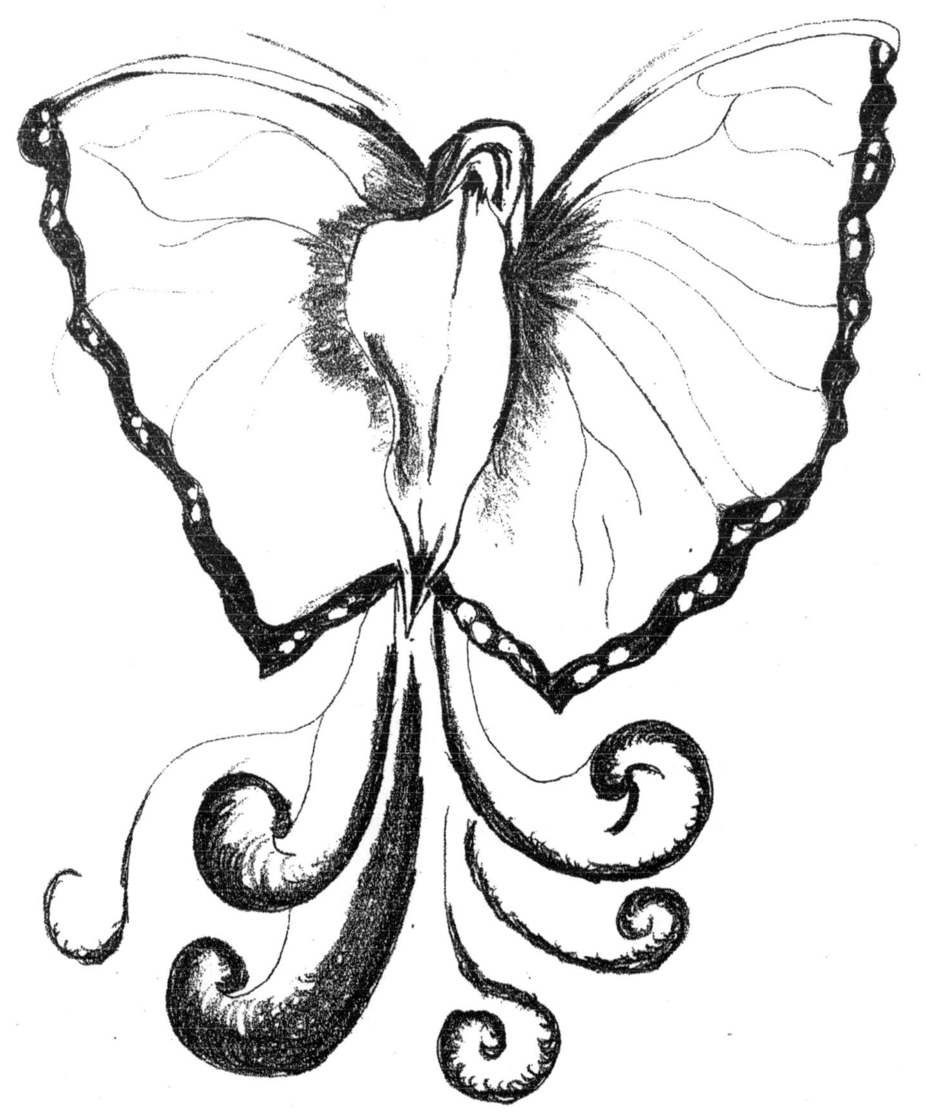

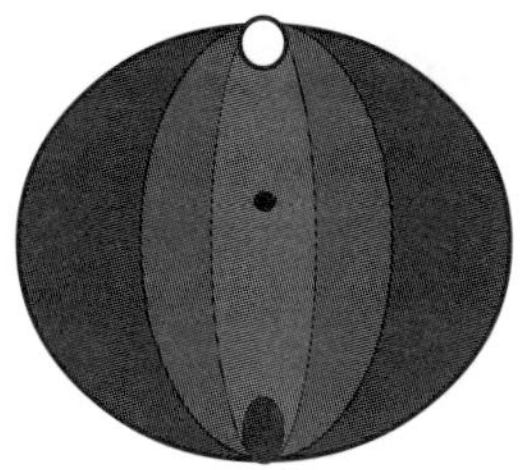

The Clitoris

I hold the center of desire. I know the vectors of satiation.

Like my brother, I grow turgid and swollen. Unlike my brother, my growth is hidden, felt rather than seen. He looks outward; I look within. He pokes his nose into things; I send out subtle feelers.

I am slow, thoughtful, contemplative. I am willing to take my time, to wait for the right moment, the perfect setting. I have strict standards and I am finicky.

Coddle me and court me. Titillate me with innuendo. Entice me with promises. Regard me with awe. Whisper to me. Sing to me of protection and permanence.

I am impetuous, wild, raging with lust. I need. I need now. I tolerate no words. All my verbs are action verbs. I am everywhere and everything. Nothing exists but my thirst, my yearning. I am insatiable, unconquerable, despotic. Cover your face. Do not look at me.

I wiggle and thrum, throb and hum. I vibrate at ever-increasing frequencies. My mantra is: More, more, more. More intense. More vibrato. Higher, broader, fuller, richer. Exquisite. Idyllic. Blissful. Boundless.

My ecstacy serves fecundity, maximizes fertility, and aids birthing. My delight gives to the future and repays the past. And beyond all that, when you assume your Crone's throne, I will remain to decorate your life with pure pleasure.

I am a bud suffused with blood. I am a sponge networked with nerves. I am your joy. I am your clitoris.

Healthy Clitoris

The clitoris is not a small penis. (*Nor is the penis a large clitoris.*)

The clitoris is the only organ whose sole purpose is pleasure.

The clitoris is a bundle of nerves. There are about eight thousand nerves in the clitoris: more than in your fingertips, lips, or tongue. And twice as many as there are in the glans of the penis.

The clitoris is quite variable, from woman to woman, in shape, size, and sensitivity. What does not vary is the shape, size, and sensitivity of an individual woman's clitoris once it is mature.

external view
front

The hormonal changes of the menstrual cycle, pregnancy, lactation, and menopause affect a woman's desire for orgasm, but not her ability to have an orgasm.

The clitoris is not very sensitive to hormones.[1] It does not get old. Once it is mature – after puberty – the clitoris remains at the peak of its power for the rest of a woman's life.[2] Your clitoris is immortal; it is unchanging and never aging.

Meet your clitoris, page 106.

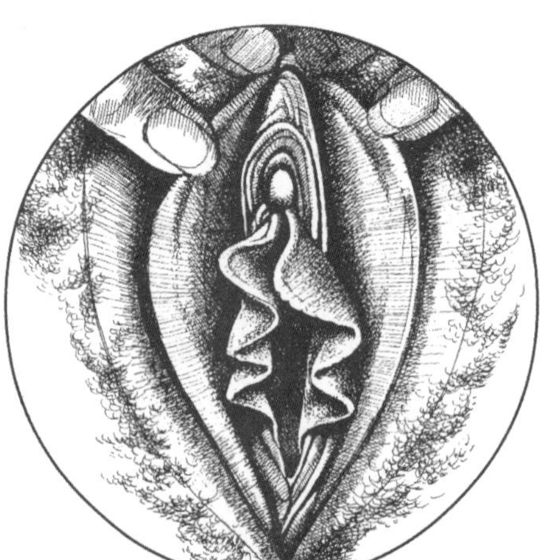

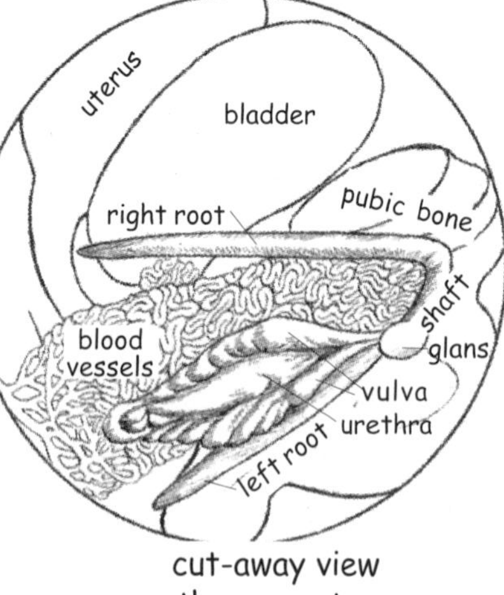

cut-away view
three-quarter

"I first met my clitoris when I was eleven. She has been my best friend ever since. She and I are inseparable." Monique

Clitoral Distresses

The clitoris is one part of "down there" that rarely has health problems, perhaps because it does not age along with the rest of the body. The clitoris does not become infected, even when there is active infection in the vagina or uterus.

Women's orgasms are easiest when they arise from clitoral stimulation. While some women find the key to orgasms easily, others don't. Without help, it can be difficult to understand **how to have an orgasm** (page 109). Then, just when you think you've got it, menopause changes the rules. **Postmenopausal sex** (page 115) can be painful or "the best sex of my entire life."

Thinking of trying a **vibrator**? Good! See page 114 for a short history of this useful "medical device."

Surgical removal of the clitoris, **clitorectomy** (page 118), is never medically justified, especially for infants.

resting clitoris
side view
uterus
cervix
bladder
rectum
vagina
pubic bone
clitoris:
root,
shaft,
glans
blood
vessels
urethra

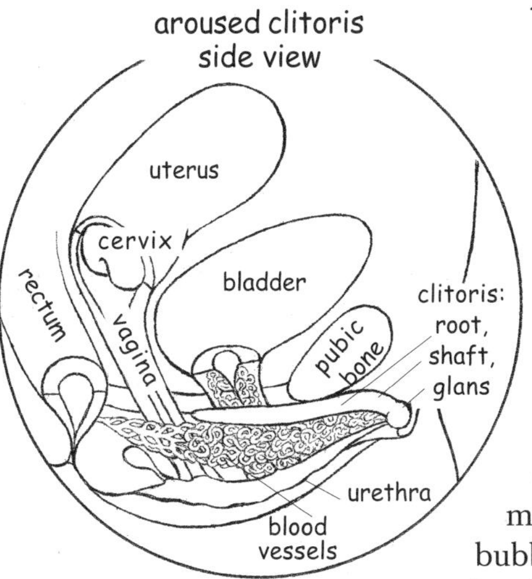

The clitoris may become **chafed** or **inflamed**. This distress is remedied by removal of the irritation: soap, bubble bath, panty hose, thongs, and tight clothing. If the problem persists, abandon underwear, enjoy a sitz bath in soothing comfrey infusion, and apply aloe vera gel generously.

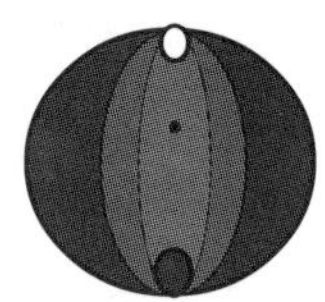

Meet Your Clitoris

> " . . . the clitoris is designed to encourage its bearer to take control of her sexuality. . . . It is versatile, generous, demanding, profound, easy, and enduring. The clitoris hates being scared or bullied . . . hurried or pushed. . . . The clitoris loves power. . . . It knows more than the vagina does, and is a more reliable counselor. . . . The clitoris is our magic cape."[3]

Step 1. *Collect Information*

• The clitoris, like the Goddess, is three: a crown, a scepter, and roots. She is covered with a fetching little hood and attended by Her ladies-in-waiting – blood-filled tissues, spongy tissues, and bundles of nerves. She sits upon Her throne: the pelvic floor.

~ Her **hood** is formed by the joining of the inner labia. Their meeting makes a little tent for crown and scepter.

~ Her **crown** is the jewel of the yoni: the **glans** of the clitoris. It looks like the tip of a tiny, smooth tongue. In some women the glans protrudes from the hood and is easily accessed. In others, the hood covers the glans and needs to be moved up and back. Many women find moving the hood against the glans very arousing; for some it is an effective route to orgasm. The **commisure** is the seam where the crown and the shaft meet. One side (often the left), rubbed smoothly and evenly, with plenty of lubrication, is, for most women, a certain path to orgasm.

~ Her **scepter**, the **shaft** of the clitoris, goes from the crown to the pubic bone, where it meets the roots. About the thickness of a chopstick, it is more easily felt than seen. Wiggle your fingers back and forth between the upper outer labia until you encounter a round springy tube. Or slide two fingers down on either side of the clitoris and press them together; the scepter is in between. (Both moves aid orgasm.) The shaft is covered in fibroelastic tissue that you can slide up and down a little if it feels good to you.

~ Her **roots**, the *crura* of the clitoris, anchor her. They are the largest and most hidden part of the clitoris. Stretching out from the base of the shaft at the pubic symphysis, these long, thin bands of firm erectile tissue spread out toward the thighs, following the line of the pubic bone down for about four inches. Gentle pressure on the spot where the roots branch (at the base of the shaft at the pubic bone) can be quite arousing.

~ The **bulbs** of the clitoris surround the roots and extend along the vagina, like parentheses just under the labia.

~ Her **erectile tissues** (and their valved capillaries) are more diffuse than His, but equal in size and weight. A clitoris, as a whole, is as large as a penis. Its erectile tissues are spread across a wider area and function as a coordinated network rather than a single unit. (After orgasm, the blood stays in the clitoris's erectile tissues, but leaves the penis's.) Engorgement is not limited to the erectile tissues: The hood, crown, scepter, roots, spongy tissues, and bulbs of the clitoris swell, stiffen, and contract pleasurably.

~ Her spongy tissues are twofold. The **urethral sponge**, sometimes called the G-spot,[4] which can be felt by placing one or two fingers in the vagina and pushing gently up and forward, toward the pubic bone. And the **perineal sponge**, which can be felt by pressing on the back side of the vagina, toward the anus.

~ Her throne is the **pelvic floor**, a collection of muscles that control the bladder and anal sphincters. Their pulsating contractions during orgasm move blood through all the structures of the clitoris and turn on the fireworks in the nerve endings.

• Unlike the penis, the clitoris does not have a venous plexus (a tight-knit group of veins that hold blood in to cause an erection). The clitoris does swell, often to twice its usual size, on arousal. But blood flows into and out of it throughout arousal and orgasm; it is not trapped and released at the moment of climax.

> "...women who will admit their lewdness call it their *gaude mihi* [great joy]."[5]

• "Clitoris" may be derived from the ancient Greek *kleitoriazein*, which means to "titillate lasciviously; to seek pleasure." Or perhaps from the Greek word for "key." Or possibly from the Greek for "to be inclined." No matter; **clitoris** (cli-TOR-is or KLIT-oris) it is in all modern European languages.

Step-by-Step Orgasm

See-through views after Suzann Gage

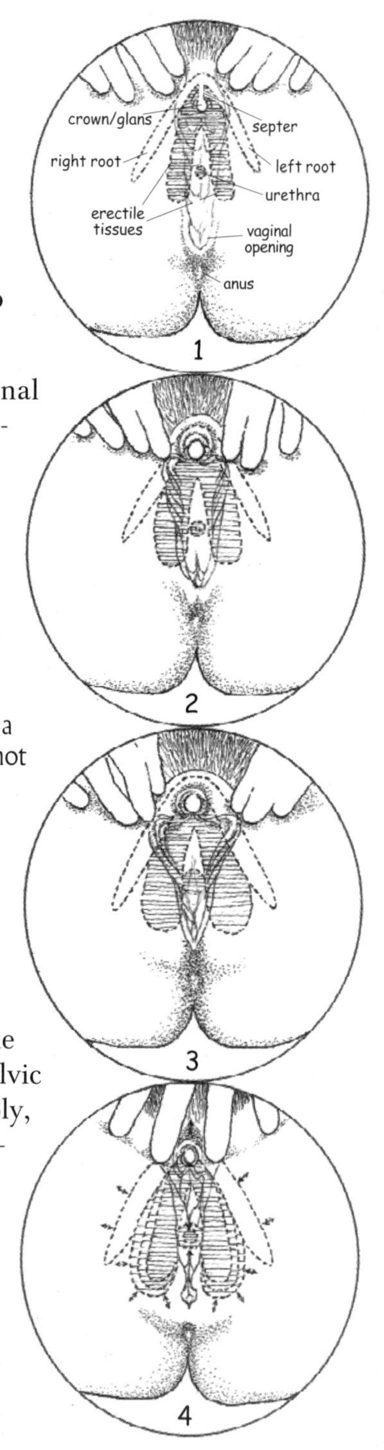

1. In the non-erect state, the crown of the clitoris is nestled in its hood, supported by the scepter and the roots, awaiting an opportunity to please you.

2. As excitement starts, the vaginal blood vessels widen, causing the entire vulva to redden or deepen in color, and the underlying spongy tissues to fill with blood. This causes pressure and tingling as the shaft of the clitoris is pulled back toward the pubic bone. The vagina sweats; pulse rate and blood pressure rise.

> "[the clitoris is] . . . a private joke, a divine secret, a Pandora's box packed not with sorrow but with laughter."[6]

3. As excitement builds, the urethral sponge and clitoral bulbs engorge with more blood, the scepter and the roots swell so much they become rigid, and the crown enlarges.

4. At orgasm, all the structures of the clitoris throb, the muscles of the pelvic floor clench and release uncontrollably, and the uterus balloons up and contracts rhythmically.

Diffuse vascularization keeps the clitoral tissues fully engorged after orgasm. Some clitorises become sensitized and need to wait a bit, though, before approaching the next orgasm.

All hail the queen!

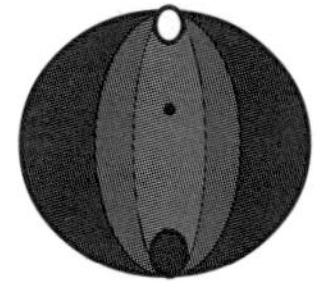

How to Have An Orgasm

"The majority of books and illustrations of female genital anatomy leave out most of the equipment responsible for arousal and orgasm. When these specialized sexual structures are omitted from our cultural images and text, they're also expunged from our mental model. The result is an ignorance that operates like a mental chastity belt; it dramatically reduces women's sexual potential."[7]

Step 0. *Do Nothing*

• Sex is more than orgasms. The clitoris is about orgasms; this section is about having them. A big gushing thank-you to Annie Sprinkle,[8] Barbara Carrellas,[9] Sheri Winston,[10] and the pioneering women of "The Clitoris: A Feminist Perspective."[11]

Step 1. *Collect Information*

• The Kinsey report on sexuality (from the 1950s) found 36 percent of women in their twenties had not had an orgasm; by the age of thirty, this figure had dropped to 15 percent.[12]

• A 1999 study found 43 percent of women experience sexual problems some times; the most common complaint is lack of libido.[13] One-third of women aged 50 and up report lack of interest in sex.[14] Half of American women are unsatisfied with sex.[15]

Perhaps we *are* unsatisfied with "sex." It usually involves penetration, which doesn't always add to a woman's pleasure. Instead, let's find satisfaction in being our own best lovers, learning how to have stupendous orgasms, and using our orgasms to heal.

• Married, conservative Christian women were the likeliest (in 1994) to say that they orgasmed consistently during sex. At every age, married women report more orgasms than single women.[16]

• Women's orgasms are triggered by nerves which originate in the clitoris, vagina, vulva, periurethral tissues, anus, and uterus.

The clitoris integrates information from these inputs, plus reports from the cerebral cortex, the hypothalamus, and the peripheral nervous system. Different women have different active nerve pathways; this changes with pregnancy, lactation, and menopause.

• It is not necessary to be in **good health** to have an orgasm, but it helps. It is not necessary to be in **a stable relationship** to have an orgasm, but it helps. It is not necessary to be in **love** to have an orgasm, but it helps. It is not necessary to have an active **fantasy** life to have an orgasm . . . but it helps.

• The anthropologist Helen Fisher reminds us that "women who are easily and multiply orgasmic have one trait in common: *they take responsibility for their pleasure.* They don't depend on the skillfulness or mind-reading abilities of their lover to get what they want. . . . [T]hey negotiate verbally or kinesthetically."[17]

• How can you know what you and your clitoris like? Masturbation and experimentation are foundational to a woman's sexual fulfillment/satisfaction. Try a vibrator (page 114).

• A recent study found women's top sexual goals are: orgasm and physical pleasure; spontaneity and flow; and closeness.[18]

• Any woman can have **multiple orgasms** – one orgasm following on the heels of another. Most orgasms last for 20–30 seconds; if they follow one another rapidly, it feels like one long orgasm. Sexual Olympians can have one hundred orgasms an hour. I'm happy to have half a dozen in half an hour. Don't fret if you have one, or none. Most women need privacy, a vibrator, and/or an attuned, attentive, trusted lover, for multiple orgasms. Most of us get better at it, much better at it, after menopause.

> "Extending and expanding orgasm is a learnable skill."
> Sex educator Sheri Winston

★ Freud claimed that clitoral orgasms were "infantile," and that "healthy, mature" women had vaginal orgasms. The clitoris gets a big laugh out of this insidious phallocentric view that penetration is needed/wanted. The vagina and the clitoris are not separate entities. The forward wall of the vagina is part of the clitoris. *All orgasms, no matter where they originate, are clitoral orgasms.*

Step 2. *Engage the Energy*

> "If you are frightened, [the clitoris] becomes numb. If you are uninterested or disgusted, it remains mute. If you are thrilled and strong, it's a taut little baton, leading the way. . . ."[19]

• Natalie Angier reminds us that the thinking part of the brain hinders orgasm, which centers in the feeling-centered hypothalamus. How to quiet the neocortex? She rejects alcohol (too numbing), and Quaaludes (not available), but finds **marijuana** "can be a sexual mentor and a sublime electrician, bringing the lights of Broadway to women who have spent years in frigid darkness."[20] Readers comment: "Makes my vagina so dry." "Helps me play."

★ Wilhelm **Reich**, one of Freud's students, disagreed with him about the value and function of orgasm. Reich believed that mental health was closely tied to orgasm; the healthier the person, the more fulfilling the orgasm, and healthy orgasm is a route to emotional health. He specified a "whole body" orgasm, one that ripples through the entire body in waves. If you're lying on your back, a whole body orgasm will cause the head and back to lift off the bed.

• **Darkness** and **silence** help the neocortex relax and allow orgasm.[21] So do happy thoughts ("I can fly!"). It also helps to tense the belly and straighten the legs until they quiver.

> "Women can have intercourse with fire, or the steaming water of a cauldron, or with the wind."[22]

Step 3. *Nourish and Tonify*

★ **Orgasms make you healthy**. They reduce stress, improve cardiovascular fitness, encourage deep breathing, fight aging, and lighten mood.[23]

What are you waiting for? Put this book down and have an orgasm right now!

Help!
Orgasm How-To

Expect results in 3–5 weeks

• Drink 3 quarts of **oatstraw** infusion a week.

• Buy a **vibrator**.

• Commit to **7 orgasms a week**, whether you are interested or not.

• Devote 15 minutes a day to doing something that **turns you on**.

★ A satisfying sexual life needs a well-nourished fantasy life. Women who are disturbed by (normal) fantasies of being overwhelmed sexually, shut off those "terrible thoughts." Then they wonder why it's so hard to get aroused and come to orgasm. Fantasy is not reality.

• Libido is missing-in-action? Lure an orgasmic mood:
~ Move your lower body – walk, dance, bike, do tai chi.
~ Take a hot bath or shower; scrub your skin all over.
~ Watch or read about loving sexual connections.
~ Explore your vulva, your clitoris, your labia.
For best results, repeat at least once a week.

★ Want stronger orgasms? **Exercise!** Twenty minutes of moderate exercise increases women's genital engorgement by 168 percent.[24] And the effect persists for hours.

• Clitoris too sensitive? You aren't alone. Do pelvic clenches (page 10) to strengthen the pelvic nerves and muscles so they aren't irritated by orgasmic increases in your root chakra energy.

• Troubled with chronic pelvic pain? Don't want sex because you hurt too much from fibroids or endometriosis? Feel too tight to have intercourse? Worried about a prolapse? Afraid you might pee on the bed when you come? Specialized physical therapists want to help. Find them at www.womenshealthapta.org.

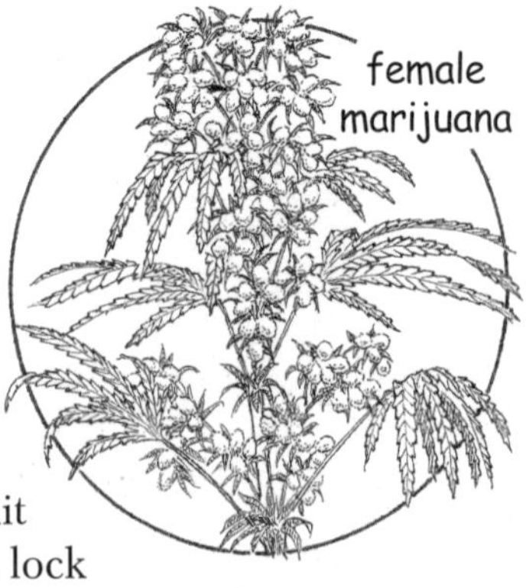

female marijuana

Step 4. *Stimulate/Sedate*

> "All the women in my immediate family learned how to climax by smoking grass — my mother when she was over 30 and the mother of four."[25]

★ A toke or two of quality **marijuana**, or **one ounce of vodka** with fruit or vegetable juice, can help you pick the lock on your "pleasure chest."

• **Women's aphrodisiac herbs** are basically the same as men's: damiana, fenugreek, ginkgo, ginseng, ginger, oatstraw, yohimbe, tribulus (*see* pages 297-99). A dropperful of **ginkgo** leaf tincture before sex relaxes blood vessels, increases blood flow, improves lubrication and engorgement, and heightens response. **Ginseng** lowers stress hormones to enhance libido. **Ashwagandha** tastes terrible and can trigger miscarriage, but its *withanolides* increase the activity of testosterone and lower anxiety. **Oatstraw** infusion increases testosterone, desire, lubrication, and enjoyment. **Tribulus** capsules give me an "itch" for orgasm.

★ Instruction in coital alignment technique (CAT) increases the number of women who have an orgasm during intercourse from 23 percent to 77 percent. Furthermore, 90 percent of all trainees (men and women) say CAT intensifies their orgasms and 60 percent say it increases their desire for more sex.[26]

Her Story

Suzanne is a retired professional.

"It was during a break in the action at a Sacred Sex weekend with Annie Sprinkle at the Wise Woman Center. The topic of female ejaculation came up. Over a third of the women said they regularly ejaculated! I vowed to learn how. It took a long time; I was really relearning how to masturbate. I enjoyed my quest, knowing I would eventually figure it out. I did. Eureka!!!"

Step 5a. *Use Supplements*

• **Vibrel** and **Zestra** (herbal oils, theobromine, and vitamins), applied topically, may increase desire and intensify arousal. The Zestra "rush" irritated my urethra and interfered with my orgasm.

• **L-arginine** relaxes smooth muscles, allowing more blood to get to the genitals. Viagra works on this principle. Creams containing L-arginine provide similar but weaker effects.

Step 5b. *Use Drugs*

★ All forms of **estrogen** increase lubrication and the intensity of orgasm. Vaginal estrogen is considered safer than other kinds.

• Drugs that counter pain, relieve allergies, ease anxiety and depression, lower blood pressure, or prevent pregnancy can depress your desire, your arousal, and even your ability to have an orgasm. NSAIDs (such as ibuprofen and naproxen) reduce lubrication, desire, and arousal. Half of those taking SSRI (selective serotonin reuptake inhibitor) antidepressants have loss of sexual interest and inhibited orgasm.[27] (Chart, page 300.)

• **Amanatadine**, a drug used against Parkinson's and respiratory infections, boosts the feel-good neurotransmitter dopamine, increasing sexual pleasure. Side effects, such as intestinal upsets and tissue swelling, are generally minor.

Vibrator Fun

Vibrators began life as a cure for "hysteria," or "moving womb," a disease prevalent among women with "pent-up sexual energy." By the late 1800s, it was estimated that three-quarters of American women were at risk.[28]

The cure? An orgasm – known by the prim medical term "paroxysm" – a prescription that dates back to medical texts from the first century C.E. (common era). Manual stimulation of the female patient to paroxysm was the cure, but it was so "time-consuming and tedious." Enter the vibrator! By the beginning of the twentieth century, health spas offering vibration therapy had sprung up like multiple orgasms.

Once "home-treatment" models were introduced, the vibrator became the fifth electric appliance – following the sewing machine, fan, teakettle, and toaster – to become a household necessity.

Hysteria was dropped from the American Psychiatric Association's list of recognized conditions in 1952.[29] But vibrators continue to be vital to women's sexual health.

Women who use vibrators experience more positive sexual function in terms of desire, arousal, lubrication, and orgasm.[30] Vibrator users are more likely to have had a gynecological exam in the previous year and to have looked closely at their genitals in the previous month, too.

In women who are quadriplegic, the earlobe can be trained to be a trigger for orgasm.

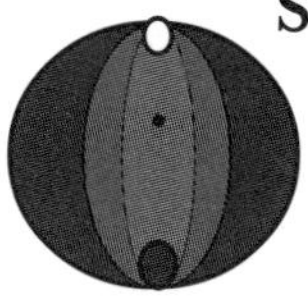

Sex After Menopause

Step 0. *Do Nothing*

> "Sex makes him feel manly and alive . . . [you can] make him feel desired in other ways besides intercourse."[31]

• The best sex for most women *during* menopause is none. Desire is down and penetration is painful. Don't force it. You *will* get interested and lubricated again when menopause is completed.

Step 1. *Collect Information*

> "[In midlife] you can have sex on your own terms . . . reinvent yourself sexually . . . explore the pleasure potential of your body."[32]

• By age 50, a woman makes only half as much testosterone – the hormone of desire – as she did in her twenties.[33] By age 65, she makes one-third as much.[34] No wonder we find ourselves forgetting about orgasms after menopause. Don't think; just do it!

Step 2. *Engage the Energy*

> "Women are turned on by most erotic acts they see. Explore!"[35]

• Imagination is an excellent way to entice desire and engage arousal. Imagining an orgasm activates the same pleasure centers as actually having one, and elicits the same physical reactions.[36]

Step 3. *Nourish and Tonify*

★ Delicious **oatstraw** infusion – 1 to 2 cups a day – frees up testosterone, increases desire, encourages lubrication, strengthens orgasm, and tonifies blood vessels and nerves. **Yoga** does too.[37]

Step 4. *Stimulate/Sedate*

• **Licorice root** suppresses testosterone – and thus libido!

• **Orgasm relieves migraines** for 50 percent of women.[38]

Step 5a. *Use Supplements*

• Dehydroepiandrosterone (DHEA), said to "enhance libido and stimulate desire," doesn't. A double-blind study of wo/men over age 60 found those taking it no randier than those taking a placebo.[39]

Step 5b. *Use Drugs*

> "The majority of herbal supplements and topical treatments lack scientific evidence supporting their effectiveness."[40]

• Drugs can ruin your sex life; see chart on page 300. Use herbs instead.

★ Hormones are often prescribed to improve arousal/desire.

~ Intrinsa, a testosterone patch, increases desire and activity, so long as you take estrogen, too.[41] After six months, there were one or two more satisfying sexual activities per month.[42,43] *Caution*: Testosterone negatively affects cholesterol; use often increases the amount of facial hair and may trigger acne.

~ LibiGel testosterone increases "sexually satisfying experiences."[44] *Caution*: The FDA requires a "black box" warning on testosterone gel; it can cause birth defects as well as numerous physical and mental problems in children exposed to it.[45]

~ Estrogen, or estrogen plus testosterone, or Viagra (sildenafil citrate) – individually, or combined with the antidepressant Wellbutrin (bupropion) – are used to strengthen desire and heighten response. *Caution*: Use of estrogen after menopause increases the risk of invasive breast cancer.[46] Limit use to six months.[47]

Her Story

Rebeka is a midwife.

"When I arrived at Bhagwan Sri Rajneesh's Osho commune, the therapist looked at me and said: 'YOU, you've got to move your sexual energy, and it starts today." After f___ing my brains out, I'm in a different space now, ten years after my last period. Sometimes sex with my partner flows; sometimes it doesn't and we don't judge. Sometimes we build energy, then stay still and almost fall asleep, but that *almost* is a twilight-meditation that is exquisite. I don't think I could have gone there if I hadn't explored as much as I did."

Her Story

Celeste is a well-educated, professional, postmenopausal woman.

"I remember my first orgasm. I was four years old. Filling the wading pool, I alternated putting the hose in the pool and down the front of my swimsuit. A photograph clearly shows the enjoyment on my face as the cold water streamed across my labia and clitoris.

"I grew older, and discovered the stream of water from the tub's faucet. It required some interesting contortions to get my clitoris in close enough proximity to the flow of water so the pressure was just right. Temperature fluctuations did cause me a few memorable moments! But it was an absolutely reliable way to have an orgasm.

"Several of my girl friends shared my physical curiosity. Exploring with them, I soon discovered, was unlikely to provoke punishment. At slumber parties and backyard camp-outs, we looked and touched and hugged and wiggled. I quickly learned that rubbing my clitoris on a warm thigh was, if not orgasmic, quite pleasurable. Rubbing my clitoris with my fingers was orgasmic, but only with patience and a lot of hard work.

"Then there were boys. Fumbling at the drive-in. My panties soaked and my clit poking out through the thin fabric with an intensity that thrilled me. My own sexuality was tightly focused on my clitoris. Their interest vacillated between parts further north and south.

"When I finally went 'all the way,' I was disappointed. Was there something wrong with me? With my 'down there'? Wasn't I supposed to have orgasms from intercourse? Maybe my clitoris was too big . . . or too small . . . or not in the right place. Maybe my vagina was too big . . . or not in the right place. Ah, the tortures of adolescence.

"I married; had a child. My clitoris remained my faithful friend; my husband didn't. Finally, in my thirties, I switched to loving women. Each new clitoris was a new territory to be investigated and cunningly coaxed into ecstasy. (My favorite band at the time was the *Cunning Stunts.*) Some women liked penetration; some didn't. Those that did, wanted the "back" of their clitoris massaged. We murdered Freud's myth of the vaginal orgasm, with great glee. We discovered female ejaculation and got the bed wet. We honored our clitorises by creating woman-centered erotica, in print and on screen.

"Menopause. The urge to reproduce completely gone. Penetration, ouch! Clitoris, as ever, ready to roll. Wet tongues. Vibrator. Lubricated fingers twirling on the spot. Seven orgasms a week keep 'down there' in good repair. I intend to do it no matter what my age.

"Now in my sixties, my partner (a man again) and I get into intercourse when we want that . . . slowly, lovingly, lustfully, sensitively.

"How will it be as I get older? My orgasmic capacity and my clit will be with me until I end, and I intend to end with joy!"

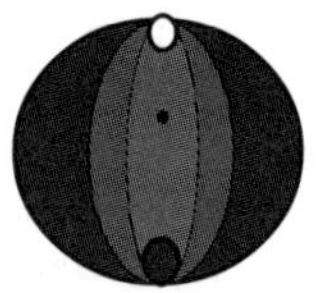

Clitorectomy

"Talk about it with angry, unbitten tongues. . . ."[48]

Step 0. *Do Nothing*

• Is it acceptable to do nothing about female genital mutilation? It occurs two thousand times a year, antiseptically, in American hospitals, and two million times a year, elsewhere, without anesthesia, with rusty razors and broken glass as surgical tools.

• Parenting a child with an enlarged clitoris? Do nothing!

Step 1. *Collect Information*

• A clitorectomy removes part or all of the visible clitoris: crown, shaft and hood. In northern Africa, it frequently includes removal of the inner labia and stitching the outer labia together.

• Throughout the nineteenth and well into the twentieth century, clitorectomy was the medical "solution" to the "problem" of female masturbation. The last recorded anti-masturbation clitorectomy in the USA was performed on a five-year-old girl in 1948.[49]

• Clitorectomies are still performed in the USA, to "reconfigure a clitoris deemed abnormally prominent (clitorimegaly)."[50]

• Pubescent girls are cut to "tame" them, keep them "innocent," and "accentuate their femaleness" (smoothness).[51,52] Over 100 million women living today in 28 countries have been cut.[53] Euphemistically called "circumcision," an equivalent cut on a boy would remove the penis entirely. In some places the "prevalence rate [of cut women] approaches 100 percent."[54]

Step 2. *Engage the Energy*

• Writer Nancy Friday suggests that modern girls are "subjected to a mental clitorectomy."[55] Little is said to pubescent girls about their clitoris. In fact, there is a medical silence surrounding the clitoris, with only two (very old) academic volumes about it.

• There are thirty times more Medline references to penis than to clitoris.[56]

Step 3. *Nourish and Tonify*

• No herbs will regrow a clitoris that has been cut off. We must take action, like Waris Dirie, the UN spokewoman for the elimination of FGM, is doing. Together we *are* working to an end of this mutilation, just as foot-binding and rib-removal were ended.[57]

Step 5. *Use Drugs*

• Women who take (or produce a lot of) progesterone during pregnancy have daughters with larger than normal clitorises.[58]

Her Story[59]

Martha is the mother of two.

"My mother took progesterone to prevent miscarrying me. I was born with a clitoris three times normal size. It wasn't a problem until my parents decided it *would* be a problem, sometime in the future.

"I was six years old when they snipped it off at the base. You can clearly see something is missing if you look at me. I am scarred emotionally, too, but not bitter. The reason is simple. I still have clitoral sensation. I'm orgasmic."

Her Story[60]

Cheryl is a computer analyst in her early forties; she is a lesbian.

"I would have preferred to grow up in a place with no medicine rather than to have had the "advantage" of surgery to "fix" me.

"I am a woman and have a double X chromosome in every cell. But I was born with a clitoris so big (and gonads) that the doctors told my parents I was a boy. A year later they realized I had a uterus, ovaries, and vagina. Oops. 'It's a girl,' they said.

"With my parents' permission, they 'reduced' the size of my clitoris by removing it at the division of the crura, where the nerves enter the clitoral shaft. I have never had an orgasm; and no doctor will even attempt to help me have one."

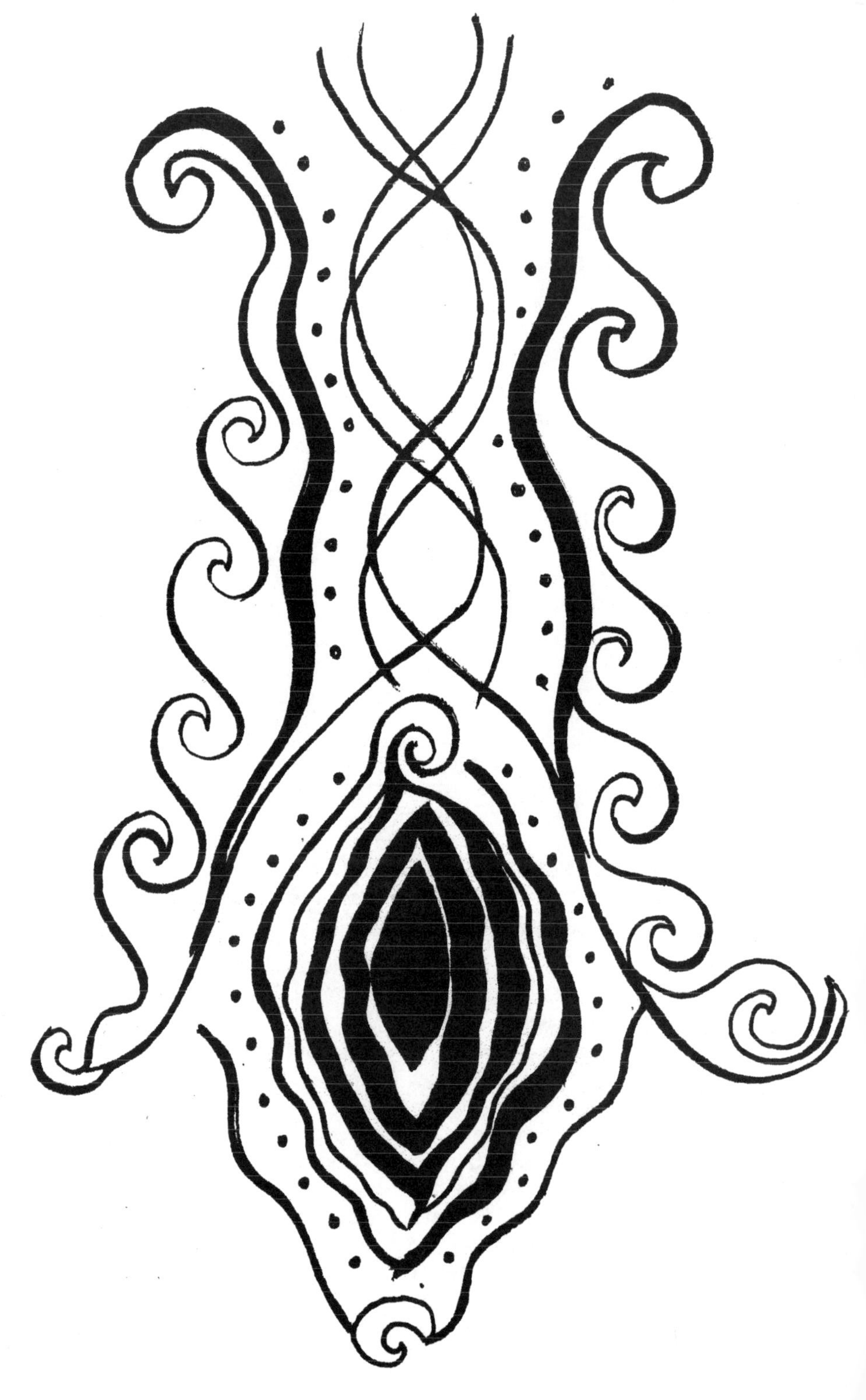

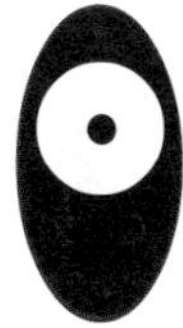

The Vagina

I am the sheath of the sword. I am toothed, armed, and ready to bite. I have the power to defend, to keep women safe. I am not passive, accepting, ready to be filled. I am aware, watchful, ready to seize what I will, what I want, and reject what I don't want.

Listen to me and I will tell you how safe we feel, you and I, right now, at this moment. When secure, I am open and receptive, moist and inviting. When threatened, I become cold and hard, hot and tight, irritated, and inflamed. If the danger is chronic, I weep, I am overrun.

In health and joy, I am a rich and thriving ecosystem: friendly yeasts, beneficial bacteria, and a generous assortment of slippery, slidey lubricants thrive in my tangy-tasting depths.

I am stretchy. I am expansive. Fill me and I yearn for more. I yield, I melt, I surrender. Yet in yielding, I deliver. I am the victor. I clench my fist and grab the prize. Mine.

Do you think that I drool? I do. Do you think that I dribble, leak, and flood? I do. I am messy. I push the boundaries. I am greedy. I am slick. I am sleek.

I lie between what is shown and what is hidden. I am both public and private. I am not visible, yet I am the identity of a woman. By my name is woman named. By my power is woman empowered. From my lips you hear only the truth. I am your vagina.

Healthy Vagina

> "Live like you have diamonds between your legs! . . . love your vagina deeply and with reverence. It is the doorway to heaven. It is the place where souls come from heaven to earth. Whether you choose to give birth to a soul or an idea, rejoice in the sacred essence of being a woman."[1]

The vagina is a muscular, mucus-lined passage that connects a woman's outer genitals with her uterus. The vagina is protected by its lips, the labia, and by its acidic mucus. It extends from the clitoris (in front) to the anus (behind). The bladder is above it, by the pubic bone. The vagina ends in a cul-de-sac at the cervix.

During sexual arousal, the vagina lengthens, opens, and – in some women – raises a sensitive inner clitoral bump often called the G-spot. When we speak of penetrative sex, it is the vagina that is penetrated; the vagina envelops the penis.

For thousands of years, men have acted as though vaginas were inert, hollow receptacles which could be filled at their will. Tens of thousands of years ago, when women told the stories, the vagina was honored, not thought shameful. (A universe of thanks to Eve Ensler and her *The Vagina Monologues*[2] for making it acceptable to say the word "vagina" out loud once again.)

The vagina is alive and sensitive, responsive and wonderfully capable of letting its wishes and desires be known. *The vagina, and its health or lack thereof, is deeply connected to a woman's sense of safety.*

Some women view their vaginas as dirty and smelly, in need of washing and deodorizing. A healthy vagina has a pleasant odor, a slightly sour taste, and is naturally "self-cleaning." A healthy vagina constantly secretes clear or milky fluids to protect its delicate tissues. These fluids are heavier and more slippery during ovulation. They change radically during sexual arousal.

A healthy vagina contains many microorganisms, some beneficial, some not. The healthy ones thrive in acidic conditions. They eat glucose from blood serum and metabolize it into lactic acid. This keeps the vagina acidic, which encourages acid-loving flora, which create more acids. This process keeps the alkaline (disease-causing) organisms from growing.

Vaginal tissues respond strongly to hormones. Progesterone gives it great elasticity. Estrogen helps it stay moist and pliable.

Vaginal Distresses

There are thirty or more bacteria, fungi, and parasites that can cause **vaginal infections** (page 144). Some live naturally in the vagina, others are introduced through intimate contact (STDs/STIs, page 143), and some are transmitted without sexual contact (HPV, page 176).

Most vaginal infections cause **discharges** (page 127), **itching**, or **burning** (page 134). Like when your nose runs during a cold and leaves the area under it raw and red, the increased volume and severe alkalinity of the fluids produced by a vaginal infection can inflame the vagina, labia, even the thighs. Other infections, like **chlamydia** (page 156), may be virtually symptomless. Untreated vaginal infections can become **pelvic inflammatory disease**/PID (page 245), a threat to fertility and your life.

A variety of reasons, including stress hormones and menopause, can cause **painful**, **dry vagina** (page 131).

If the vaginal tissues become alkaline, if they receive too much sugar, or if there are too few beneficial flora, then innate microorganisms such as **candida/yeast** (page 146) and **gardnerella** (page 154) can overgrow. Having an innate infection makes it much easier to "catch" other sexually transmitted diseases/infections (STDs, STIs) – including **gonorrhea** (page 164), **syphilis** (page 166), **trich** (page 150), and **herpes** (page 160).

If you have a vaginal infection, it is likely you have multiple concurrent infections. In one European study, 30 percent of the women diagnosed with trichomoniasis also had gonorrhea.[3]

Celibacy, lesbianism, and mutual monogamy reduce the number of infectious organisms introduced into the vagina. But nuns, lesbians, and monogamous women can still get vaginal infections or **non-specific vaginitis** (page 136), **vaginal ulcers** (page 140), or **Bartholin's gland cysts** (page 138).

Women who had an episiotomy – a cut made in the perineum during childbirth – may have painful vaginal and perineal **strictures**, which can be eased with comfrey sitz baths or applications of aloe vera or vitamin E oil. Less common, but more dangerous, is **vaginal cancer** (page 141), which is of special concern to DES daughters (page 202).

★ Vaginal problems/infections can be caused by fear. ★

A woman who feels insecure in her life or uneasy in her home produces stress hormones. This leads to vaginal infection in two ways. One, it changes the pH of her vagina, killing beneficial acid-loving organisms while allowing problematic alkaline-loving ones to grow freely. Two, it thins the mucus coating which protects the vagina from infection, literally eroding the vagina's safety net.

When a woman is frightened, her vaginal muscles tighten. Forced penetration tears the tight tissues. Stress or trauma, but especially the combination, allows all manner of unwelcome guests to thrive in the vagina.

Her Story

Shelia was 33 years old and nursing a child when I met her.

"My first child was born dead. There was no reason. I was devastated, but I got pregnant again the very next month.

"After the birth of my second child my vagina remained inflamed and painful. All tests for infection were negative. My doctor told me the pain was all in my mind and prescribed steroids, which I refused to take.

[I gently asked Shelia about her feelings of abandonment, of betrayal, of deprivation. I asked her if she was angry at her baby for being born dead.]

"I was horrified when Susun asked me if I was angry. How could I possibly ever be angry at my innocent baby? I felt so guilty; I had failed her. I couldn't even imagine being angry. I burst into tears at her words and could hardly answer her."

[While I believed her denial of anger, I believed her vagina more. She herself described it as "angry." I urged her to get in touch with her anger. Meanwhile, applications of yogurt and slippery elm mixed with honey could ease her vaginal pain.]

"I went back to see Susun over and over, hoping for some other answer. She insisted that I deal with my anger at the death. I could hardly believe it was possible at first, but the deeper into my heart I looked, the more it seemed to be true. How could I be so awful, so uncaring? Gradually I began to understand that my anger is part of my caring. Finally, after fourteen months, I accepted my anger. Susun listened, encouraged me, sat with me as I raged and cried. Like a miracle, the pain in my vagina disappeared. Oh my gosh!

"p.s. I'm feeling sexy again, too. Smile!"

Guided Meditation for A Secure Vagina 

♥ This meditation is designed to improve the health of the vagina, to thicken the protective mucus lining, and to restore ease to vaginal muscles. It is both preventative and curative medicine.

♥ *Women who have a history of sexual abuse may wish to do this meditation in stages on a daily basis; build gradually and continue until it is real in your mind and body, psyche and spirit. Women who have chronic vaginal infections will find it useful to do this meditation every time they menstruate. Other women may use it as the occasion arises.*

♥ *Preparation:* Find a safe place, outside or inside, to be alone for thirty minutes. You will need a blanket that completely covers you. If you wish, you can write the statements "*I will protect you. I am holding you.*" on a card or piece of paper for reference.

♥ *Guided Meditation*: Sit comfortably. Sigh audibly as you breathe out and lower your head toward your chest. Slowly raise your head as you inhale. Continue for about a minute. Then imagine your vagina is breathing in and out. Continue to sigh. Allow emotions – sorrow, rage, confusion, joy – to arise.

Be present with your feelings. Wrap your blanket around youself as tight as you can and still feel comfortable. Continue to breathe. Say out loud: "I will protect you. I am holding you." Say it again and again. Let tears come if they will. Let anger come. Let ecstasy come. Be compassionate with your confusion and fear.

Pay attention to any physical reactions that accompany your feelings. Pay no attention to words and stories that arise. Let go of blame; let go of shame.

When you feel ready, move one or both hands between your legs. Hold your vaginal area (*yoni*) firmly but gently. Repeat, out loud: "I will protect you. I am holding you." Say it again and again, observing and feeling any emotions, without blame, without shame, without guilt. Hold yourself tenderly. Be the protector you long for. Breathe.

♥ *End*: Slowly, mindfully, unwrap yourself. Breathe in. Sigh out loud ten times. Let it be wordless; no need to write it down or speak about it. Stay with your feelings; let go of the reasons.

♥

 Alkalinizers 

These make the vagina more susceptible to infections

- Male ejaculate, including sperm and seminal fluid
- Birth control pills
- Menopausal and postmenopausal hormone therapy
- Diabetes, high blood sugar
- Antibiotics
- Unusual stress, even positive stress; anxiety, fear
- Bubblebath
- Washing your vagina with soap
- Anything that allows feces into the vagina
- Douching regularly
- Feminine hygiene spray
- Artificial sweeteners, diet soda
- Raw fruit, fruit juice
- Saliva and other sexual lubricants
- The hormonal changes that precede menstruation
- The menstrual fluids themselves
- Pregnancy
- Lochia (the flow that follows childbirth)

 Acidity Restorers 

These make the vagina resistant to infections

- Yogurt orally and vaginally
- Acidophilus inserted in the vagina
- Ascorbic acid inserted in the vagina
- Salt water sitz bath
- Sitz bath, finger bath, or douche with:
  - ~ handful of salt in a quart/liter of warm water, *or*
  - ~ 2 tablespoons/30ml of vinegar in one qt/ltr of water, *or*
  - ~ 1 cup hydrogen peroxide in 3 cups/750ml water, *or*
  - ~ oak bark or any astringent herb (page 130), *or*
  - ~ 2 tablespoons/30ml of Betadine iodine in 1 qt/ltr water.

    Note: Betadine dries out vaginal tissues.

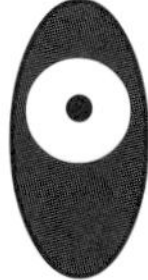

Vaginal Distresses

"Don't try to sit on your distress, dearest daughter," cautions Grandmother Growth. "It will prove to be a hot, itchy, prickly, miserable seat, I can promise you.

"Your vagina knows the truth. You may try to deny what upsets you, you may sugarcoat your rage and drug your anxieties away, but your vagina will tell you the truth. You can use your sexuality to please others and be sensitive to the needs and feelings of everyone else, but your vagina won't let you ignore your own needs forever. It will get irritated and sore.

"If you fear for your own existence and for those you care for, if you are filled with tension and stress, your vagina will be distressed too.

"And it will distress you. Your vagina will speak with discharges and smells, pain and burning, dryness and inflammation. Be gentle with yourself, my darling. Be gentle with your vagina. Your vagina is not your enemy. It is your friend. It is your guardian. It speaks to you with pleasure. It speaks to you through pain. If it is hurting, it is reminding you to honor your womanhood, to honor your body. Your vagina is the passageway to your sacred inner mystery. Ancient wisdom has spiraled through the ages to coil in your vagina, to empower you.

"Sit down and eat a bowl of yogurt. Trust your vagina. Listen to it."

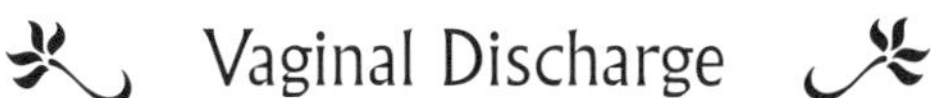

Vaginal Discharge

Step 0. *Do Nothing*

• **Vaginal discharge is normal**. The amount and texture of discharge varies from one vagina to the next, and changes throughout one's life. Most days vaginal discharge is white or clear; around ovulation it becomes cream-colored. Discharges contain healthy mucus produced by the cervix, dead cells from the vaginal walls, and secretions from the vagina. As ovulation approaches, the vaginal fluids change, becoming more obvious and more copious, either thinner or thicker in texture, slipperier, stretchier, and wetter. As menstruation nears, and after menopause, vaginal fluids diminish, becoming drier, tackier, and darker/lighter in color.

Step 1. *Collect Information*

• When the discharge is thick, curdy, foul smelling, and strangely colored, the vagina and/or the cervix are warding off an overgrowth of: chlamydia (page 156), gardnerella (page 154), gonorrhea (page 164), herpes (page 160), trichomoniasis (page 150), and/or yeast (page 146). Pelvic inflammatory disease (page 245) or cervicitis (page 174) could also be to blame.

Step 2. *Engage the Energy*

• **Homeopathic remedies** are not first aid for vaginal infections. Instead, they heal the underlying causes, thus lessening the chance of recurrences. For best results, use herbs or drugs as needed to counter infection plus a homeopathic remedy.

~ *Alumina*: discharge itchy, burning, chronic, thick; worse in latter half of the menstrual cycle.
~ *Borax*: discharge thick, white, irritating.
~ *Conium*: discharge burns, itchy; emotional bruising, numbness.
~ *Graphites*: discharge itchy, burning.
~ *Kreosotum*: discharge itchy, burning, yellowish, smelly, irritating, stinging; weak overall.
~ *Mercurius solubilis*: discharge offensive greenish-yellow, itchy, thick, with fever or chills; follows antibiotic use.
~ *Nitric acid*: discharge thick, cloudy, itchy; vulva burned and fissured; comes after antibiotic use.
~ *Pulsatilla*: discharge acute, burning, hurts thighs; worsened by menstruation, pregnancy; comes after antibiotic use.
~ *Sepia*: discharge acute burning, itchy, smelly, yellowish; low pelvic pain, exhaustion. (If you have these symptoms, see page 245.) Can't express feelings, pregnant.
~ *Sulphur*: chronic, bad-smelling, burning, yellow discharge; worse in morning or with intercourse.

Her Story

Kanji is a young black woman who lives in the inner city.

"To know our own tastes and smells and fluids is powerful. The book that really helped me tell the difference between 'normal' and 'abnormal' vaginal discharges and odors was *Taking Charge of Your Fertility*.[4] I looked. I sniffed. I even tasted. I gained intimate familiarity with my vaginal fluids and how they changed with my cycles. I even learned something new: to touch my cervix and experience its changes.[5]

"I used to think any vaginal discharge was wrong, any change was bad, and any vaginal fluid that wasn't clear meant infection. I confused tacky cervical fluid with the "curds" of a yeast overgrowth. Now I know better.

"I wish we all had a more intimate relationship with this part of our own bodies and each other's too."

Step 3. *Nourish and Tonify*

• Reduce uncomfortable vaginal discharges by using condoms consistently (but see below), or by chosing celibacy, monogamy (with a monogamous mate), or lesbianism.

★ Since irritating vaginal discharges are caused by inherent, as well as sexually-transmitted organisms, it is important to have a well-nourished immune system (page 162) and an acidic vagina (page 126) for optimum health.

• Condoms, especially those with lubrication or spermicide, can upset the vagina's pH. Inherent organisms then overgrow and make itchy discharges.

★ Soap is alkaline. Wash your vagina with plain water.

• The **camel pose** opens the pelvis, increases circulation to the vagina, and normalizes pH. Kneel on a mat, flex your feet, lean back, and reach for your heels. Hold for three breaths. Fold forward and breathe. Repeat.

Help!
Vaginal Discharge

Expect results within 1–2 weeks

• Get tested for infections/overgrowths.

• Do an **oak bark sitz bath** daily, for at least ten minutes.

• Take a dropperful of **yarrow tincture** three times a day.

• No intercourse for two weeks.

Step 4. *Stimulate/Sedate*

★ Western herbalists call an unwanted vaginal discharge *leucorrhea* ("the whites"). Eastern herbalists call it a "damp disorder." Both agree that **astringent herbs** used in sitz baths (page 368) dry up discharges and restore the vagina to a healthy state. If there is still a discharge after ten days of sitz baths, consider oral use of an anti-infective herb (page 165) and getting tested for infectious organsims. Astringent herbs include:

~ **American cranesbill** (*Geranium maculatum*) root is especially effective against bloody discharges.

~ **Avens** (*Geum urbanum*) roots and leaves counter inflammation.

~ **Bistort** (*Polygonum bistorta*) herb shrinks hemorrhoids, too.

~ **Comfrey** (*Symphytum uplandica x*) root/ leaf, strengthens, soothes, and heals everything down there.

~ **Meadowsweet** (*Filipendula ulmaria*) leaf/flower is a powerful agent of change for achy, sore, weepy vaginas. Relieves pain fast, really, really fast.

~ **Witch hazel** (*Hamamelis virginiana*) bark or leaf eases pain and eliminates itchy discharges.

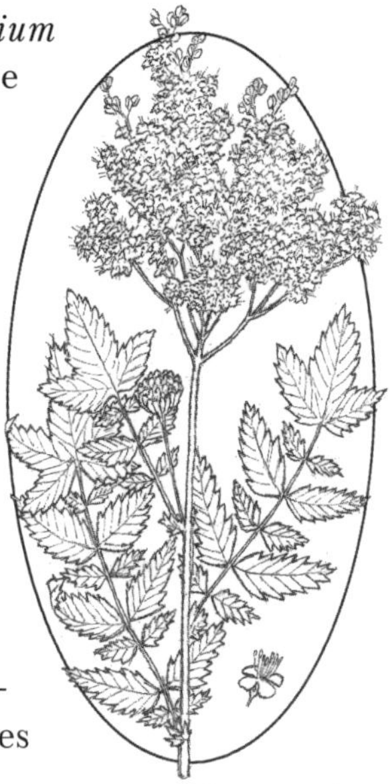

~ **White pond lily** (*Nymphaea odorata*) root counters swelling and reduces profuse discharges.

meadowsweet

★ **Oak bark** is an astringent herb with antibacterial and antiviral properties. This makes it especially helpful for women plagued by chronic infections/discharges. Oak bark sitz baths of at least 10–15 minutes duration will kill infections, re-acidify the vagina, normalize discharges, and help heal inflamed/irritated tissues.

Step 5. *Use Drugs*

• Antibiotics, antibacterial soaps, and essential oils can kill protective vaginal microorganisms. Taking antibiotics doubles the risk of developing a vaginal infection.[6]

Vaginal Dryness, Vaginal Pain

Step 1. *Collect Information*

• Vaginal dryness can be mild or so painful it interferes with daily life. It can be caused by birth control pills, breast-feeding, aging, and/or lack of mucus-producing cells. It may occur at all times, or only when attempting intercourse. It is normal for the vagina to be drier when conception is unlikely, such as after menopause or during the first months of breast-feeding. About half of postmenopausal women are quite bothered by vaginal dryness.[7]

• About two-thirds of American women experience pain before, during, or after vaginal penetration at some point in their lives.[8] This pain is called "dyspareunia."

• If you are experiencing general pain "down there," it may be vulvodynia (page 93), or chronic pelvic pain (page 15).

• Doctors describe postmenopausal vaginal dryness as *atrophic vaginitis* or *lichen sclerosus et atrophicus.* These terms – and others, like *crone crotch* – insult women; I do not use them.

• The non-drug remedies suggested in this section are safe for women who are breast-feeding or pregnant.

Step 2. *Engage the Energy*

★ Safe vaginas are wet; frightened ones are dry. The meditation on page 125 helps your vagina feel safe, and moist. Connect your heart and womb. Call forth your guardians! Claim your space!

• Menopausal and postmenopausal women find intercourse less painful if they have an orgasm first.

Help! Vaginal Dryness

Expect results in 3–10 days

• Apply **chickweed oil** to the labia and vagina, as far in as you can comfortably reach, 1–2 times a day.

• Eat at least 1/2 cup of **yogurt** a day.

• Eat more **phytoestrogenic** foods, like lentils, red clover infusion, whole grains, and cooked root vegetables.

• Give yourself **7 orgasms** a week.

- **Homeopathic remedies** for women with dry vaginas include:
  - ~ *Lycopodium*: desires sex but coition increases distress.
  - ~ *Nat.-mur.*: adverse to coition; vagina painful, very dry.
  - ~ *Sepia*: adverse to coition, chilly overall; vagina painful.

Step 3. *Nourish and Tonify*

★ Keep your vagina moist (and sexy) by eating half a cup of **plain yogurt** a day (a quart a week).

★ Inserting an acidophilus capsule (or two) will make your vagina drool. Be forewarned: wear protection or do it at night.

★ **Pelvic floor exercises** (page 10) increase blood flow to, help restore the elasticity of, increase tissue thickness in, and bring moisture to the vagina, especially for postmenopausal women.

★ **Phytoestrogens** help prevent and treat vaginal dryness without increasing cancer risk. All roots and seeds, nuts, beans, and whole grains are good sources. Freshly-ground flax seeds are a source of phytoestrogens; flax oil isn't.

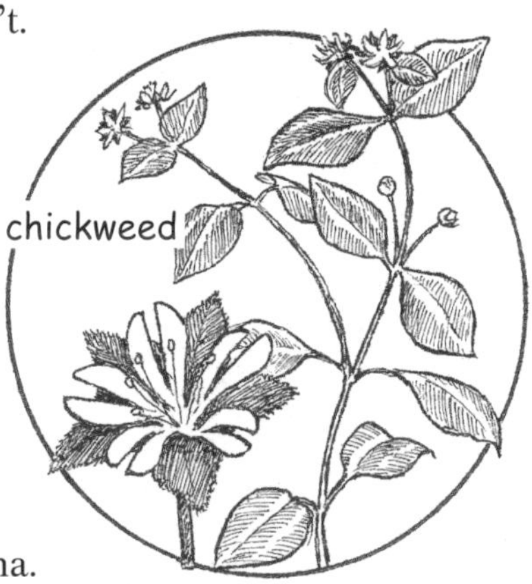

★ **Chickweed oil** used directly on dry vaginal tissues is highly effective for restoring lubrication and flexibility due to its lavish supply of slippery saponins. It heals, soothes, and stops itching. (Make it: page 367, or buy it already made.)

• **Mallow** root sitz baths lubricate, ease pain, plump up tissues, and restore healthy circulation to the vagina. (Make it: page 368.)

★ **Oatstraw** (or hay) baths are a classic curative used in the Alpine regions/Switzerland. They relax and soften vaginal tissues and restore health to the nerves. Make a gallon of oatstraw infusion, strain the liquid, heat, and add to a hot bath. Save some to drink. One woman swears that drinking oatstraw infusion for two weeks turned her desert "down there" into a flowing oasis!

Step 4. *Stimulate/Sedate*

★ **Red clover infusion** and phytoestrogenic foods can help reverse vaginal dryness. So can 2–4 dropperfuls of **chasteberry tincture** taken daily for 2–3 months.

> "Sexual activity helps maintain a healthy vaginal epithelium (the cells lining the vaginal walls), increases vaginal elasticity, and improves lubrication. . . . It also helps keep the vagina more acidic, providing some protection against infection."[9]

• A small piece of solid **coconut oil** or **shea butter**, inserted vaginally, will melt and coat, heal and moisten; it's antifungal, too.

• Drugstore sell **glycerin**, which plumps up tissues, and **ascorbic acid powder**, which acidifies and prevents infections.[10] Mix them together and apply, or buy it ready-made as KY Liquid.

Step 5. *Use Drugs*

★ **Replens** contains pilocarpine, which continuously moisturizes for 48–72 hours and restores vaginal pH, helping prevent yeast. Use is limited to no more than three times a week. Alternate with healing herbal oils like chickweed or calendula.

★ If your vagina is so dry it hurts to walk, sit, or lie down, and the remedies you've tried haven't worked, and you *are not pregnant*, vaginal **estrogen** (cream or insertable tablets) will help. Use for up to a year appears safe.[11] Use the smallest amount that works for you; try one-eighth of an applicator.[12] Are so-called bio-identical hormones such as Tri-Est cream safer? I don't think so, the FDA doesn't think so, feminist health advocacy groups don't think so.

• Five drops of **chamomile** or **yarrow** essential oil mixed into two ounces of olive oil and applied to the vulva and vagina bring fast relief. Essential oils can disrupt vaginal flora, and can irritate some women, so go slowly. Limit use to no more than ten days.

Step 6. *Break and Enter*

• Avoid super-absorbent tampons. They dry out vaginal tissues and cause small injuries that can attract bacterial and viral infections.

Vaginal Itching/Burning

Step 0. *Do Nothing*

• No douching. No soap; no bubble bath. No shaving; no waxing. No spermicides. No tampons; no condoms. No underwear, tights or pantyhose, or cut the crotches out. No intercourse.

Step 1. *Collect Information*

• Itching and burning may be caused by surgery, drugs, radiation, sexual assault, yeast (page 146), trich (page 150), herpes (160), and HPV (page 176). Itching is also common when vaginal tissues are very dry (page 131).

Step 2. *Engage the Energy*

• **Homeopathic remedies** for women with itchy, burning vaginas: *Alumina, Arsenicum album, Caladium, Calcarea carbonica, Kreosotum, Mercury solubilis, Nitric acid, Pulsatilla, Sulphur, Sepia.*

Step 3. *Nourish and Tonify*

★ If you already eat a quart of **yogurt** a week, continue. If not, go right out and buy plain yogurt. Eat some. Then put some "down there" for instant relief. Be sure to get some *in* there, too. Ahhhh!

• **Aloe vera gel** is a soothing remedy for burning vaginal tissues. Fresh aloe vera gel is superior to the bottled version which is preserved with an acid that can sting.

★ **Mallows** are your ally if your vaginal itch is traumatic. Gelatinous substances in their roots and leaves quell itching. Mallow sitz baths are deeply healing and restorative.[13] (Make it: page 368.)

Help!
Vaginal Itching

Expect results immediately

• Apply **plantain oil** or **plain yogurt** to the labia and vagina hourly.

• Eat at least ½ cup **yogurt** a day.

• Avoid all spicy, peppery foods.

• Visualize **cool water** flowing over and through your labia.

Step 4. *Stimulate/Sedate*

★ **Witch hazel** extract, available at drugstores, stops itching fast. Refrigerate, then pour some on a cloth and apply.

★ **Chamomile oil/ointment** soothes and heals as rapidly and as well as drugs. Make it: page 367.

★ **Plantain** is the anti-itch champion. For fast relief, try leaf oil/ointment. For deeper healing, soak a spoonful of fresh or dried seeds (of big-leaf plantain) in cold water overnight. It makes a slippery gel that relieves itching anywhere, even inside the vagina. The gel is also antifungal, so it's especially helpful in relieving itchiness from yeast overgrowth.

plantain (inset: seeds)

• Made crazy by a chronic vaginal itch, one woman applied Noxzema ointment lavishly to her labia. I winced, but she swore it was the only thing that worked.

Step 5. *Use Drugs*

• If you're in anguishing pain, and herbs haven't helped, you may wish to try:

~ Non-steriodal anti-inflammatory pain killers (NSAIDs)
~ Oral or injected cortisone
~ Estrogen cream (page 133)

Don't Douche!

Douching makes the vagina "dirty," not clean. *Don't douche!* It pushes harmful bacteria up into the uterus, increasing your chances of getting a vaginal infection.[14] *Don't douche!* Women who douche are four times more likely to get pelvic inflammatory disease.[15] *Don't douche!* Three-quarters of women of color douche.[16] Tell your sisters: *Don't douche!* Lower income women douche the most.

Be wise! Don't douche!
Instead, practice your Kegels in the bathtub.

Non-specific Vaginitis

Step 0. *Do Nothing*

★ Do not share hot tubs, towels, or underwear if your vagina is itchy or inflamed.

Step 1. *Collect Information*

• Non-specific vaginitis is a catch-all term used when no one organism explains the vagina's inflamed, irritated state. There is often an overgrowth of several infections in sub-clinical amounts.

• Is it vaginitis or bacterial vaginosis (page 154)? Or perhaps it's pelvic inflammatory disease (page 245)?

Step 2. *Engage the Energy*

• **Homeopathic remedies** for non-specific vaginitis:
 ~ *Caladium*: vulva itchy, dry; sex, pregnancy worsens.
 ~ *Kreosotum*: discharge very itchy, yellow, stinky; vulva raw; menses, pregnancy worsen.
 ~ *Pulsatilla*: discharge greenish-yellow, bland, thick or thin, burning; moodiness, weeping.
 ~ *Sepia*: vagina raw, burning, itchy; discharge white, yellow, bloody, lumpy, slimy, worse by day, fine at night.

• Women with chronic vaginal infections form a "sisterhood of women who battle the inevitable return of their infections. This war bonds us together; but . . . in a destructive, rather than constructive way, as our community exists only so long as we have a problem. There is a lot of unexpressed anger among us."[17]

These Kill Infectious Micro-organisms on Contact

❖ **Garlic** suppository
❖ **Myrrh** finger bath or sitz bath with tincture or tea
❖ **Yarrow** finger bath or sitz bath with tincture or infusion
❖ **Berberine-rich** plants, orally and topically (page 137)

Step 3. *Nourish and Tonify*

★ Feminist health clinics find women clear non-specific and chronic vaginitis more quickly when they combine **pelvic floor exercises** (page 10) with their other treatments.

Step 4. *Stimulate/Sedate*

★ **Berberine-rich herbs** include barberry, Oregon grape, goldthread, and goldenseal. Use them as tinctures, sitz baths, or teas.

★ Old wives, their daughters, and their granddaughters cherish this remedy. Combine one quart of **oak bark** infusion and one quart of berberine-rich herbal infusion and sit(z) in it. It does it all: acidifies the vagina, kills a wide variety of unwanted infectious organisms, tones tissues, eases pain, counters inflammation, and makes your "down there" smile.

• **Acupuncture** based on a Five-Element diagnosis has proven helpful for some women with chronic non-specific vaginitis.

Step 5. *Use Drugs*

• Vaginitis can be caused by a contraceptive sponge or a pessary left in the vagina more than 24 hours.

★ The Wild Rose Clinic in Geneva cultures the vaginal discharges of women with non-specific vaginitis, then tests different **essential oils** against the cultures. "Different oils, even different batches of the same oil, have different abilities against different organisms."[18]

Essential oils are strong medicines; they can damage tender vaginal tissues and disrupt flora. Be cautious!

Help!
Non-specific Vaginitis

Expect results in a month

• Sitz in **oakbark** infusion twice a day for at least ten days.

• Eat at least ½ cup **yogurt** a day.

• Take 10–20 drops of a **berberine-rich herb** twice a day for 30 days.

• Wear loose **organic cotton** or **silk** underwear; better yet, wear none.

• **Love your vagina**. No douching, no washing. **Exercise it.**

Bartholin's Gland/Vestibular Cysts 

Step 0. *Do Nothing*

• Cysts or infections in the vestibular glands rarely spread or cause any damage, so it is not necessary to treat them.[19]

Step 1. *Collect Information*

• Two glands – called the vulvovaginal, vestibular, or Bartholin's glands – lie at the entrance to the vagina, one on each side. Once thought to produce lubrication, these small glands, like the vermiform appendix, currently have no known function.

• Nonetheless, cysts and abscesses can occur in them, swelling them from their usual soft lima bean size to the bulk and rigidity of a walnut. That can make your vagina very uncomfortable.

Step 2. *Engage the Energy*

• **Homeopathic remedies** for women with vestibular gland cysts include *Aconitum, Rhus toxicodendron, Serenoa serrulata, Baryta carb., Lycopodium,* and *Pulsatilla.*

• How is this cyst your ally of health? Is there something entering or trying to enter your vagina that you need protection against?

Step 3. *Nourish and Tonify*

• Nourishing herbal infusion of **oatstraw** or **red clover** help normalize hormones, and calm vestibular gland distress. (Make it: page 367.)

Step 4. *Stimulate/Sedate*

• Dissolve vaginal cysts with **hot sitz baths**/compresses of **comfrey** leaf, self-heal herb, slippery elm, oak bark, or **green clay**.

Help! Vestibular Cysts

Expect results in a week

• Apply a **hot towel**, hot herbal **compress**, or **softening oil** to the cyst twice a day.

• Take one drop of **poke root tincture** daily for 7–10 days.

• Do the **Guided Meditation for A Secure Vagina.**

★ A **comfrey leaf compress**, applied directly, eases swelling, relieves pain, softens skin and dissolves cysts. Its astringent constituents tone and strengthen vaginal tissues, too. Compressing often produces better results than a few lengthy applications.

To make: Boil fresh comfrey leaves in water to cover until soft (15–45 minutes), fold them into a cotton or linen towel, and apply to the cyst. If you don't have fresh comfrey, pour a quart/liter of boiling water over an ounce/30mg of dried comfrey leaf. Infuse for four hours; strain. Drink the liquid; compress with the leaves.

• Shrink infected or abscessed vulvovaginal glands with frequent (8–12 times daily) large (2 or 3 dropperfuls) doses of **herbal anti-infectives** such as **echinacea** or **usnea** tincture. For greater effect, add one drop of **poke** root tincture, once a day.

• Twice daily application of a **softening herbal oil** can eliminate a vestibular cyst with little effort. My favorites include red clover oil, comfrey root oil, and plantain oil. (Make it: page 367.)

Step 5. *Use Drugs*

• **Oreganol**, the essential oil of oregano, can burn off cysts – and burn sensitive vaginal tissues. Ouch!

Step 6. *Break and Enter*

• An MD can lance your cyst. But why bother? A hot comfrey sitz bath or compress works as well, with much less risk of infection.

Her Story

Elise is a French-Canadian mother of two.

"For the first thirty-two years of my life, my vagina was simply a mechanical part of my body. I wanted it to be moist, sexy, orgasmic, open, inviting, clean, and good looking. Instead, it was lonely, sad, dry, dead, afraid, uninviting, and way too bushy!

When I became pregnant, my relationship with my vagina changed. I took time to listen to her. I discovered she can be feisty, quiet, sleepy, tender. She has been there all along, waiting for me.

My vagina is a powerful place! When I am tempted to ignore her, I remember she is my friend. I do the *Sheila Na Gig* meditation in the *Goddess Oracle*[20] to help me stay in touch with her."

Vaginal Ulcers

Step 1. *Collect Information*

• Vaginal ulcers – sores that won't heal – are rare. There may be slight persistent bleeding and pain, often on intercourse. A sensitive vagina may be ulcerated by tampons, diaphragms, or intercourse; infections can also break down and ulcerate tissues.

• If your mother, grandmother, or great-grandmother might have taken DES (page 202), that "ulcer" may be a cancer.[21]

Step 2. *Engage the Energy*

• Envision cool blue or green light healing your ulcer.

• **Homeopathic remedies** for women with vaginal ulcers include *Hydrastis canadensis*, *Mercurius solubilis*, and *Sepia.*

Step 3. *Nourish and Tonify*

★ **Comfrey** leaf infusion, internally and externally, strengthens vaginal tissues, heals current ulcers and prevents future ones.

Step 4. *Stimulate/Sedate*

★ Astringent herbal sitz baths – especially **oak bark** – heal ulcerated tissues and help prevent recurrences. Make it, page 368.

Her Story

Frances is an olive-skinned actress, always on the road.

"For five years I was bothered by painful growths down there. I visited doctor after doctor in town after town. Most told me I had cysts in my Bartholin glands. Antibiotics and lancing relieved the pain and swelling, but only for a short while.

"I never saw the same doctor twice; yet I left my health totally in their hands. I never even looked in the mirror to see what was up down there. Perhaps my story would have had a different ending if I had had consistent medical care, or if I had actively cared for myself. The lumps weren't cysts, but cancer, metatastic when finally diagnosed. I'm doing all I can now, but it's a little late, huh?"

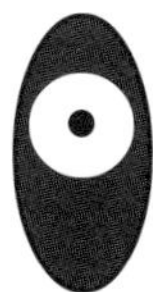

Vaginal Cancer

Step 1. *Collect Information*

• Vaginal cancer is extremely rare. Only five women per million will have it; those whose mother or grandmother took diethylstilbestrol (DES) are at much greater risk.[22] If you think there is something growing in your vagina, especially if you are postmenopausal, seek experienced advice. Vaginal cancer can kill.

• One out of one thousand DES daughters will be diagnosed with vaginal cancer, usually a very aggressive form, and often before the age of twenty.[23] Risk does diminish with age, but never falls to zero. (More on DES, page 202.)

• DES daughters need to be especially vigilant about the health of their vaginas. Be sure your annual Pap smear includes cells from your vagina so any cancerous changes are seen early on.

• If your mother, or even your grandmother, took DES, tell your daughter. When mice are given DES, tumors occur in the reproductive tracts of their daughters *and* granddaughters.[24]

Step 2. *Engage the Energy*

• Trained classical homeopaths use nosodes to help counter genetic patterns that lead to cancer. **Homeopathic** diethylstilbestrol is a **nosode of DES**. One dose, taken once, is said to reverse the genetic damage that sets the stage for vaginal (and other) cancers in DES daughters and granddaughters.

Help!
Vaginal Cancer

Expect results in 2–3 months

• Drink **red clover** infusion.

• Consider a **macrobiotic** diet.

• Experiment cautiously with **poke** root tincture.

• Use **milk thistle tincture** before chemotherapy; drink **carrot juice** before radiation.

Step 3. *Nourish and Tonify*

★ A weekly quart of **red clover infusion** helps prevent, and reverse, hormonal cancers. DES daughter? Drink two a week.

★ **Burdock root**, infusion or tincture, is a proven ally for DES daughters who want to prevent or eliminate vaginal cancer.

Step 4. *Stimulate/Sedate*

• Tiny doses of **poke** root tincture – 1–4 drops taken 2–3 times a day – have helped some women beat vaginal cancer.

Step 5. *Use Drugs*

★ If you are a DES daughter, consider having your daughter(s) vaccinated with the controversial agent Gardasil; it protects against vaginal cancer, too. The abnormal cell growth that precedes vaginal cancer is *vaginal intraepithelial neoplasia* (VIN). None of the 9000 women who received Gardasil developed VIN; while 24 among the 9000 women who received placebo injections did.[25,26]

Step 6. *Break and Enter*

• Investigate laser surgery, cryosurgery, radiation treatments, topical chemotherapy, and light therapy. Every woman and every cancer is unique.

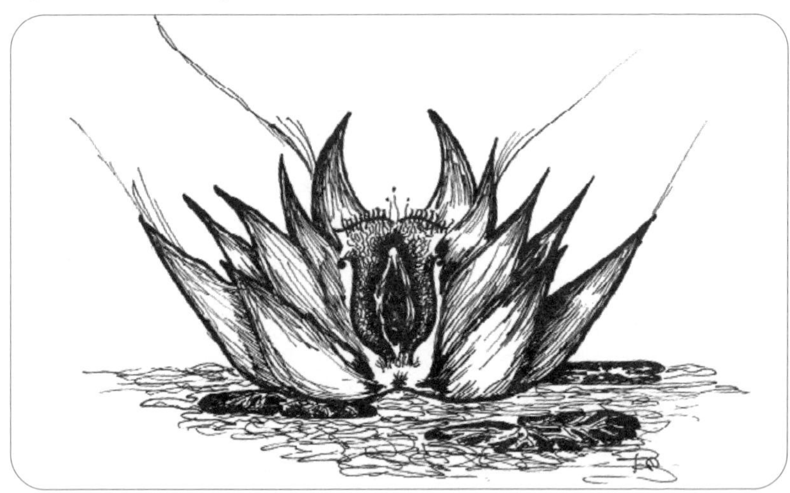

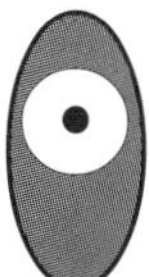

Vaginal Infections: STDs/STIs

"The world is filled with life, dear granddaughter," says Grandmother Growth as you walk together. "And some of that life can distress you. Your vagina is filled with life, dearest granddaughter, and some of that *life can distress you, too.*

"When you are too sweet, life can run over you. Bacteria, fungi, and parasites thrive on your sweet acquiescence. They like it when you always say 'yes,' when you always agree. When you put your needs aside and let others have their way, the life in your vagina magnifies your decision. It is wisest to stay a little on the sour side, like me," she says, sticking her tongue out rudely.

"What you term an 'infection,' I call a 'reminder,' a reminder to care for yourself. Do you need a time-out from your responsibilities? Do you need to re/create safety in your life? I can help. Come with me."

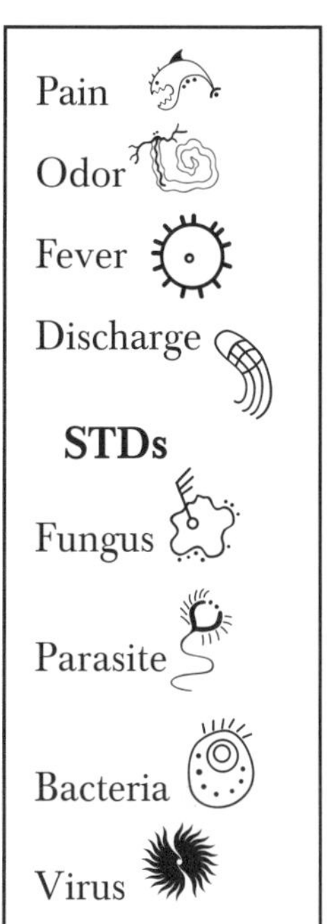

• Embarrasment about problems "down there" can ruin your health. Be aware of changes in your and your partners' genitals. Demand safe sex. Speak openly with your health care helper about your concerns and experiences. Planned Parenthood is there to help: confidential, compassionate, and at a price you can afford.

• Used correctly, condoms are 98 percent effective at preventing STD/STI (sexually transmitted disease/infection), and 97 percent effective at preventing unwanted pregnancy.[1] For the health of your vagina, choose ones without spermicide. (More on page 291.)

• In 2008 the Centers for Disease Control and Prevention found 50 percent of black teens and 20 percent of other teens were infected with an STD.[2]

STDs/STIs

The most common sexually-transmitted diseases/infections are yeast (page 146), *Trich* (page 150), *Gardnerella* (page 154), *Chlamydia* (page 156), *Herpes* (page 160), gonorrhea (page 164), and syphilis (page 166).

Other STDs/STIs

Cytomegalovirus[3] (sigh-tow-MEG-a-low-VI-rus), or CMV, is transmitted through all body fluids: saliva, semen, blood, cervical and vaginal secretions, urine, and breast milk. It is the most common mother-to-fetus infection in America. Between 40–80 percent of children become infected with CMV before puberty from other children's saliva. There are no symptoms with the first infection. The virus remains active in the body for life. Reinfection with CMV, or another STD, can cause CMV to become active, resulting in swollen glands, fatigue, fever, weakness, nausea, diarrhea, vision loss, hearing loss, mono-nucleosis, even mental retardation. *There is no protection and no cure,* though antibiotic drugs and herbs can control symptoms. Adults with weakened immune systems may become mentally disordered or blind from CMV.

Human immunodeficiency virus (HIV) can cause AIDS, the fifth leading cause of death for young American wo/men.[4] Incidence in older Americans is increasing. Hourly doses of St. Joan's wort tincture can slow the progression of HIV. Tests for HIV generate a high rate of false positives (50 percent), so retesting any positive result is strongly advised.

Human papilloma virus; page 176.

Lice; page 91.

Molluscum contagiosum (mo-LUS-kum con-tay-gee-OH-sum) is a common viral infection that is passed by nonsexual and sexual contact.[5] Symptoms – small pink, waxy, round growths in the genital area or on the thighs or abdomen – generally appear within 12 weeks of infection, but may not appear for years. The growths may be removed with caustic herbs (like celandine), chemicals, freezing, or lasers; or they may be left untreated.

Scabies; page 91.

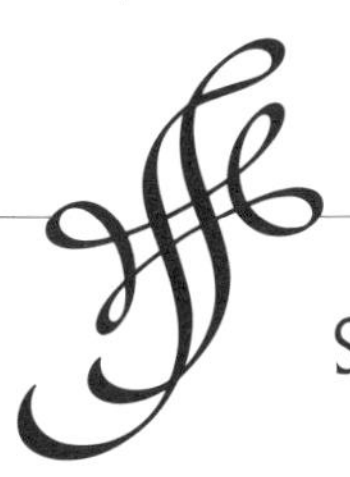

STD/STI Symptoms

Some sexually-transmitted diseases/infections have symptoms, some have few or none. This list can be used to help match distresses in the genitals to possible/probable causes.

Seek help if the remedies you are using don't relieve symptoms promptly. Some STDs may become life-threatening. Some make infection with HIV more likely. Some cause infertility.

If untreated, 20–40 percent of women infected with chlamydia and 10–40 percent of those with gonorrhea will develop PID and tubal scarring that may lead to infertility, ectopic pregnancy, and chronic pelvic pain.[6]

- **abdominal pain**: chlamydia, gonorrhea, PID, UTI
- **bleeding/spotting**: chlamydia, gonorrhea, PID, trich, UTI
- **blisters or sores**: gonorrhea, herpes, syphilis, *lichen planus*
- **discharge, white**, with yeasty odor: candida, yeast
- **discharge, colored**, with bad odor: BV, chlamydia, gonorrhea, PID, trich, desquamative inflammatory vaginitis, epididymitis
- **fever**: chlamydia, herpes, lice, PID, syphilis, UTI
- **glands swollen**: herpes, syphilis
- **intercourse painful**: chlamydia, gonorrhea, herpes, PID, vaginal dryness, yeast
- **itching**: herpes, HPV, lice, scabies, trich, yeast
- **nausea**: chlamydia, PID
- **rectal pain**: chlamydia, hemorrhoids, herpes
- **testicular pain**: chlamydia, herpes
- **urination burning** or frequent: chlamydia, gonorrhea, herpes, PID, trich, UTI, epididymitis, yeast
- **vaginal/vulvar pain**: BV, CPP, gonorrhea, herpes, lice, PID, scabies, vulvodynia, yeast

Vaginal Yeast (*Candida albicans*)

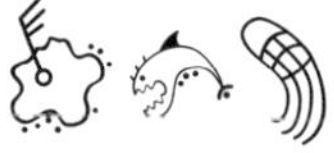

Step 0. *Do Nothing*

• Most women are adverse to intercourse when their vagina is disturbed by a yeast overgrowth. This is wise, as the friction of penetration can worsen the symptoms.

• Pretend you're a wild starlet and throw away your underpants, pantyhose, leotards, tights, and girdles. This well-known cure for diaper rash – omit the diaper – counters vaginal yeast too. If you must wear undies, cotton only and cut out the crotch.

Step 1. *Collect Information*

• Virtually every woman alive has had one or more run-ins with vaginal yeast. *Candida albicans* is a single-celled organism, a kind of fungus, which lives in our vaginas with its sister, *Lactobacillus acidophilus.* When the vaginal pH is acidic, *Lactobaccillus* rules. When the vaginal environment is alkaline, *Candida* proliferates.

★ Candida is also known as monilia, moniliasis, yeast, the whites, and leucorrhea. It is characterized by a thick, white, yeasty-smelling, lumpy, vaginal discharge which is highly irritating to the vulva. It may cause painful urination and itching, too.

• Candida infections can also live on the skin, nails, mouth, lungs, and feet (athlete's foot).

• Candida is part of the flora of a healthy vagina and of healthy intestines. The vaginal one is genetically different from the intestinal one, however.[7] A vaginal yeast infection implies nothing about Candida in the gut.

Candida albicans

Step 2. *Engage the Energy*

★ A yeast infection is a good way to say "no" to intercourse. Do you have any other way to say it?

• **Homeopathic remedies** for vaginal yeast overgrowth.
 ~ *Calcarea carbonica*: vulva burns, very itchy; discharge yellow or milky; worse before/after menses.
 ~ *Graphites*: vagina, labia sore; worse before menses.
 ~ *Kali-carb*.: vagina sore, itchy; coitus painful; warm worsens.
 ~ *Kreosotum*: discharge offensive; vulva irritated, itchy, burns.
 ~ *Lachesis*: vulva burns; worse if pregnant, before menses.
 ~ *Lycopodium*: vulva irritated, itchy; stress, menses worsen.
 ~ *Mercurius*: vulva irritated, itchy, burns; stress worsens.
 ~ *Natrum muriaticum*: vagina itchy, burning, painful; stress worsens symptoms.
 ~ *Nux vomica*: stress, warmth, menses, pregnancy worsen.
 ~ *Pulsatilla*: vagina burns, painful; watery discharge.
 ~ *Sulphur*: vulva very itchy, painful; worse before menses.

Step 3. *Nourish and Tonify*

★ Prevent vaginal yeast overgrowth with **plain yogurt** or other fermented milk. Women who consume a cup a day have only one-third as many yeast infections as women who consume none.[8]

• Yogurt applications ease pain and itching and remain the favorite home remedy for relieving the distress of a yeast infection.

> "Douching with yogurt may be harmless, but it won't cure a yeast infection."[9]

• **Maitake** are mushrooms that specifically inhibit and destroy candida. Women with chronic infections benefit the most. A dose is ½ gram daily for a month, increasing by ½ gram a month to a maximum of 3 grams daily.[10] A cup of fennel seed or ginger root tea will relieve the severe gas pains that will result from use of maitake.

Help!
Yeast Overgrowth

Expect results in 3–5 days

• Apply **plain yogurt** to the labia and vagina four times a day.

• Eat at least ½ cup **yogurt** a day.

• Drink a cup or more of **chamomile** or **goldenrod tea** daily.

• Sitz in any **antifungal** herb (page 148) *or* use **boric acid** capsules vaginally, daily.

• Counter yeast by inserting 1–2 **acidophilus capsules** high in the vagina to soothe, heal, and restore pH.

Step 4. *Stimulate/Sedate*

★ A **garlic suppository** kills candida,[11] gardnerella and non-specific vaginitis. Peel a clove of garlic, oil it, and insert well up into the vagina. Use a fresh clove every 8–12 hours for two weeks. To remove: Squat and bear down; use your fingers to help. *Note*: Your breath will reek of garlic almost as soon as you do this!

★ Before resorting to antifungal drugs, try one of these safe and effective **antifungal herbs**.

~ **Black walnut** husk tincture, internally and externally, is extremely effective against candida.[12]

~ **Cranberries** and blueberries contain the candida-killer *arbutin.*[13]

~ **Chamomile** flower tea, sipped and sat in, destroys candida.[14] It is ideal for women who are sensitive, timid, and afraid of their own sexuality, according to Swiss herbalists Barbara and Peter Theiss.[15]

~ **Goldenrod** flower tea/sitz prevents and cures inflamed urogenital yeast infections say German researchers.

~ **Goldenseal** root sitz baths are anti-yeast.

~ **English ivy** leaf washes kill candida.

~ **Licorice** sitz baths kill candida.

~ **Pau d'arco** salve or sitz bath also kills candida.[16]

~ **Garden sage**, tinctured or infused, used internally and/or externally, restores pH and dries up yeast.

• White flour and white sugar and sweets – not just soda pop and candy, but raw fruit and fruit juices too – may (or may not, depending on whom you ask) promote yeast overgrowth.

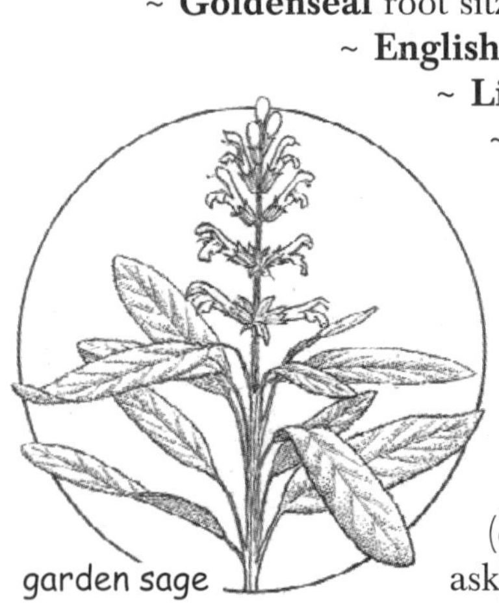

★ Herbalist Dr. James Duke says **echinacea** root tincture prevents and treats yeast infections. It stimulates the production of white blood cells, which love to snack on yeasties. It works alone or *with* antifungal drugs. In a German study, 60 percent of women who took an antifungal drug had a recurrence, while only 10 percent of those who took echinacea *and* the drug, did.

★ *The Journal of Reproductive Medicine* reports that **boric acid** cured 98 percent of women with chronic, drug-resistant yeast infections. To use: Fill 00 gelatin caps (sold at health food stores) with boric acid USP (sold at drugstores). Insert one in the vagina nightly before bed for two weeks.

★ **Sunlight** kills yeast. Spread 'em! Be inventive; be discreet.

• **Moxibustion** – the burning of *Artemisia* – is used with acupuncture to tone the vagina and prevent further yeast overgrowths.

• Chronic yeast infections from birth control pills? Help yourself with soothing **aloe vera gel** or **Crotch Cream** (page 370).

★ Recurring yeast may be symptomatic of Type 2 diabetes.[17]

Step 5a. *Use Supplements*

• Counter chronic yeast infections by getting more B vitamins from meat, whole grains, beans, and red clover or oatstraw infusions. Supplements – 100mg daily of B_1, B_2, and B_6, plus 200mg of B_3, taken daily for no more than 60 days – are far less effective.

★ A single drop of **tea tree oil** diluted in a 2 ounces/60ml of oil and applied to the vagina can kill fungal infections.

Caution: All essential oils are highly concentrated and require great care in their use. Tea tree oil can burn sensitive vaginal tissues, inflame the cervix, and devastate the protective bacteria and yeasts in the vagina. *If you buy a prepared cream, be sure it is no more than one percent essential oil.*

Step 5b. *Use Drugs*

• Yogurt, whether taken orally or applied vaginally, does *not* prevent yeast infections in women taking antibiotics.[18]

• One dose of an oral prescription antifungal quells yeast. But topical antifungal drugs are as effective and have fewer side effects. Look for suppositories of nystatin (Mycostatin) or miconazole nitrate (Monistat), or a tioconazole ointment.

★ Before you use any antifungal drug, remember: Not every vaginal infection is a yeast infection, and yeast infections can hide other infections. Broad-acting herbs are better allies than systemic antifungal drugs if you don't know for sure it's only yeast.

• Postmenopausal women with chronic yeast infections find 1–2mg estrogen or testosterone cream applied topically, twice a week, to be of great benefit.

Trich (*Trichomonas vaginalis*)

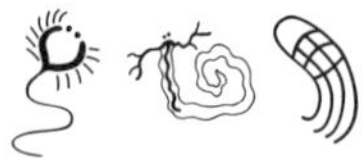

Step 1. *Collect Information*

> "Herbal remedies for *Trichomonas* are among the least impressive home remedies. None are more than 50 percent effective."[19]

• Trich ("trick") is *Trichomonas*: a single-celled, four-tailed, protozoan parasite. About five million new cases of trich are diagnosed yearly in the USA.

• Trich is normally present in the vagina, intestines, and rectum without causing problems. Overgrowths are hard to counter without using drugs.

• Trich is an STD and can be spread by intimate contact. But sex is not required. Hardy trich can live in wet, warm places like toilet seats, towels, underwear, and swimsuits. In fact, trich may be smarter than we are; it has three times as many genes as its human hosts.[20]

Trichomonas vaginalis
(inset: one cell)

★ Women with trich infections have a thin, foamy, itchy vaginal discharge that is yellowish-green or gray in color and foul/fishy in odor. Infected men are often symptom-free.

• It is easy to become reinfected with trich if your partner(s) is not treated at the same time so all the trich is eliminated at once. (Just for men: Tips on eliminating trich on pages 293 and 374.)

• Trich can move up into the bladder. If you have a UTI that won't respond to treatment, it might be trich.

• Like candida, trich is pH sensitive. An acidic vagina will resist infection, but trich can easily overwhelm healthy flora in an alkaline vaginal environment. (*See* page 126 for ways to acidify the vagina.)

Step 2. *Engage the Energy*

• **Homeopathic remedies** for women with green discharges.
 ~ *Arsenicum*: bad smell; vulva irritated, burning.
 ~ *Carb. veg.*: bad smell; vulva burns, itches, cracks open.
 ~ *Nitric acid*: bad smell, vulva burns, itches, is irritated, ulcerated, cracked; worse after menses.
 ~ *Sanicula*: fishy, briny smell; desires salt, bacon, icy milk.
 ~ *Sepia*: very bad smell, vagina, vulva itches, smarts, burns, ulcerated; pregnancy, stress worsens.

Step 3. *Nourish and Tonify*

• **Dessicating agents** dry out the trichomonads and kill them.

~ **Oak bark** powder is antimicrobial.

~ Finely powdered **charcoal**, the kind used against poisoning, smothers trich. It also makes a black mess on everything, from your underwear to your sheets.

~ **Clay** powder, such as kaolin or green clay, makes life tough for trich.

Help! Trichomonas

Expect results in 14–20 days

• Take 15–25 drops of any herbal tincture containing **berberine sulfate** (page 152) 3–4 times a day.

• Use a **desiccating agent** vaginally every day.

• Get into **hysterical hygeine**.

~ **Slippery elm** bark powder has been used for hundreds of years against all vaginal disorders.

For best results, use desiccating agents once a day for 3 weeks. Mix herbs with coconut oil and insert vaginally, or put 3–6 capsules of powdered herb well up into the vagina, against and behind the cervix. Showers only – no baths – during treatment cycle.

Step 4. *Stimulate/Sedate*

★ The alkaloid **berberine sulfate** – present in the tinctures of the roots of barberry, gold thread, goldenseal, Oregon grape, huang-lian (*Coptis*), and yellowroot – is an antimicrobial agent shown to inhibit the growth of, and to induce morphological changes in, *Trichomonas*.[21,22] In a study done in India, 90 percent of those who took berberine sulfate and 95 percent of those who took a drug were trich free in two weeks. At the one-month follow up, 83 percent of the berberine group and 90 percent of the drug group were still clear. The study's authors noted the lack of side effects in those receiving berberine.[23] The dose of any berberine-rich tincture is 10–20 drops several times daily for 3–4 weeks.

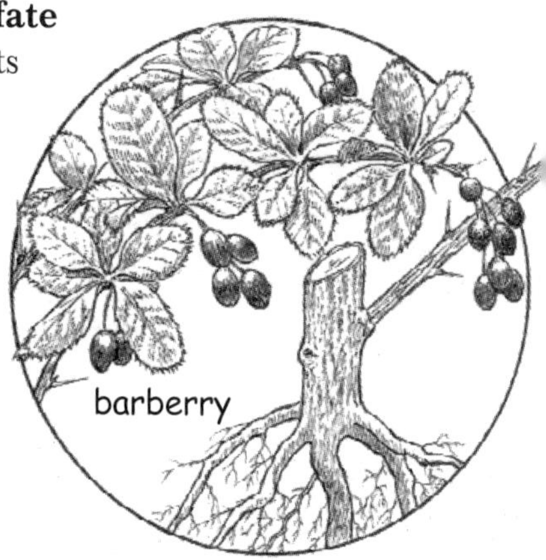

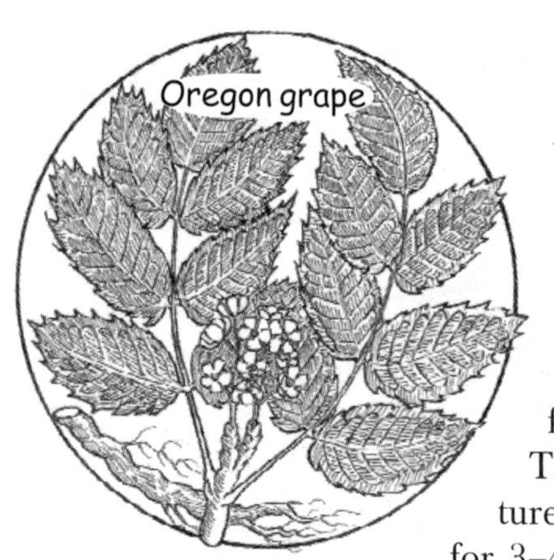

• Several weeks of **hysterical hygiene** are called for when dealing with a trich infection. Strip your bed and your bathroom and wash everything, using bleach or vinegar. Wash your hands after toileting. Swab off the toilet seat with dilute bleach. Remember, trich is persistent and hard to kill.

Her Story

Flagyl is not safe for the children of lactating moms. Six weeks after I gave birth, at my scheduled check-up, my OB/Gyn thought my cervix looked "bubbly." I was complaining of some postpartum vaginal irritation, it's true. But I never expected he would write a prescription for Flagyl for me, a nursing mom.

I was upset enough to get a second opinion. The midwife who checked me out "down there" found a yeast overgrowth. She suspected that my estrogen levels were low, too. I never filled the prescription. Home remedies healed me and kept my baby safe.

Step 5. *Use Drugs*

• MDs use the drugs inidazole and metronidazole (Flagyl) – a "highly toxic drug that is often ineffective due to resistance, particularly by *Trichomonas*. . . ."[24] (*see* below) – to kill trich. A single 2g dose eliminates 95 percent of trich infections. Clotrimazole, a milder drug with fewer side effects, is only 60 percent effective. Ampicillin, Terramycin, and sulfa drugs are not effective.

• Herbalist and healer Joy Gardner says regular use of spermicidal jelly can help prevent trich (but not other) infections.

• European herbalists use essential oils – 5 drops tea tree, 4 drops cypress, 8 drops lavender, plus 3 drops red thyme – to kill trich.[25] To use: dilute four drops of the blend in a carrier – such as two cups water, a cup of yogurt, or 2 ounces/60ml of olive oil – and apply freely to the inside of the vagina. (*Caution*, page 149.)

Flagyl

❖ What is it? A very strong antiprotozoal/antibiotic drug.

❖ *Not safe* for pregnant or nursing women, or those with blood diseases, peptic ulcers, or central nervous system disorders.

❖ Common side effects: lowering of white blood cell count, nausea/vomiting, headache, diarrhea, joint pain, flushing, metallic taste in the mouth, numbness in the extremities.

❖ Side effects worsened by alcohol, vinegar, and mayonnaise.

❖ If you take it, eat yogurt throughout and for 6 weeks afterwards.

Bacterial Vaginosis (*Gardnerella vaginalis*)

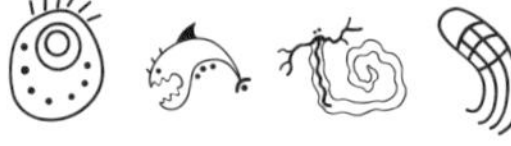

Step 0. *Do Nothing*

• Abstain from sex and wear underpants to bed while dealing with *Gardnerella.* This breaks the cycle and gives non-drug remedies a better chance to work.

• The cure rate is the same whether partners are treated or not.

Step 1. *Collect Information*

> "BV occurs due to an overgrowth of normal vaginal organisms with a mixture of *Gardnerella vaginalis* and other oxygen-intolerant bacteria. BV can arise spontaneously or be sexually transmitted."[26]

• Bacterial vaginosis (BV) is the leading cause of vaginal complaints in the USA.[27] It is often confused with yeast; it is mistakenly called leucorrhea, bacterial/chronic/non-specific vaginitis, hemophilus. Half of all affected women have no symptoms.[28]

• *Gardnerella* (and its friend *Atopobium*) are anaerobic bacteria which live in the vagina. In an alkaline environment (pH over 4.5) they overrun healthy flora. "Vaginosis" means no infection.[29]

★ Symptoms of BV range from none to intense itching and irritation of the vagina and vulva accompanied by a grayish white discharge; the rank smell distinguishes it from yeast.

Help!
Bacterial Vaginosis

Expect results in 7–10 days

• Eat **yogurt**; apply some vaginally.

• Take a dropperful of **yarrow tincture** twice a day.

• Try a **garlic suppository** (pg 148).

• If it's chronic, try MAM (pg 209).

• Chronic BV can cause adverse cervical changes according to the Santa Cruz Women's Health Center. BV itself does not spread into the uterus, but it has been linked to an increased risk of HIV infection, PID (pelvic inflammatory disease), and complications of pregnancy.[30]

> " [Of the] three most common vaginal infections — trichomonas (a one-celled organsim), candida (a yeast), and bacterial vaginosis — the third is the most prevalent and the most difficult to treat. It tends to come back again and again."[31]

Step 2. *Engage the Energy*

- Homeopathic **calendula gel** soothes irritated vaginas.
- **Crab apple** flower essence counters chronic BV.

Step 3. *Nourish and Tonify*

★ Keep vaginal acidity high (page 126) to prevent and treat BV. **Plain yogurt**, eaten and applied vaginally at least once a day, is a highly effective acidifier. Do this even if you take antibiotics. Taking acidophilus increases the effectiveness of Flagyl.

★ Researcher Sharon Hiller isolated lactobacilli from the vaginas of healthy women, put them in capsules, and used them vaginally to cure women who had *Gardnerella* infections.[32] Easier: insert one or two **acidophilus** capsules high in the vagina every other day for two weeks. (You'll drool; do it at night or use a pad.)

Step 4. *Stimulate/Sedate*

★ **Yarrow** is the self-defense queen. She'll help you bid "farewell" to BV. For best results, mix a quart of yarrow infusion or tea with a cup of vinegar and use daily for 2–4 weeks as a sitz or finger bath. The tincture, in dropperful doses, may be taken 2–3 times a day as extra insurance.

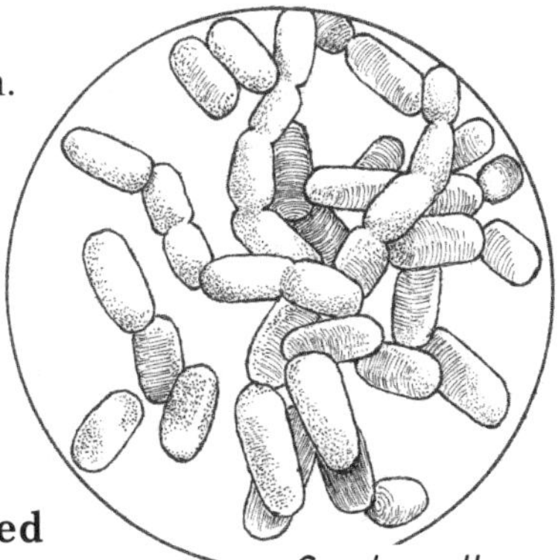

Gardnerella

• Bag Balm, a stiff, **sulphur-based ointment** used on the udders of cows is an old-time remedy. It stinks, but works against hard-to-clear surface bacterial infections like *Gardnerella*.

• A sitz bath or finger bath with **meadowsweet** leaf infusion is recommended by herbalist Terry Willard, PhD to counter "chronic vaginitis with leucorrheal discharge."[33] Meadowsweet's astringent and analgesic properties help restore vaginal pH and ease irritation and pain.

★ That old stand-by, **garlic**, works wonders for women with BV. Insert a whole clove into the vagina and leave overnight.

Step 5b. *Use Drugs*

• The drugs of choice for eliminating *Gardnerella* are:

~ Clindamycin (Cleocin), used vaginally or systemically.

~ Topical Flagyl – MetroCream – used for five days, is as effective as, and has fewer side effects than, oral Flagyl.

~ Flagyl (metronidazole), taken in multiple small doses several times a day for a week, clears 80 percent of cases.[34] Be sure to take probiotics during and after treatment. (Cautions page 153.)

~ Tinidazole, a newer drug, is a Flagyl spin-off; same cautions.

Chlamydia (*Chlamydia trachomatis*)

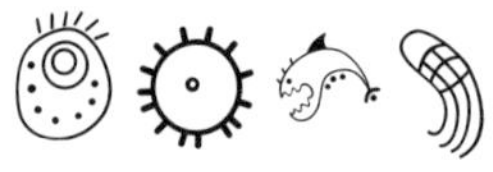

"*Chlamydia* too often goes unnoticed because something else seems to explain the symptoms; it should be considered whenever other genital infections are found."[35]

Step 0. *Do Nothing*

• Undiagnosed and untreated chlamydia infections are the main cause of infertility worldwide. In men, it scars the tubes that deliver sperm. In women, it scars the egg tubes. Chlamydia can lead to chronic pelvic pain (page 15), PID (page 245), and ectopic/tubal pregnancies (page 269).

Step 1. *Collect Information*

"Sexually-transmitted chlamydia leaves most of its victms unaware of their infections until the damage is irreversible."[36]

• Chlamydia (kla-MIH-dee-uh) is a parasitic bacterium. It is the world's most common STD, with 3–4 million new cases annually in the USA[37] (up from 600,000 cases in 1998[38]). More than 800 million people worldwide are currently infected, with 90 million new infections each year.[39] Up to 85 percent of infected women and 40 percent of infected men have no apparent symptoms.[40]

• A 1998 study of 13,000 female U. S. Army recruits found one in ten had *Chlamydia*, with more infections in those from Southern states. That same year, 24 percent of 3000 sexually-active young women (12–19) tested positive for chlamydia.[41]

★ It is strongly recommended that sexually-active women under the age of 25 have safe sex *and* be tested yearly for chlamydia.

• *Chlamys* is Greek for cloak, an apt name. Chlamydia cannot grow outside a cell; it must dress, or cloak itself, in another cell in order to multiply. And, chlamydia is hidden, or cloaked, from the immune system when it has made itself at home inside a cell. Because patroling T-cells cannot recognize and destroy them, *Chlamydia* can linger for decades without obvious symptoms.

• When the immune system does see chlamydia, it sets up an "enthusiatic" inflammatory response, which damages tissues.[42] Symptoms of a chlamydia infection may flare up months or years after it has apparently disappeared.[43] They include abnormal vaginal discharge and vulvar itching in women, and painful or burning urination, urethritis, urinary tract infections, and abdominal pressure and pain in men and women.

★ Chlamydia is "the silent STD." *Few men or women have symptoms; many become infertile; some die.*[44, 45]

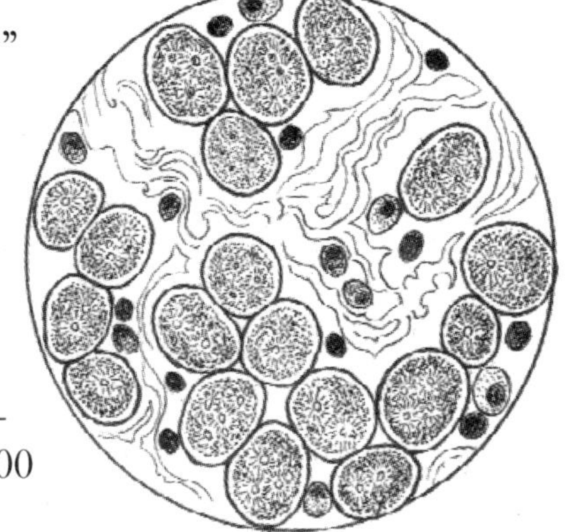
Chlamydia

• Chlamydia can infect the eyes as well as the cervix, ovaries, egg tubes, epididymis, urinary tract, rectum, and throat. It is responsible for *trachoma*, a chronic, often blinding, eye infection affecting about 500 million people in the Third World.

• *Chlamydia pneumoniae* causes colds, bronchitis, and pneumonia. It has tentatively been linked to atherosclerosis, as well.[46]

• Untreated, chlamydia often makes its way from the vagina to the endocervical glands, where it enters the cells and can linger for many years, irritating and inflaming the cervical tissues. About half of all cases of cervicitis are caused by chlamydia infections.[47] If it makes its way into the uterus, endometrium, tubes or ovaries, it can silently damage these delicate organs, causing fertility problems and ectopic pregnancies.[48] It can also become PID.

• About three-quarters of infected mothers will pass *Chlamydia* to their baby during birth,[49] increasing the child's risk of pneumonia and eye infections. Rates of spontaneous miscarriage, fetal death, and pre-term delivery are higher among women with active chlamydia infections.

• Chlamydia is diagnosed by a variety of tests; cultures are still considered most accurate. Delaying diagnosis delays treatment and can give chlamydia time to do permanent damage.

• A 2002 study in Baltimore found 8 percent of 600 adults between the ages of 18 and 35 had an undiagnosed and untreated chlamydia and/or gonorrhea infection. About 15 percent of women of color were affected, as were 1.3 percent of other women, 6.4 percent of men of color, and 2.8 percent of other men.[50] Undiagnosed cases were more numerous than diagnosed cases!

Step 2. *Engage the Energy*

• **Creative visualization** can allow you to uncloak the chlamydia and make it visible to your immune system so drugs have a better chance of working. Close your eyes, breathe deeply and evenly, and imagine removing their cloaks.

Help!
Chlamydia

Expect results in 7–10 days

• Integrate your medicine: Use anti-infective herbs (page 159) with **antibiotic** drugs.

• Take **probiotics**, too.

• Try a **creative visualization**.

Step 3. *Nourish and Tonify*

• It is nearly impossible to defend ourselves against an organism that hides inside our own cells. Even drugs have a hard time getting at chlamydia. Protect yourself: Have penetrative sex only with uninfected partners or always, always use a condom.

Step 4. *Stimulate/Sedate*

• Neither herbs nor drugs are strongly effective against chlamydia, but both together are better than either alone. A dropperful of the tincture of **echinacea**, **pau d'arco**, **St. Joan's wort**, **usnea**, or **yarrow**, or 2–3 drops of **chaparral**, taken 3–4 times a day with an antibiotic can improve your chances of getting rid of chlamydia. Please use tinctures; I think herbs in capsules are ineffective, overpriced, and often dangerous.

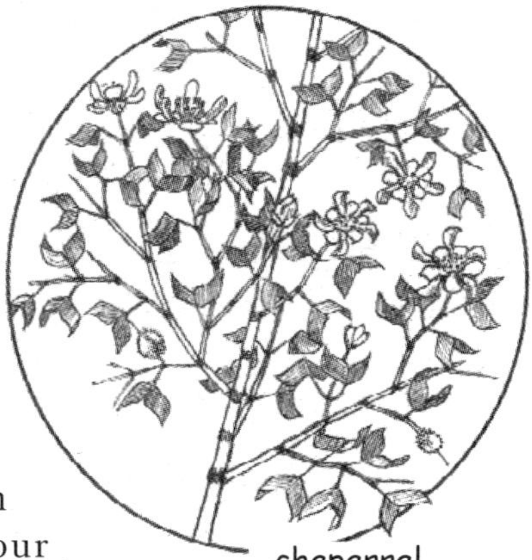

chaparral

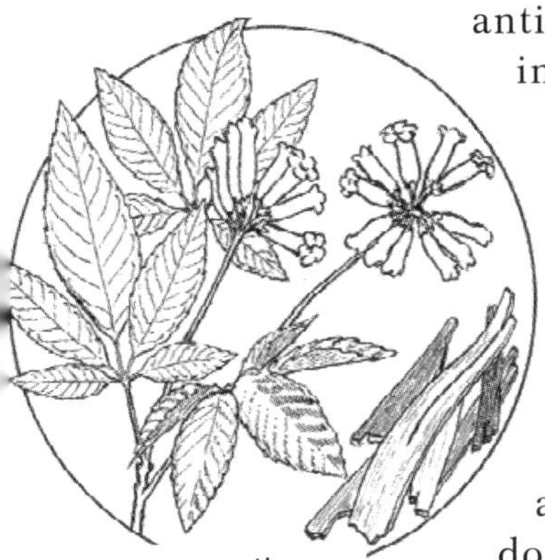

pau d'arco

Step 5. *Use Drugs*

• The most effective **antibiotics** against chlamydia are azithromycin (one dose) and erythromycin (for pregnant women). Chlamydia can be resistant to treatment, but it appears unable to become resistant to drugs. (Its genome has remained essentially the same for millions of years.[51]) Take *every* dose of antibiotic, refrain from intercourse during the entire treatment, get treatment for all partners concurrently, and use complementary medicines.

• Nonoxynol-9, a spermicide, does **not** protect women against chlamydia, gonorrhea, or HIV infections.[52,53] Some health-care activists believe using nonoxynol-9 *increases* the risk of getting an STD because it inflames and irritates vaginal and cervical tissues.

Genital Herpes (*Herpes Simplex Virus Type 2*)

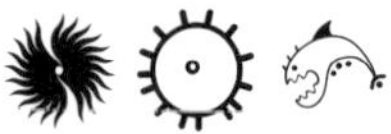

Step 0. *Do Nothing*

• There is no cure for genital herpes or *Herpes simplex* virus type 2 (HSV-2). Once you have it, you have it. Currently, about 30 million Americans have it.

Step 1. *Collect Information*

• *Herpes* comes from the Greek word, "to creep." This virus creeps into the nerves through the skin and mucus membranes, most easily if there are cuts or tears. Once inside, it migrates to the spine, where it lurks, awaiting sufficient stress to activate it into an eruption of painful lesions (sores).

• Vaginal, anal, and oral sex, even with protection, can pass HSV-2 to a partner. And herpes can be spread even in the absence of sex. It requires only bare skin contact to transmit.[54]

• Genital herpes infects over 25 percent of adults in the USA and Europe, with one million new cases annually in the USA.[55,56,57]

• HSV-2 isn't restricted to the young. Researchers looking at blood samples from relatively affluent suburbanites outside six major cities found HSV-2 infection in 36 percent of women 40–49 and nearly 30 percent of women 50–59. At all ages, more women than men were infected.[58]

• More than half (53 percent) of women of color aged 18–24 with a history of STDs are also infected with HSV-2, while 24 percent of those without a history of STDs are infected.[59]

• Almost a third (31 percent) of women who have only one partner, ever, will become infected with HSV-2.

Help!
Genital Herpes

Expect results in 2–4 days

• Apply **St. Joan's wort oil** to all sores as often as possible.

• Take a dropperful of **St. Joan's wort tincture** 4–8 times a day.

• Supplement with L-lysine.

• There is a reliable blood test for herpes, both HSV-1 and HSV-2.

• Symptoms of HSV-2 can be painfully obvious: an aching sore on the genitals, vulva, anus, or thighs – sometimes accompanied by vaginal discharge, back pain, and urinary discomfort. The sore often breaks open, leaving a slow-healing, painful ulcer.

• Or there may be no symptoms. About 80 percent of infected people don't know it.[60, 61] Those already carrying HSV-1 (oral herpes) are most likely to remain symptom-free with HSV-2.

• The first outbreak of HSV-2 is always the worst. There may be five or more outbreaks the first year, but the number declines as the infection matures.[62] In those with strong immune systems, there may be no further outbreaks after the first year or two.

• Because herpes creates breaks in the protective mucosa of the genitals, it triples the risk of contracting HIV (the AIDS virus).[63]

• Women with HSV-2 – unless in the midst of a first outbreak – can safely give birth vaginally because they have already passed herpes antibodies to their baby. To help prevent lesions during the stress of labor, make an infusion with one ounce each burdock and echinacea roots in a quart of boiling water. Steep for eight hours. The dose is a cup or more a day throughout the last month of pregnancy.

Step 2. *Engage the Energy*

• Genital herpes hides in the nerves "down there." Any major change, desired or not – such as fatigue, trauma, hormonal changes, excessive exposure to sunlight, new job, new home, new sexual relationship, travel, illness, surgery, sexual guilt, tight clothes – can trigger HSV to become active and create lesions.[64]

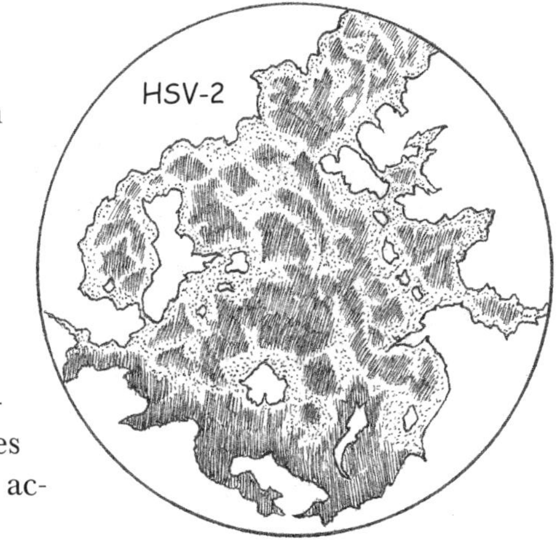

- **Homeopathic remedies** for those with genital *Herpes* include:
  - ~ *Capsicum*: genital rash red, itchy, burns; cracked skin.
  - ~ *Dulcamara*: genitals stinging, itchy, burning when rubbed; worse on exposure to cold or damp, before menses.
  - ~ *Graphites*: painful red sores, clear or straw-colored ooze, itchy not burning
  - ~ *Nat-mur.*: pearl-like blisters, hot, swollen; genitals very dry.
  - ~ *Petrolatum*: genitals itchy, red, dry/moist, cracked, bleeding, includes thighs and perineum.
  - ~ *Psorinum:* chronic outbreaks, itchy, weak; heat helps.
  - ~ *Rhus tox.*: genitals burn, itchy; cold/damp worsen.
  - ~ *Sepia*: eruptions better in the evening or after exercise.
  - ~ *Sulphur*: chronic outbreaks worsened by heat.
  - ~ *Sempervivum*: genital area painful, bleeding, worse at night.

Step 3. *Nourish and Tonify*

★ **Avoid nuts** during a herpes outbreak. Hazelnuts, Brazil nuts, peanuts, walnuts, and almonds contain large amounts of arginine, an amino acid that worsens herpes symptoms.[65]

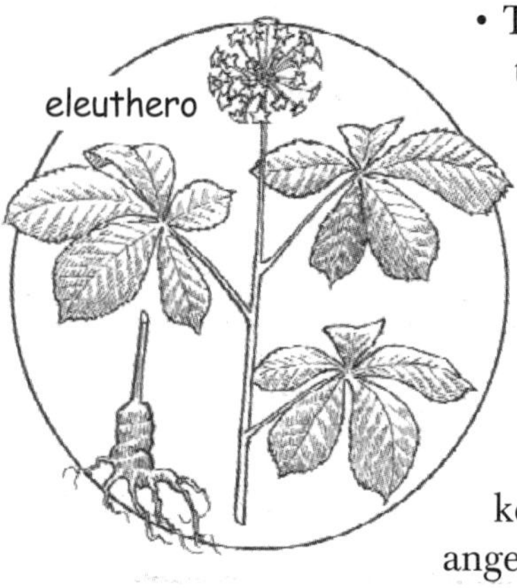

eleuthero

• To prevent outbreaks of herpes, keep the immune system strong. Use tonifying herbs daily, as tinctures or cooked into foods: My favorites are the berries of **schizandra** or the roots of **astragalus**, **burdock**, **dandelion**, **eleuthero**, or **yellow dock**. Also, drink nourishing nettle and red clover infusions (make it, page 367) and eat lots of mushrooms, kelp, and cooked vegetables (red, orange, yellow, and dark green).

★ Consistent use of **burdock** and **echinacea** root infusions – the dose is 1–2 cups a day for at least six weeks – seems to eliminate herpes. I pour 1 quart/liter of boiling water over 1 ounce/30g of each root and steep overnight. To avoid reinfection, be certain all sexual partners – even if they are asymptomatic – imbibe daily for the full six weeks.

• **Black currants** – fresh fruit, jam, juice, or extract – prevent the herpes virus from attaching itself to cell membranes, halving its ability to replicate. They are tart, but tasty.

Step 4. *Stimulate/Sedate*

★ **St. Joan's wort** is a stellar remedy for both preventing and relieving herpes outbreaks. Prompt and liberal use of the **oil** can prevent sores from forming, heal lesions, and reduce pain. Dropperful doses of the **tincture** taken hourly, relieve pain. Repeated use can eventually eliminate outbreaks altogether.

★ A polysaccharide in **self-heal** has specific activity against the herpes virus, at least in lab animals. In cell-based tests, glycyrrhizic acid from **licorice** homed in on the herpes virus and caused it to self destruct. Dropperful doses of either tincture, may help.

• For an anti-herpes **salve**, combine equal parts of fresh or dried herbs – including anti-infective echinacea or grindelia, lymphatic movers/tonics cleavers, calendula, or burdock, anti-viral St. Joan's wort, lemon balm, or self-heal, and berberine-rich Oregon grape or barberry – into a healing oil. (Make it like Crotch Cream, page 370.)

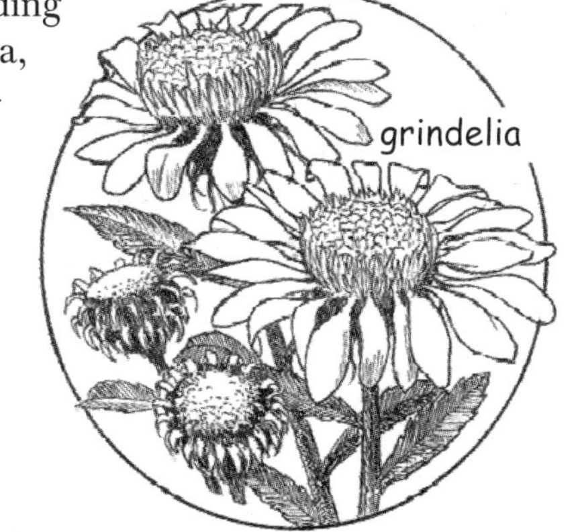

• **Salt water** dries herpes sores.

Step 5a. *Use Supplements*

• **L-lysine** – in food, supplements and creams – helps relieve and prevent herpes outbreaks. Best food sources (mg in ½ cup): halibut or white fishes (920), chicken (740), goats' milk (520).[66]

Step 5b. *Use Drugs*

• High doses of famciclovir reduced genital herpes outbreaks to an average of one a year in those newly infected. Those who took a placebo had at least six outbreaks that year.[67]

Gonorrhea, The Clap (*Neisseria gonorrhoeae*)

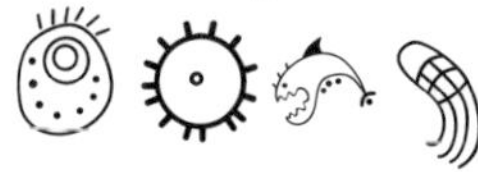

Step 0. *Do Nothing*

• An untreated gonorrhea infection vastly increases a woman's risk of pelvic inflammatory disease (PID) and ectopic pregnancy. It also contributes to arthritis, heart, brain, and skin problems.

Step 1. *Collect Information*

• Gonorrhea is an ancient bacterium. It is one of the oldest known STDs. Mesopotamian healers described it over 7000 years ago, and it's still common. There are about 1.4 million new infections yearly in the US, down from 2 million in the 1990s.[68,69]

• Since the 1300s, gonorrhea has been known as "the clap." Infection is slangily referred to as "a dose."

• Under twenty and sexually active? You are twice as likely to get a dose as those 20–24.

★ Unprotected intercourse or oral sex, once, with an infected person will result in the partner getting a dose 80–90 percent of the time.[70] (Yes, you can get gonorrhea of the throat.)

• If you have symptoms of a gonorrhea infection (and most women don't), you could have a vaginal discharge, pain when urinating or defecating, spotting, pain or bleeding during intercourse, and/or fever.

• About **80 percent of women with gonorrhea have no symptoms** at all.[71] Ninety percent of men have a milky discharge from the penis within 10–14 days of infection.[72] (If you have gonorrhea, your partner/s will too; if they have it, so do you.)

Help!
Gonorrhea

Expect results in 7–10 days

• **Take drugs**. Really.

• During and after your course of antibiotics, eat lots of **yogurt**.

• Take an antibacterial herbal tincture (page 165), too; four or more dropperfuls a day.

• Diagnosis of gonorrhea is simple for men, but complicated for women. The bacteria hide in the cervix among many other similar organisms, so only a tissue culture can give a clear result.

• Half of the women who have gonorrhea also have chlamydia.

• Undiagnosed and untreated gonorrhea infections are a major cause of PID and infertility.[73] In rare cases, it is fatal. A serious chronic vaginal discharge may indicate gonorrhea.

Step 2. *Engage the Energy*

• The **homeopathic remedy** for watery, cold discharges from the pelvis is the tissue salt *Natrum muriaticum.*

★ Homeopaths use *Medorrhinum*, the gonorrhea nosode, not to treat gonorrhea, but to restore and insure genetic health, to protect progeny, and to counter ancestral gonorrhea. (See page 167.)

Step 3. *Nourish and Tonify*

★ Barriers provide excellent protection against gonorrhea.

Step 4. *Stimulate/Sedate*

• The Heroic anti-gonorrhea/syphilis formula on page 373 is an example of a "blood-cleansing" herbal combination that will, no doubt, make you run to the bathroom, but won't, alas, cure a bacterial STD. Lavish, hourly doses of herbal antibiotic, antibacterial tinctures such as usnea, echinacea (page 342), yarrow, or myrrh, could help. As could antibiotics *and* herbs.

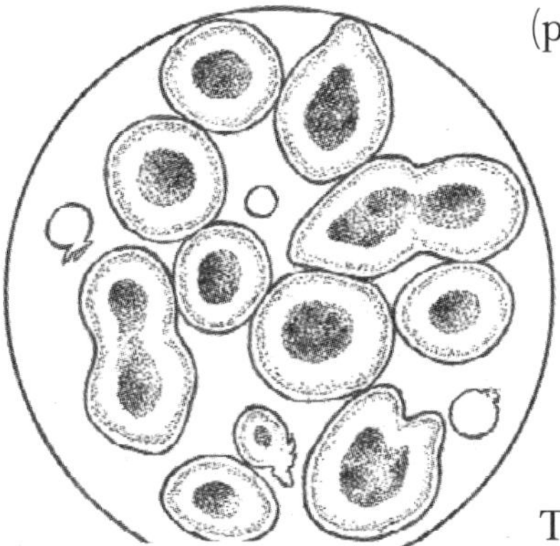

Gonorrhea

Step 5. *Use Drugs*

"This is a 'bad bugs–no drugs' issue."[74]

• Most strains of gonorrhea are now resistant to most antibiotics such as penicillin and tetracycline. They have recently become resistant to ciprofloxacin and fluoroquinolones, the previous drugs of choice. Only injected cephalosporins remain effective.[75] Spectinomycin (Trobicin) is used when gonorrhea infects the throat.

Strains of gonorrhea currently found in Asia, Indonesia, and Hawaii are frequently resistant to virtually all antibiotics.

Syphilis (*Treponema pallidum*)

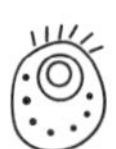

Step 1. *Collect Information*

• Syphilis is a spiral-shaped bacterium or spirochete. It is an ancient STD whose symptoms were accurately described by Chinese healers more than 5000 years ago.

★ There are only two ways to contract syphilis: from penetrative sexual contact or from a transfusion of infected blood.

• According to the Centers for Disease Control and Prevention, there were a total of 40,920 Americans with syphilis in 2007.[76] Men who have sex with men account for 64 percent of these.[77] Syphilis infections peak in cycles of 8–11 years. Infection rates dropped between 1990 and 2000, then began to move up again.[78]

• Diagnosis is by blood test, but a negative test is not reliable until three months after initial exposure.

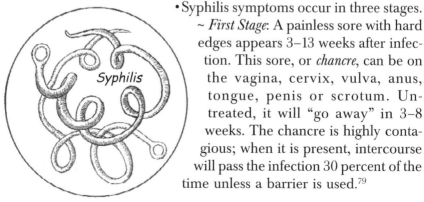

• Syphilis symptoms occur in three stages.

~ *First Stage*: A painless sore with hard edges appears 3–13 weeks after infection. This sore, or *chancre*, can be on the vagina, cervix, vulva, anus, tongue, penis or scrotum. Untreated, it will "go away" in 3–8 weeks. The chancre is highly contagious; when it is present, intercourse will pass the infection 30 percent of the time unless a barrier is used.[79]

~ *Second Stage*: An itchless whole body rash (even the soles of the feet are affected), swollen lymph nodes, sore throat, headache, hair loss, weight loss, and general distress caused by syphilis in the blood. Genital sores can reappear. Untreated, all these symptoms also "go away" – deeper into the organs – in 2–6 weeks.

~ *Third Stage*: Two-thirds of those infected will suffer no further symptoms.[80] But 20–30 percent will have their eyes, liver, kidneys, heart, bones, and brains damaged – some will go insane, some will die.

Step 2. *Engage the Energy*

• Homeopaths believe infections from syphilis, gonorrhea, and TB reverberate through the generations. Geneticists have recently confirmed that our DNA can be influenced by things that happen to our parents *before* they conceive us. *Syphilinum*, the **syphilis nosode**, helps prevent past/future generational syphilitic effects.

Step 3. *Nourish and Tonify*

• Those with strong immune systems are less likely to be adversely affected by syphilis. More seaweed! More mushrooms!

Step 4. *Stimulate/Sedate*

• According to herbalist Michael Castleman, historically, "remedies [used to treat syphilis] were known euphemistically as blood purifiers." No one wanted a remedy for venereal disease (VD), as that would imply – correctly –that they had "a case." Finally, I understand what all those blood-cleansing herbs are really meant to do: Get rid of syphilis. Aha!

Help!
Syphilis

Expect results in 10–20 days

★ **Take drugs**. Really. And while you are taking them also:

• Eat lots of **yogurt**.

• Take a dropperful of **astragalus** tincture daily for a month.

• Take 1 drop of **poke** root tincture daily for two weeks.

• Consider *Syphilinum* (above).

• Every powerful herb in the world has been used to counter syphilis, often with gratifying results. Most infected individuals remain reasonably healthy (often despite treatment). Lacking blood tests, previous healers had no way to know if the herbs – or the odds – were in their favor.

★ Syphilis is a high-risk infection. *Antibiotics are the best medicine.* If you wish to try herbs, be sure to have blood tests at least every three months to gauge your progress.

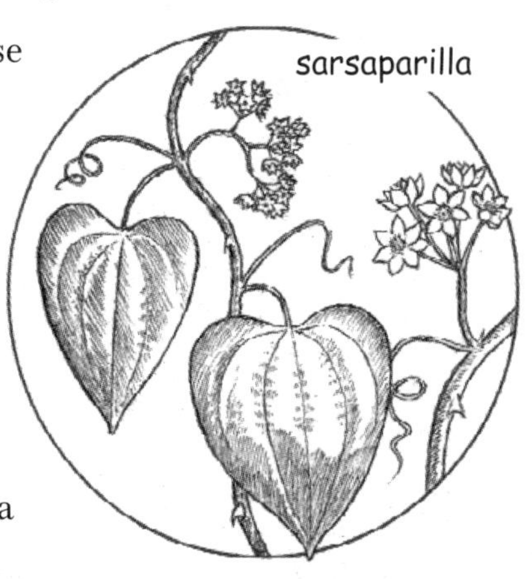

• Heroic herbalists treated those with syphilis by "cleansing" them with powerful cathartic herbs and decoctions of **burdock**, **barberry**, **Oregon grape**, **white pond lily**, **poke**, **sassafras**, and **sarsaparilla** roots.

Sarsaparilla is not anti-syphilitic, despite being listed as such in the *U.S. Pharmacopoeia* from 1820 to 1882. Poke root may be, but as a fresh root tincture, not as a tea.

• More "use-at-your-own-risk" herbal remedies – chosen from those listed in Christopher Sauer's *America's First Book of Botanic Healing,* published serially from 1762 to 1778 – for countering "the French pox" (syphilis):

~ **Colocynth melon** (*Cucumis colocynthis*)

• To use: Pour white wine over half a fresh melon in a glass vessel. Let stand, well covered, overnight. Pour off the clearest part, warm, and drink. "Continue for six days, while doing, avoid cold air, and in this manner be freed of this nasty affliction sooner than by any other method."

~ **Fumitory** (*Fumaria officinalis*)

• To use: Chop and infuse in goat's milk; drink a tumblerful day and night for six weeks.

~ **Lignum vitae** (*Guaiacum off.*) • To use: Combine 8 ounces lignum vitae with 2 ounces *Smilax* or burdock, 2 ounces sassafras, 1 ounce fennel seed, and 1½ ounces each powdered antimony and Zante currants. Add to one gallon water and boil for several hours. Strain; take one-quarter cup day and night.

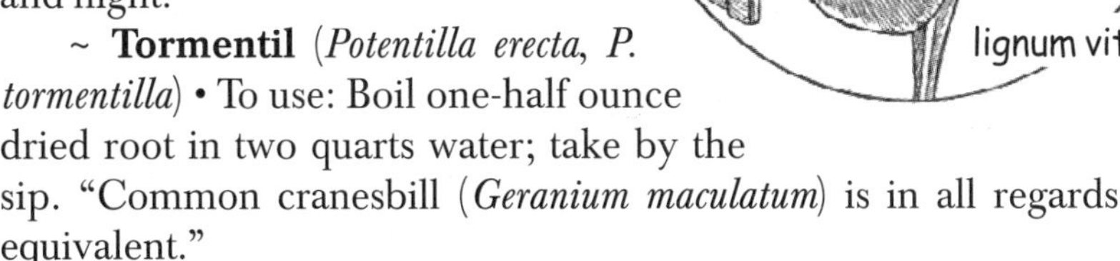

~ **Tormentil** (*Potentilla erecta, P. tormentilla*) • To use: Boil one-half ounce dried root in two quarts water; take by the sip. "Common cranesbill (*Geranium maculatum*) is in all regards equivalent."

★ Complementary medicines enhance the effects of antibiotic drugs, helping to prevent recurrences. For optimum results, I use a dropperful dose of one **immune-strengthening herb** – such as **astragalus** root, **eleuthero** root, **schizandra** berries, or medicinal **mushrooms** – plus a dose of one **infection-fighting herb** – such as **echinacea** root (3 dropperfuls), **yarrow** herb (1 dropperful), or **poke** root (1–4 drops) – taken 2–4 times a day.

Step 5. *Use Drugs*

★ Treatment of syphilis with penicillin during the first two stages is 98 percent successful. Other antibiotics have a 90 percent cure rate. A brief, but severe, flu-like reaction, which can cause miscarriage or early labor, is an expected result of treatment.

Step 6. *Break and Enter*

• If you are in the third stage of syphilis infection, your doctor may recommend a spinal tap to check for infection in the nervous system. Consider carefully; spinal taps carry risks.

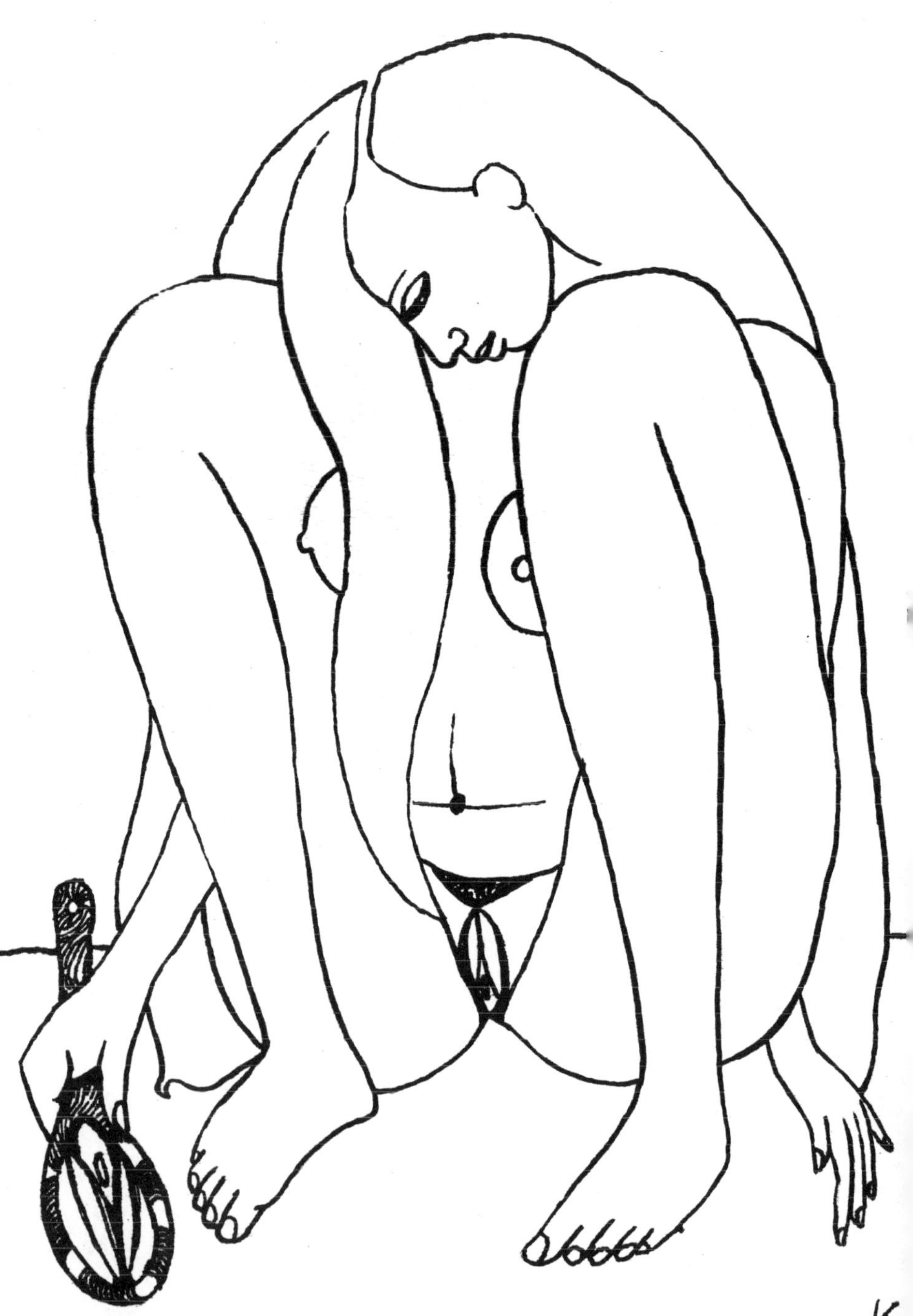
K

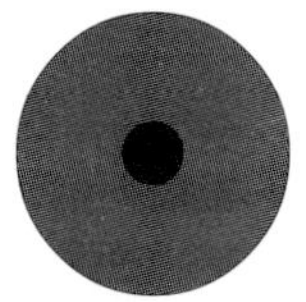

The Cervix

I am the portal; I am the door. I connect inside to outside, outside to in. I determine; I decide. I open; I close. I reveal; I conceal. I preface the passage of birth. I mark the boundary. I pulse within you.

I am the window; I am the porthole. I am the guardian; I am the gate. Neither mucus nor blood, slime nor semen, may pass without my consent. None may leave, and none enter, except by my grace. I hold the wise blood. I hold the growing babe. Until it is time to open. Then . . . blood flows! Sperm swims! Babe is born!

I am the mark of the sun. Dare you reach inside to touch my hidden mystery? I am but a finger's length away.

Put the tip of your finger upon me, withdraw it and observe. Can you pull strings of fertile mucus from thumb to finger? Do your fingers stick together a little? Is there blood?

Trust my judgment. I am not innocent, now or ever. I am sensitive as the best hound's nose, authoritative as the wisest crone. My knowledge is deep and certain. My single eye sees true. (Women in India maintain that I have two eyes, and both see true.) Trust me, and I will teach you much.

I know how to be firm and potent. I know how to stand strong. I know how to be loose and soft. I know how to efface myself and make way, how to stretch wide in sweet surrender. Trust me to know the difference. Trust me to guide you.

I am the mouth of your womb. I am your cervix.

Healthy Cervix

Your cervix is the neck of your uterus. It lies in the upper part of the vagina. It looks like a pink donut, a donut with a smiling hole if you've given birth vaginally.

A thin layer of cells, called the epithelium, covers the cervix. The epithelium has two kinds of cells: ones that grow in columns, and ones that are flat and scaly. The columnar cells make up the inner surface of the cervix (the donut hole) and are red, like facial lips. The flat squamous cells make up the outer surface (the donut) and are pink, like the inside of facial lips. The place where they meet is the squamo-columnar junction, or transition zone.

A healthy cervix is full of changes. Sometimes it is closed and high in the vagina. Other times, it drops down and opens slightly to let menstrual blood out and sperm in. During ovulation it produces fertile (stretchy) mucus to aid fertilization. The cervix thins during labor and opens wide (10cm) so the baby can move through it.

Medical opinion holds that the cervix is "insensitive to pain," an opinion that I, and every woman who has read this book in manuscript form, challenge with our personal experiences. My cervix feels both pain *and* pleasure. Does yours?

Look at Your Healthy Cervix

Imagine how difficult it would be to keep your lips, eyes, chin and cheeks healthy and looking good if you never looked at them. Though it may seem odd, looking at your cervix and touching it, at least once in your life, is important to your health.

Touch your cervix by squatting – or by placing one foot on a chair – and inserting your fingers into your vagina. The cervix feels like a nose. If you wish, you can wiggle it from side to side.

Looking at your cervix gives you clues to your overall health as well as an early warning of infections. (You'll also see normal wear and tear from childbirth, intercourse, or surgical procedures.)

It's easy to look at your cervix.

You'll need a mirror, a flashlight, a plastic speculum (to open the vagina), lubricant, and some private time and space (though I have done this in groups). Insert the lubricated speculum, lean back, shine the light on the mirror and angle it so the light reflects up into the vagina. There's your cervix. Wow!

A healthy, fertile cervix is pink with a small, round, red mouth, the os, in the center. Before puberty – when pink squamous cells grow across it – the entire cervix is red. After a vaginal birth, the os curves into a smile. After menopause, it is small and tight.

If your cervix is infected, irritated, or abnormal, it will look lumpy, bumpy, red, and weepy. If HPV has colonized it, it will look fine unless you paint it – using a long-handled watercolor brush – with acetic acid (vinegar), which turns HPV lesions white.

A reference book – such as *A New View of a Woman's Body*[1] – can help you interpert what you're seeing.

How do you get a speculum? Ask for the one they use the next time you have a gynecological checkup. Or simply ask for a mirror and look at your cervix right there in the doctor's office!

> "Learning to look at my cervix was one of the most empowering things ever. I kept looking until the speculum broke."[2]

Keeping your cervix healthy is a lot like keeping your whole self healthy. Give it loving attention: regular visual and tactile inspections, freedom from trauma, and a diet well supplied with protein and healthy fats. The cervix is part of the uterus. Keep it healthy with uterine tonics such as raspberry leaf infusion, motherwort tincture, cooked leafy greens, and pelvic floor exercises.

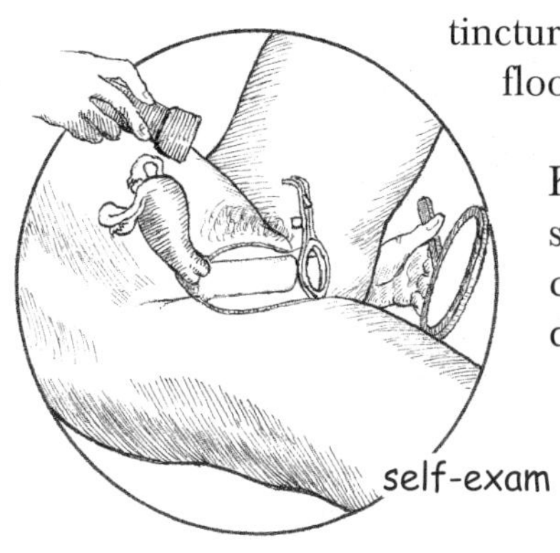

The cervix is part of the vagina. Keep it infection-free with vaginal safeguards like yogurt, safe sex, discriminating taste in lovers, and freedom from constricting clothing.

The cervix is a doorway and a teacher. Take the time to listen to, and heed, its messages.

Cervical Distresses

Although generally tough and hardy, the cervix is vulnerable to abrasion and infection. If yours looks red, you may have: an STD (page 143), **acute** or **chronic cervicitis** (below), **eversion** or **erosion** (next page), **HPV** (page 176), **dysplasia** (page 189), even **cancer** (page 196). **Pap smears** (page 184) can catch cervical cancer early, but often lead to unnecessary and harmful treatments.

Cervicitis

Acute cervicitis is any sudden, intense reddening, swelling, or bleeding of the cervix. Symptoms – if they are present – include pain with intercourse, genital itching and burning, and/or a vaginal discharge. Acute cervicitis can follow a difficult birth, surgical procedures, or trauma. It can be triggered by hormonal drugs such as birth control pills or by irritation from an IUD string. Most often, however, cervicitis is caused by infective organisms such as trich, candida, or hemophilus. Treatments that counter these infections will eliminate the cervicitis.

In the absence of infection, daily application of **aloe vera gel**, **honey**, or **vitamin E oil** directly on the cervix for 2–3 weeks is generally effective. (Use your fingers or a tampon.)

Chronic cervicitis is a persistent, recurring inflammation of the cervix. Years of untreated, unchecked cervical infections and irritations cause the cervix to thicken, cysts to grow and protrude, and scars from childbirth and gynecological procedures to weaken and become vulnerable to deep infections. Symptoms – such as abdominal discomfort, a foul-smelling discharge, or deep pelvic pain – may come and go.

Surgery, antibiotics, or harsh herbs are the most common treatments; they clear away inflamed cervical tissues, like using heavy machinery to scrape the land bare, making way for something new. Instead, like careful gardeners, we can counter infections (page 143), reverse precancerous changes (page 189), and increase the health of the woman and her cervix. Surgery and drugs are a last resort if 12 months pass without improvement.

Cervical Eversion and Erosion

Cervical eversion and erosion are so similar they are frequently confused, even by doctors. In both, the red, inner-surface (columnar) cells of the cervix grow too quickly and push aside the pink, outer-surface (squamous) cells. Cervical eversion requires no treatment. If it is confused with erosion, a precancerous change, unnecessary and potentially harmful treatment is likely.

When the cervix is **everted**, or turned inside out, it has a clear line between the red and pink cells. Eversion may be caused by prescription hormones; the cervix will return to normal if they are discontinued. Congenital eversions are present from birth and may be prominent during pregnancy, but generally disappear after menopause. Eversion is not a problem; there is no remedy.

A cervical **erosion** lacks a clear dividing line between the red and pink cells. Any red cervix may be deemed "eroded." "[Erosion] conjures up a frightening picture of the cervix wasting away like bare earth after a heavy rain, [and] is not only erroneous, but absurd."[3] Nothing is sloughing off; there is no erosion. Just the opposite: cells are growing too rapidly, jostling for space, creating dysplasia (page 189). Fear of cancer causes doctors to push birth control pills and surgery as treatments. Instead, try daily applications of honeysuckle tincture (page 200), comfrey leaf sitz baths, and 1–3 quarts of red clover infusion weekly for at least a month.

Before You Agree to Surgery

Any fast-growing or abnormal cells could be, or could become, cancer. That's why you'll be urged to have surgery to remove "eroded" cervical tissue, genital warts, or dysplasia.

Give yourself some time to try the successful alternatives gathered here.

Surgical procedures – including endometrial biopsy, D&C, aspiration extraction of the contents of the womb, radiation implantation, cone biopsy, cryosurgery, and laser ablation – can *cause* cervicitis or cervical erosion, especially if there is a concurrent, untreated cervical/vaginal infection.

Genital Warts
Human Papilloma Virus (HPV)

"I am Grandmother Growth. I nourish and protect all growing things. I am the Grandmother of all life. I am the Grandmother of plants and animals, fish and insects. I am your Grandmother. And I am the Grandmother of bacteria and viruses, too.

"Feel the life throbbing in your body – your blood, your breath, your nerves and muscles. Now feel the other lives that live with you, in you, on you. There are more bacteria in your gut than there are cells in your body.

"When you are healthy, these bacteria and other microorganisms vibrate with you. They add to your health; they become part of the dance that is you. When your rhythm falters, they falter too. Bacteria and viruses that interfere with your health thrive and take over. Unless your immune system takes action, they can usurp the dance of your life.

"Your immune system is nourished by true pride. It falters, and may fail, when fed blame and shame and guilt. Healthy genitals are proud genitals. Healthy sexuality is about loving oneself as well as another. Be pleased with what is between your legs, dearest one. Be secure in yourself.

"Walk tall. Laugh often. Be flexible. Fill yourself with life and you will have little to fear from most viruses."

Help!
Genital Warts/HPV

Visible warts: results in 2 weeks

- Apply fresh **celandine sap** or **thuja oil** (caution) daily to wart.

Cervical lesions: results in 2–3 months

- Take a dropperful of **St. Joan's wort** tincture 2–4 times a day.
- Drink/cook with **astragalus**.

Step 0: *Do Nothing*

★ ". . . for women who exhibit the earliest signs of HPV infection, the best prescription may be no treatment at all," says Karyn Herndon. "Three out of four women . . . lost their flat warts . . . suggesting that the body's immune system can drive the virus into a dormant state."[4]

• Having an HPV infection is "like having the sniffles," according to Anna-Barbara Moscicki, MD. "It's an infection your body can usually handle . . . and get rid of."[5] Seventy percent of infections are gone within one year; 90 percent are gone in two years.[6]

• In a ten-year study of sexually-active women aged 13–21, half became infected with HPV. Seventy percent of those women (105) did not develop lesions or warts at all. Of those who did (45), only 10 percent (4.5) were diagnosed with cervical cancer.[7]

• The more sexual partners a woman has, and the younger her age when she begins, the more likely she is to become infected with human papilloma virus. However, even virgins can get genital warts (from toilet seats or wet towels). So much for not doing it! Neither celibacy nor oral sex (HPV infects the throat, causing cancer there, too) will protect you. Read on!

Step 1: *Collect information*

• Medically, warts are *papilloma*; they are caused by papilloma viruses. There are more than one hundred known papilloma viruses. Some are generalists, causing warts anywhere on the skin or mucus surfaces, but most are quite specific and fussy about where they'll live.

Prevent Genital Warts/HPV

• HPV can live in, and be passed from, the skin of the scrotum, the perineum, and the anus – areas left uncovered by male condoms. **Female condoms**, which cover the vulva (outer tissues) as well as the vagina, offer better protection.[8] HPVs can be spread via oral sex, genital-to-genital contact, intercourse, and frottage.

• **Lesbians**, **nuns**, and women whose sexual partners are **circumcised** have the least HPV, genital warts and cervical cancer.[9]

• Gardasil, a genetically-engineered serum, triggers antibody responses against four cancer-promoting HPVs. It is expensive, well-tested,[10] controversial, and effective only if given *before* infection with HPV occurs. Gardasil does not protect against all HPVs.

• Many of the papilloma viruses are noncontagious, but some – especially those that give rise to plantar warts and genital warts – are not only contagious, but widespread and stealthy. The large group of human papilloma viruses are resilient enough to live outside the body. In a warm, moist place, skin cells containing them can remain infectious for several days.[11] Symptomless people can infect others.

• Genital warts caused by HPVs are the ones we get "down there." Genital warts are also called *condyloma acuminata*, *cervical warts*, *venereal warts*, or *moist warts*. Genital warts infect men and women equally, but are more commonly diagnosed in women. (Babies can be infected, especially orally, during the birth process if the mother has cervical or vaginal warts.[12]) Some of the HPVs that cause genital warts are benign; others can give rise to deadly cancers.

• HPVs primarily infect the tissues of the vagina, cervix, penis, urethra, anus, and throat, causing visible warts on the external genitalia and invisible warts elsewhere, such as on the cervix, usually within nine months of infection.

• Warts on the labia and inside the vagina are noticeable, but generally don't itch or hurt. Warts on or in the cervix, anus, urethra, and throat are invisible as well as painless. They are usually detected only by medical professionals searching for them.

The genital warts we can see are nothing to worry about.
It's the ones we can't see that are the troublemakers.

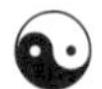 Especially for Men 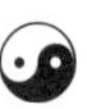

If a woman has genital warts, the Centers for Disease Control and Prevention do *not* recommend testing her male sexual partners for HPV, since "there is no cure," and more than 80 percent of men already carry it in their urethra, or on their penis/scrotum.

HPVs living in the rectum can initiate anal/rectal cancers. Ninety-five percent of HIV-positive men living in cities are infected with anal HPV, as are 60 percent of urban men who are HIV-negative.[13]

• Genital warts can be flat, smooth, tall, stalked, or even cauliflower-like. They often grow in clusters, but may occur singly.

• HPV is the most common sexually transmitted disease in the USA and Europe. There are more than six million new cases a year in the USA.[14] At least 50 percent of all sexually active people will be infected over their lifetime. During a three-year study, 40 percent of a group of female college students got HPV infections.[15]

• Of the twenty types of HPVs which colonize the genital area, four are known to initiate cervical cancer, the leading cause of death from cancer for women in Africa, Asia, and India.[16] HPVs also cause penile and anal/rectal cancers, and aggressive squamous-cell cancers of the throat, head, neck, and tonsils.[17] Fortunately, only a small percentage of HPV infections do this. And we can do much to insure we aren't in that small percentage.

Once infected with human papilloma virus, you are infected for life.
There is no known cure.
The best strategy is to nourish the immune system.

Step 2: *Engage the energy*

★ Swiss herbalist Rina Nissim considers homeopathic *Thuja* the "ground remedy" for the genitals. It is especially indicated when there are genital warts.[18] Higher dilutions, such as 30C, are best.

• Reiki keeps the cervix healthy. (Self-administered is fine.)

Step 3: *Nourish and tonify*

• Well-nourished immune systems clear HPV infections. The stressed immune systems of those who are pregnant, smoke, are poor or malnourished, have a systemic infection or cancer, or are HIV-positive may allow an HPV infection to go on to cancer.

• **Nourish immunity** with whole grains, cooked greens, roots, cabbage-family plants, organic dairy products and meats, onions, garlic, seaweed, mushrooms, and nourishing herbal infusions.

★ **Astragalus root**, taken daily or every other day as a tincture (a dropperful or more), or cooked into food, is a tasty, effective immune system tonic. Herbalist Anne McIntyre uses herbs that target abnormal cervical cells – burdock, calendula, plantain, myrrh, and rose – along with astragalus, nettle, and dandelion.[19]

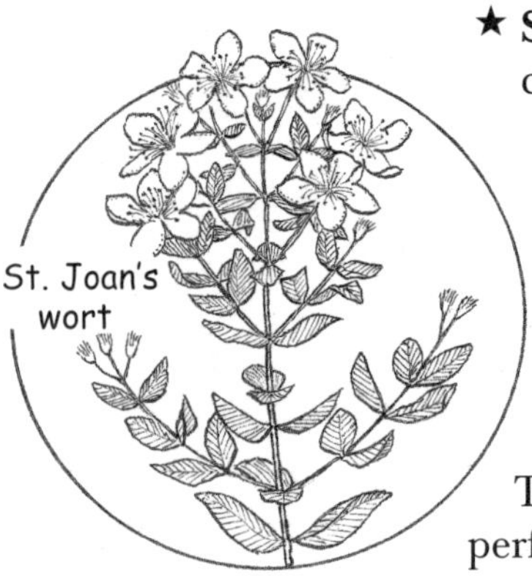

St. Joan's wort

★ **St. Joan's wort** has antiviral actions that can interfere with a wide range of viruses including HPV and HIV. Tincture of the fresh plant – even when taken in large, frequent doses for many years – kills viruses without triggering sun sensitivity. But use of tea, capsules, or isolated alkaloids can cause solar hypersensitivity.

To *prevent* a viral infection, I use one dropperful of St. Joan's wort tincture in a little water three or four times a day for a few days. To *treat* viral infections, I take a dropperful in water every 1–2 hours until symptoms abate, and continue with less frequent doses until I no longer need it. *Possible drug interaction*: Large or frequent doses of St. Joan's wort improve liver function so much that pharmaceutical drugs may be eliminated too quickly to be effective. **Do not use if you have an organ transplant.**

★ **Lemon balm** and/or **hyssop** ointment is effective against both venereal warts and herpes. (Make it: page 367.)

Step 4: *Stimulate/Sedate*

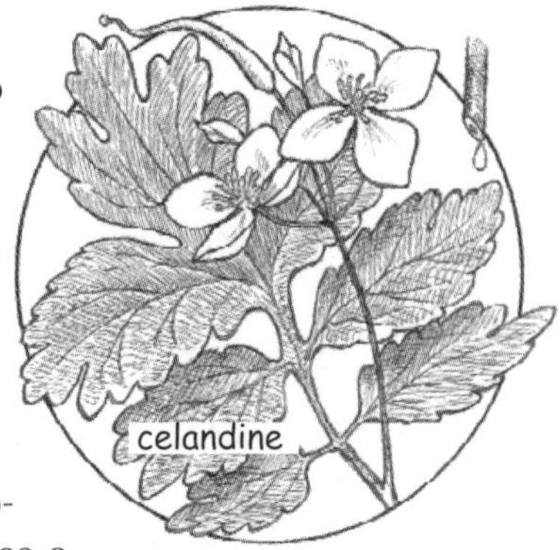

★ **Celandine** is my favorite herb for removing external warts. Application of the bright yellow/orange sap is safe, painless, and easy, for those who live where it grows. I've found this evergreen plant in vacant lots and open spaces in temperate-zone cities around the world. **Fresh sap** from leaf stalks or the roots is applied directly to the wart at least once a day until it is gone. Topical applications of tincture can be used, but with much less effect.

celandine

★ **American mandrake** is the queen of external genital wart removal when used in a concentrated form – podophyllin – as a topical treatment. Podophyllin has severe side-effects: burns that leave scars; death; and birth defects or fetal death if used while pregnant. All skin except for the warts must be thoroughly covered with petroleum jelly before application, and the podophyllin wiped off before it penetrates too deeply, usually in 1–4 hours. Weekly treatments over six or more weeks are the norm. A less concentrated, safer form – podofilox – is available by prescription for use at home. Celandine sap is even safer and more fun; trichloroacetic acid (page 182) is safe, too.

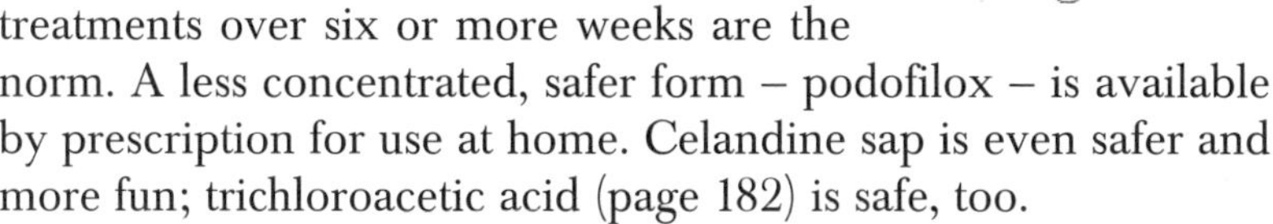

• Women who applied an ointment containing a protein found in **breast milk** reduced their HPV lesions by 75 percent. The protein – alpha-lactalbumin – "selectively induces apoptosis [cellular death] in tumor cells."[20] Perhaps fresh breast milk would work too?

Her Story

Zes is a 24-year-old disabled lesbian.

"I had a large cluster of genital warts above my clitoris and several smaller ones around my anal and vaginal openings. Atypically, they were itchy and bothered me, perhaps because I was also infected with the skin parasite scabies. My diet is generally inadequate in protein and fat, although I do make an honest effort to eat well on a very limited budget.

"I purchased some celandine tincture last winter and applied it to my warts three times a day. Within a week they were noticeably smaller. Despite faithful applications for several more weeks, the warts shrank no further. Then the snow melted and I found a patch of celandine growing right by my back door!

"The first application of fresh sap turned the warts almost black. Three days and six applications later, the main group was very dark and crisp at the edges, while the warts in the moister areas turned white. On the sixth day of treatment, the large group of warts peeled off and the others were clearly disintegrating. Good-bye to my warts!"

• **Thuja** tincture or essential oil (EO) applied cautiously to genital warts can "burn" them off. Herbalist Deb Soule mixes 25 drops of thuja EO into one ounce of infused calendula, comfrey, and/or St. Joan's wort oil.

• Other "burners" include the sap from papaya, figs, or dandelion stems.

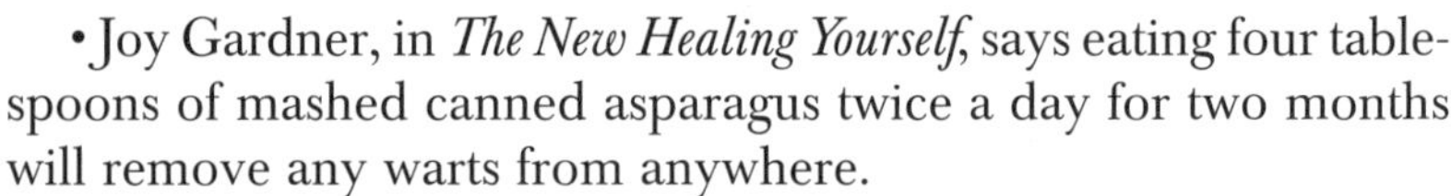

• Joy Gardner, in *The New Healing Yourself*, says eating four tablespoons of mashed canned asparagus twice a day for two months will remove any warts from anywhere.

• HPV infections peak during the summer. Sunlight somehow helps it colonize tissues, and may make it more cancer-causing.[21]

Step 5: *Use drugs*

★ **Trichloroacetic acid**, applied in the doctor's office weekly for six weeks, is as effective as podophyllin in removing warts, but less likely to leave scars; and it is safe to use during pregnancy.[22]

• Aldara (5% topical cream) clears genital warts from 50 percent of those who apply it every other day for three months. There are few adverse effects and a low recurrence rate. (Warts grow back 72 percent of the time with other treatments.[23])

Step 6: *Break and enter*

> "It is not known how many women who have had expensive [painful] laser surgery or . . . cryosurgery are informed beforehand that the treatment is purely cosmetic and has a high recurrence rate."[24]

★ Women treated with laser removal of cervical warts were *twice as likely* as untreated women to have precancerous and cancerous changes occur in the following years.

• If a colposcopy shows warts or lesions, standard practice is to remove them. Read on before allowing *any* invasive procedures, even a biopsy, even if it seems "minimally" invasive.

• Colposcopy is a harmless close examination of the cervix with magnifying binoculars. But the vast majority of doctors will assume you've agreed to a biopsy if you agree to a colposcopy. Biopsy forceps "chomp" out pieces of cervical tissue for a pathology exam. You can refuse the colposcopy; or clearly refuse a biopsy with it. Ask for an HPV-DNA test instead. (*See* next entry.)

★ Testing cervical cells for DNA from cancer-causing HPV strains is as reliable as a biopsy, and less expensive. Screening every women over twenty every two years for HPV-DNA would reduce the number of cervical biopsies by 60 percent.[25] Any woman whose cervical cells are negative for HPV – and about 45 percent do – does not need a colposcopy. Even if her test is positive for HPV, there's still only a 10–20 percent chance she'll need treatment.[26]

★ Invasive treatments are detailed on page 194. Before you agree to any procedure, remember: Surgery doesn't cure HPV. **Removal of infected tissues does not remove the virus.** HPV remains in the body, ready to recur when the immune system is at an ebb. In fact, surgery is a major stress to the immune system, and can increase the chances that a given lesion will progress to cancer. Give Wise Woman ways a chance first.

> "Regardless of treatment, one in four HPV-infected people will have a recurrence within three months."[27]

Her Story

Sarina is a young inner-city mom of four.

"When my yearly Pap smear revealed abnormal cells, I was frightened. One of my friends died of cervical cancer just last year.

"The specialist I consulted said I should have a colposcopy and a biopsy. I trusted the doctor's opinion, so I did it. I was positive for HPV, so I followed the doctor's advice and had cryosurgery.

"In fact, I had cryosurgery 7 times in 3 years, but the HPV kept recurring. Then they told me I needed to have a cone biopsy. I finally stood up and said 'No! No more.' They'd led me to believe that cryosurgery was a cure. No one said my HPV lesions would just come back.

"Now I'm really taking care of myself: eating well, paying attention to myself and my needs. I've stopped fooling myself; screening tests don't make me healthy. I make me healthy."

Pap Smear

"Who can be trusted?" says Grandmother Growth with a warm smile. "Who will tell you if there are abnormal cells growing down there? Can you trust a test? Can your trust yourself?

"You can trust yourself. Your inner wisdom is trustworthy. Tests are a linear reading of a spiraling process. They may or may not tell the truth. Listen to yourself. Honor yourself. Trust yourself.

"Yes, it takes some practice to trust yourself. Yes, it is not easy to tell the difference between unreasonable fear and a distressing truth. Your Wise Healer Within is on the job, ready to tell you how you are. This voice, like mine, is here to help you. It will tell you what you need to tend to. It will visit you in dreams. It will bring memories. And, if you take the time to listen to your inner wisdom, it will warn you long before cancer can threaten.

"This test cannot harm you. But your fear of cancer may push you to agree to harmful treatments. Trust your inner voice. Be confident in yourself. If the test results differ, either way, from your inner knowing, disregard the outer information and pay attention to the inner wisdom.

"If your inner wisdom says something is amiss, investigate further, no matter what the test results. If, however, you know that all is well, yet you test positive, refuse further tests and treatments; retest later."

The pathologist George Papanicolaou pioneered the Pap smear, a non-invasive screening test for cervical abnormalities, in the 1920s. A Pap smear neither diagnoses cancer, nor gives assurance that there is no cancer. False negatives occur 10–20 percent of the time.[28]

A Pap smear is a sample of the tissues of the cervix (and sometimes vagina). It is most convenient for the sampler if the samplee lies on her back and puts her feet up in stirrups. This position is psychologically distressing for some women. If it is for you, you can let the examiner know you want to put your feet down on the examining table or to draw your knees up and hold them with your hands. Breathe deeply and relax. With the knees lifted and spread, the vulva is visible and a speculum can be gently fitted into the vagina, allowing the cervix to be seen.

Cells are collected from the outer surface of the cervix, as well as from inside the cervical os, with a small blunt implement and a tiny brush. This is akin to using your fingernail to scrape cells from the inside of your cheek. It is non-invasive and there is rarely any bleeding. Depending on the sensitivity of your cervix, you may have sensations that range from "didn't feel a thing" to "ouch, that hurt!"

The collected cells are either preserved in liquid (best) or smeared directly on a slide and sent to a lab. Liquid preservation is required for HPV-DNA testing. At the lab, a pathologist (or a computer) "reads" Pap smears by looking at your cells under microscopic magnification. Any abnormal cellular changes are noted. Because people are different, having a smear read by a different lab may give different results.

To get the truest reading, keep your vagina in its natural state for at least one, and up to three, days prior to having a Pap smear: avoid douching, intercourse, spermicides, vaginal hygiene products and sprays, and the insertion of boluses, pessaries, or hormonal creams. If you are menstruating or have had vigorous sex the night before, cancel your Pap smear. It won't be accurate.

The original Pap smear classifications confused both patients and doctors, resulting in hundreds of thousands of women being frightened into harsh, and unnecessary, treatments.[29]

In 1988, the new Bethesda classifications were introduced with the goal of reducing overtreatment. The number of categories of results was increased to provide more specific information about the cells in the smear. Unfortunately, the new categories have doubled the number of women receiving abnormal results.[30] Thus, instead of fewer needless hysterectomies and drug prescriptions, twice as many women are now overtreated. Protect yourself. Read about dysplasia (page 189) before agreeing to any treatment.

> "Unfortunately, informed consent rarely enters the Pap test equation. . . . The need to be fully informed about the risks as well as benefits is even stronger for anyone undergoing a screening test, which by definition is given to healthy people without symptoms."[31]

• There are at least thirty different variations in the spectrum from healthy to cancerous cervical cells.

• There is controversy about what level of abnormality requires further tests or treatment, and also about how often women need to have a Pap smear done.

• The Bethesda classifications, in order, from the best to the worst [*with conservative treatment guidelines in brackets*]:

Negative for lesions [*do nothing*]
Organisms present [*do nothing*]
ASC-US (Atypical squamous cells of undetermined significance) [*retest in 3–6 months, or colposcopy*]
ASC-H (Atypical cells, some high-grade) [*colposcopy*]
LSIL (Low-grade squamous intraepithelial lesion) [*colposcopy*]
HSIL (High-grade squamous intraepithelial lesion; dysplasia; cervical carcinoma in situ) [*colposcopy*]
AGC: Atypical glandular cells [*colposcopy*]
CIN II/III (cervical intraepithelial neoplasia) [*colposcopy*]
AIS: Endocervical adenocarcinoma in situ [*surgery*]
Squamous cell carcinoma [*surgery*]
Adenocarcinoma [*surgery*]

Pap Abnormalities — What to Do?

> "For every person who benefits from early detection, many more are diagnosed with a [non-threatening] cancer they did not need to know about [or treat]."[32]

★ If your Pap report is "bad," depending on how bad it is, it's safe to **wait 1–6 months and then redo it**. You don't have to agree to any treatment or even any more diagnostic tests. Up to two quarts of **red clover infusion** a week helps normalize cells.

• Conservative guidelines say all women with ASC-US need a colposcopy.[33] Using a HPV-DNA test to distinguish between those with ASC-US who are HPV-positive and those who are HPV-negative, positions only positives to colposcopies. Negatives are monitored with repeat Pap smears; 99.5 percent of women with abnormal cells who are negative for HPV-DNA are cancer-free.[34]

• Classifications between ASC-US and CIN II/III denote increasing risk of cancer. Ask your Wise Healer Within if you can wait and watch (and drink red clover infusion), or if you need to take action now.

• Women with CIN II/III do need a colposcopic examination, and probably a biopsy, but may wish to use alternative treatments additionally. Only half of those with CIN III will progress to cervical cancer in a five-year period.[35] Be in the other half!

• Women dealing with cervical dysplasia or cervical cancer (including *endocervical adenocarcinoma in situ, squamous cell carcinoma,* and *adenocarcinoma*) will find help starting on page 196.

Pap Smear — How Often?

• The American Cancer Society says *all* women under the age of 65 should have a *yearly* Pap smear. This includes women without a uterus (one-third of hysterectomies done in the USA leave the cervix) and even those without a cervix. (Smears from the vagina can reveal vaginal cancer.)

• With the onset of puberty, as part of a young woman's rite of passage, schedule a Pap smear. Remember, it isn't necessary to have sex to be infected with HPV or to get cervical cancer.

• In countries with socialized health care, Pap smears are done every third year since cervical cancer grows so slowly. This is becoming the norm in the US as well, especially for women over thirty who have had three clear smears in three years.

• Pap test results are notoriously inaccurate, both in missed cancers and in false alarms. Yearly testing "makes up" for this. New biomarker tests "identify 50 percent more precancerous lesions than Pap smears," but are only 88 percent accurate.[36]

• Computerized screening (PAPNET) promised to correct false results from human-read Pap smears, but has actually increased ambiguous findings and overtreatment.[37]

• The **safest** and most conservative plan – for sexually-active women who are under the age of 25, for sexually-active women of any age who have multiple partners, and for any woman whose sole partner has other partners – is to have regular, yearly Pap smears.

• However – given that women who have annual Pap smears are the most likely to be overtreated – the safest course may not be the healthiest thing to do! If your doctor wants to follow up on your Pap smear by doing invasive tests or treatments, **protect your health**, refuse. Schedule another smear – or two or three – taken at least three months apart, before doing anything else.

> "Based on solid evidence, regular screening with the Pap test leads to additional diagnostic procedures (e.g. colposcopy) and [surgical] treatment for low-grade squamous intraepithelial lesions (LSIL), with uncertain long-term consequences on fertility and pregnancy. These harms are greatest for younger women, who have a higher prevalence of LSIL, lesions that often regress without treatment.
>
> "Additional diagnostic procedures were performed in 50% of women undergoing regular Pap testing. Approximately 5% were treated for LSIL. The number with impaired fertility and pregnancy complications is unknown."[38]

★ For those, like myself, who prefer to avoid doctor visits, a visual examination for HPV is as good, maybe better, than a Pap smear. Nurse-midwives in Zimbabwe were asked to take a Pap smear, then to swab the cervix with a mild vinegar solution and (with the aid of a flashlight) to check for white areas that signal abnormal cells. While 77 percent of the positive vinegar tests were accurate, only 44 percent of the positive Pap smears were.[39] To check yourself, follow the instructions on page 173, then paint your cervix with white vinegar and a long-handled watercolor brush or cotton swab. Lesions are immediately visible.

• Of 2,763 postmenopausal women who had Pap smears annually for four years, 110 had abnormal results, but only one woman actually had cervical cancer.[40]

> "Even in the context of a major clinical trial, which would presumably employ the most skilled pathologists, these specialists disagreed with one another's diagnosis [of Pap smears] at an alarmingly high rate."[41]

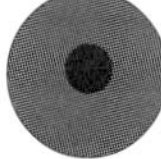

Cervical Dysplasia

"I am always changing," confides Grandmother Growth with a smile. "And so are you. Change is the essence of life.

"But some of my changes, and some of yours, are not in the best interests of your life. Guardians oversee the changes, watching for what is new and different, alert to what might change your life to death.

"Feed your guardians well, give them all they need to be robust and strong, and you have little to fear as the years change you. But let them starve, deprive them of your care, irritate them, harass them, choke them with tobacco smoke, let viruses and bacteria colonize your cells, and the changes can overwhelm even the fiercest of guardians.

"Listen to me, my daughter. Listen to your own wisdom. Listen closely. Learn to flow with change, then you can choose the changes you desire."

Step 0. *Do Nothing*

★ Study after study finds that most low/moderate grade cervical dysplasias (LSI) will regress to normal without treatment.

• How many is most? In one study, 96 percent (300 of 314) of women with mild/moderate dysplasia had a normal smear at a later examination.[42] In another study, four percent (9 out of 235) of untreated women with mild/moderate dysplasia progressed to cancer; all were successfully treated and are cancer-free.[43] A 1992 study at UCLA found 80 percent of those with low-grade dysplasia had normal Pap smears nine months later.[44] In a 1999 study, only one percent of cervical dysplasias became malignant.[45]

• Untreated high-grade dysplasias also spontaneously revert to normal more than half the time. Of women with HSIL, CIN II or CIN III, about 38 percent will return to normal without treatment. About half of the remaining 62 percent (or one-third of the original group) will progress to cancer.[46] Watchful waiting, with frequent repeat Pap smears, can alert you to changes that require action. Meanwhile, you may wish to use the many suggestions in this section to prevent progression.

> "[When a woman has cervical dysplasia] . . . the risk [of missing cancer] with careful observation is virtually nil. I think we are needlessly scaring a lot of women."[47]

• Conservative care standards for women with dysplasia who refuse treatment include repeat Pap smears, and – if needed – yearly colposcopic examinations, until all cells are normal.

★ Women who wish to be more pro-active while waiting will find 1–4 dropperfuls of St. Joan's wort tincture and 1–2 cups of red clover infusion daily, plus a diet rich in anticancer foods (page 191) helpful in guiding cells toward normalcy quickly and safely.

Step 1. *Collect Information*

★ Ten percent of all annual Pap smears done in the USA find abnormal cells. Of these, only one percent will progress to cancer.[48] The other 99 percent – millions of women every year – are frightened into making poor decisions about their health.

★ *If your mother took hormones while she was pregnant with you – this applies to men as well as women – your risk for cancer is very high.* Women whose mothers took DES (page 202) are vulnerable to aggressive cervical (and vaginal) cancers that grow quickly and metastasize rapidly. Regular consumption of red clover infusion and burdock tincture can help prevent these cancers.

Step 2. *Engage the Energy*

• Can repressed grief, rage, and resentment set the stage for reproductive problems, even cancer? Many believe it to be so.

★ Practitioners of Chinese Medicine/Five-Element Theory say that unexpressed anger and grief generate "evil heat" that can damage the health of the reproductive system. (More about this, page 192.) You don't have to commit to years of therapy to find and release buried feelings. Even a few sessions of bioenergetics, art therapy, or gestalt will help.

• Fresh **wheat grass juice** was popularized by Anne Wigmore as a way to prevent and treat cancer. Since it is *not* a source of nutrients,[49] I consider it an (expensive) energy medicine. To reverse dysplasia, it is drunk by the ounce and/or used as a douche.

Step 3. *Nourish and Tonify*

★ **Eat more cooked cabbage-family plants, have less cancer**. More and more studies agree. The compound at the heart of the benefit seems to be indole-3-carbinol (I3C). Find it in high amounts in cooked Brussels sprouts (470 units in 100 grams), collards (165), kale (102), cauliflower (104), and broccoli (72).[50, 51]

Half of the women who took pills of I3C in a recent study had complete regression of their CIN II-III lesions, while none of the women in the placebo group did.[52]

★ In a study of one hundred non-Hispanic black women, those whose diets were highest in **lycopene** and other vitamin A precursors were one-fourth to one-third less likely to have dysplasia.[53] (Those whose diets contained less than 5000 IU of vitamin A daily had triple the risk.) Enrich your diet with cooked tomatoes, sweet potatoes, winter squash, pumpkin, carrots, and dark leafy greens.

★ **Folate**, also called **folacin**, is a B vitamin that helps prevent dysplasia. Women with high levels are five times less likely to have dysplasia than those whose levels are medium or low.[54] The best sources are nettles, leafy greens, lentils, beans, seeds, whole grains, and nuts. **Folic acid** (page 193) is the synthetic form.

★ Low vitamin C is connected to higher levels of dysplasia.[55] (Eating less than 30mg a day increases risk by a factor of seven.) Don't reach for a pill though. **Food forms of vitamin C** are far more effective.

Help!
Cervical Dysplasia

Expect results in 2–6 months

- Eat more **red**, **orange**, and **green** foods . . . at every meal!
- Drink infusion or take tincture of each of these often: **dandelion**, **red clover**, and **burdock**.
- Relax. Avoid **evil heat** (page 192).
- Retest in 3–12 months.

• **Carotene**-rich foods, not supplements (page 201), force abnormal cells to return to normal.[56] Tomato sauce, sweet potatoes, spinach, kale, nettles, winter squash, and cherries are great sources.

• Opt for **more protein**, especially from organic meat, milk, yogurt, and cheese. Animal proteins kick the liver into high gear and helps it "remove [cancer-promoting] estrogen entirely on the first pass."[57] Perhaps that's why a metastudy of 61,500 Britons found **vegetarians twice as likely to be diagnosed with cervical cancer** as meat eaters.[58]

Step 4. *Stimulate/Sedate*

★ In Chinese medical theory, **evil heat** is deep, hidden inflammation, often caused by deep, hidden emotions. Evil heat (and inflammation) can trigger abnormal cell growth. Accordingly, avoid hot spicy foods when dealing with abnormal or cancerous cells. That means no black pepper, no cayenne, jalapeño, or other peppers, and only a little ginger, cinnamon, nutmeg, or cloves.

• Women who smoke cigarettes have a 60 percent greater risk of cervical cancer compared to nonsmokers.[59]

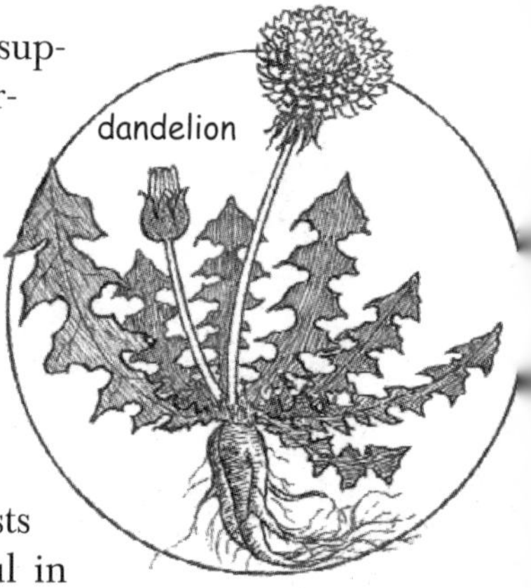

• Herbalist Brigitte Mars says vaginal suppositories made from powdered chaparral mixed into melted cocoa butter – plus regular use of **dandelion**, **burdock**, and **red clover** (the anticancer trio) teas or tinctures – eliminate dysplasia 70 percent of the time.[60] (Remember, 80 percent of dysplasias revert to normal if nothing is done.)

• Herbalist Rosemary Gladstar suggests the "dubious-sounding, [but] successful in normalizing dysplastic cells"[61] Eclectic Institute *Vaginal Depletion Pack*.[62]

• Naturopathic physician Dr. Luthra says cervical dysplasia is easily reversed by eating lots of fruits, vegetables, and whole grains rich in vitamins A, D, E, and folate.[63] She notes that low-grade bacterial infections can cause dysplasia. My favorite anti-infective is **echinacea root tincture** (page 342).

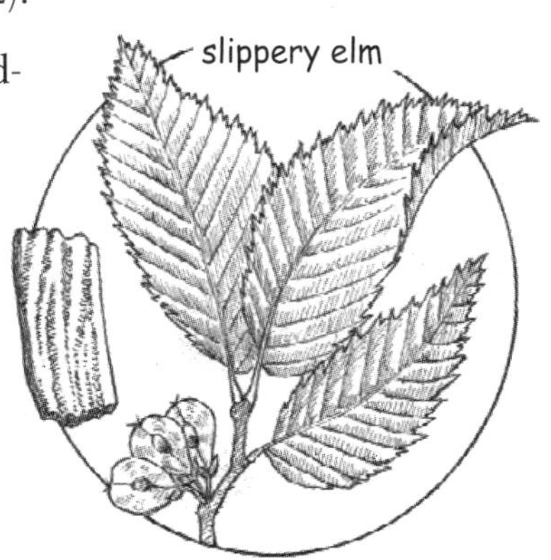

• Some herbalists, following the modern medical model, believe that injuring the cervical tissue enough to cause it to slough off will result in healthful regrowth. **Red clover tar** is used as "do it yourself" surgery. (Make it: page 379.) Follow with applications of soothing, healing herbs such as slippery elm bark or marshmallow root.

Step 5a. *Use Supplements*

• Naturopaths treat women who have cervical dysplasia or carcinoma *in situ* with high doses of supplements, herbs (page 375), and a restricted diet. After a year of treatment, of 43 women, none were worse, two were the same, and the rest returned to normal or improved.[64] *Women with mild to moderate dysplasia who do nothing at all get the same results, at considerably less expense.*

• Women with precancerous cervical lesions who took very high doses of beta-carotene (50,000 units a day) and/or ascorbic acid/ vitamin C pills (500mg daily) were just as likely to go on to full-blown cancer as those who took no supplements.[65]

• Some women swear **folic acid supplements** reverse their dysplasia and their cells become abnormal again when they stop taking it. The upper limit is a daily dose of 400 micrograms.

Caution: Folic acid supplements impair your ability to absorb zinc, a critical nutrient for immune health.[66]

Step 5b. *Use Drugs*

• Long-term use – over 8 years – of birth control pills (oral contraceptives) quadruples the **risk of cervical cancer**.

• **Retin-A** applied to the cervix prompted complete regression in 43 percent of those with moderate dysplasia but none of those with high-level dysplasia.[67,68] (Twenty-seven percent of those treated with a placebo also regressed.) Retin-A was applied once a day for four days via a cervical cap holding a sponge, and repeated after three and six months.

Step 6. *Break and Enter*

> "A logical step before having a cone biopsy or any surgery for diagnostic purposes is to exhaust other options first. A suspicious Pap smear needn't panic a woman into consenting to traumatic . . . or unnecessary operations."[69]

• "Aggressive therapy on low-grade lesions has gotten out of hand," says gynecologic oncologist Arthur Herbst of the University of Chicago.[70] Be sure the diagnostic tests and treatment you accept are specific to your individual situation and problem. Too many MDs believe that even low grade, easily reversible cervical cancers are best dealt with by a hysterectomy. *Most cervical cancers are slow-growing and don't require immediate surgery.*

• If you choose to have dysplastic cervical tissues destroyed or removed, you'll be offered a variety of ways to do that: electrical cauterization, laser ablation, freezing, and cone biopsy. All have about the same rate of success, but with greater or lesser pain, more or less cost, and varying healing times after the procedure.

~ **LEEP** (Loop Electrosurgical Excision Procedure) is more a biopsy than a treatment. A low-voltage electrified wire cuts from the cervix a button-sized specimen, which goes to the pathology lab. Because it is inexpensive, fast (about four minutes), easy to do, and avoids repeat visits by the patient (diagnosis and "treatment" are combined), LEEP is widely overdone. It leaves a wound that takes three months to heal. LEEP is not a cure for HPV.

~ **Laser** ablation vaporizes tissue. It is expensive and painful, but the cervix heals in two weeks. It can damage the cervical cells and make detection of future dysplasia difficult. Tissue is neither examined for cancer nor preserved.

~ **Cryosurgery** is less expensive and less painful, both during the 3–5 minutes it takes to freeze the cervical cells and the 3–8 weeks it takes for the cervix to heal. The frozen cells melt and slough off, causing a profuse watery discharge. The procedure can destroy mucous glands in the cervix necessary for pregnancy or so stiffen the cervix that normal delivery is hindered, and the freezing agent "spreads out in all directions and may even bury the transitional zone more deeply, leading to potential problems in follow up. . . ."[71] Tissue is neither examined nor preserved.

~ **Cone biopsy** (page 203) is a hysterectomy alternative. It creates scars that compromise conception and childbirth.

~ **Hysterectomy** (page 235) is the conservative recommendation for women with severe dysplasia and *carcinoma in situ.* Recurrence and metastatic disease are virtually eliminated, but this is serious surgery, with serious repercussions.

• Schedule surgery for the last day of your menses so you'll have the most time to heal before menstruating again.

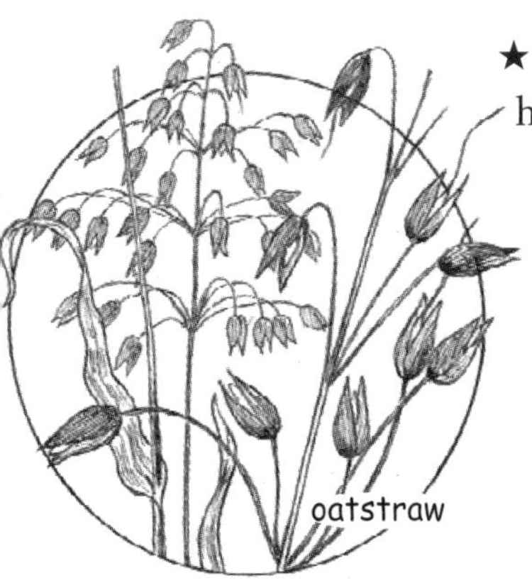

★ Prepare for surgery (and help yourself heal after) with **potassium-rich foods**, such as nourishing herbal infusions of nettle, oatstraw, or red clover. The Ithaca Women's Health Care Collective says the watery discharge that accompanies healing from cervical surgeries is high in potassium, and eating lavish amounts insures good healing.

Her Story

Claudia lives in Manhattan; she is in her thirties.

"When my Pap smear came back 'abnormal,' my gynecologist referred me to a specialist.

"That doctor was up there with his microscope [doing a colposcopy] for what seemed like forever. He didn't see anything abnormal. Instead of suggesting that I wait and have another Pap, he told me I needed to have a cone biopsy.

"I was scared. I trusted him. I had it done. The biopsy found nothing abnormal.

"But that isn't the end of my story. Two years later, my pregnancy ended abruptly in my eighteenth week when I went into labor and gave birth to a perfect, whole fetus. It died during the delivery. There was nothing wrong with me or the baby. My cervix had been rendered 'incompetent' by the cone biopsy.

"I know now I should have waited a few months and had another Pap smear taken instead of agreeing to surgery. I hope my story can save another woman the heartbreak I endured."

Cervical Cancer

"How many ways of being are there, sweet friend?" asks Grandmother Growth warmly. You sense this is a serious question and you fear you don't know the right answer.

"Between the yin and the yang, between the dark and the light, between normal and abnormal, there are infinite shades and numberless ways of being. Without lines, they arise and change, drift away or settle in, some promoting your well being, some eroding it. An erosive change is almost upon us daughter. How will we meet it?

"Cells are changing in your cervix. They are changing quickly; they are speeding; they are growing too fast. They are making a sloppy mess, growing without order, without symmetry. Can you keep up with it? Or is it tearing you loose from your moorings and setting you adrift? Is it freedom? Or is it chaos?

"Cells are changing too fast for the guardians of your immune system to deal with them. Before the guardians are overwhelmed and overrun, you must find help, dearest granddaughter. Ask for aid. Call out for assistamce. Invoke health.

"What are the steps to your dance with cancer? What do you need to do to stop it now, before these wild cells escape and become lethal?

"The guardians of your life may still prevail. Call them up! What is your vision of health? Call it forth! What nourishing herbs are your allies? Ingest them! Must you fight? Then prepare yourself for battle!

"Your choices are uniquely yours, my dearest one. Let them arise from the deep well of your own inner wisdom. Trust yourself. I'll hold your hand in the dance . . . follow or lead, fast or slow, as you will. Let's go!"

Step 0. *Do Nothing*

★ Do you actually have cervical cancer, or one of its precursors? This is an important distinction. Current practice tends to overtreat women with abnormal cells, dysplasia, hyperplasia, or *in situ* carcinomas. In nine out of ten cases, these conditions do not progress to cervical cancer, even if left untreated.[72]

> "Physicians could confidently monitor patients for [amount and types of HPV] virus with currently available tests for several months before deciding to treat [the cervical cancer] . . . more aggressively."[73]

Step 1. *Collect Information*

• Cervical cancer kills about 4,000 American women and almost 300,000 women worldwide every year.[74] It is symptomless in the early stage, but a Pap smear may find it.

• Each year five million American women are told their Pap smear reveals dysplasia, or abnormal cells. Most will be treated as though they have cancer. Only one percent of them – the 45,000 new cases of cervical *carcinoma in situ* diagnosed yearly – have anything to worry about. Only .002 percent – the 10,000 new cases of invasive cervical cancer – have a real problem. [75]

★ Cervical cancer *in situ* is generally **very slow-growing**. Untreated, half will regress and half will, over a period of 10–30 years, progress to invasive cancer.[76] About 10 percent of women (the incidence is increasing) have *fast-growing* cancer which becomes invasive within a year.[77] Cervical cancer is most common in women 40–60 years of age, but also occurs in younger women.

• Black women and other women of color are twice as likely to be diagnosed with cervical cancer and almost three times as likely to die of it as white women. They are generally older at the time of diagnosis and have very abnormal cervical cells, but are less likely to receive aggressive treatments.[78]

• Fifty percent of the women in the USA diagnosed with cervical cancer had a clear Pap test within the past five years; the other 50 percent haven't had a Pap smear in five years.

• Women without access to Pap smears are four to five times more likely to die of cervical cancer than women who do. Women in countries where Pap smears are not routinely accessible – including Brazil, India, and much of Africa – are also much more likely to lack indoor plumbing, be malnourished, live in poverty, and be forced into intercourse and childbirth before the age of 18. All these factors increase the risk of a cervical cancer diagnosis.

• Cervical cancer is more likely if you smoke tobacco (triples risk), take birth control pills (over 8 years quadruples risk), have multiple sexual partners (more than 5 quadruples risk), are in a relationship with a man who is uncircumcised and who has had more than 25 partners, engaged in (or were forced into) intercourse before the age of 18 (triples risk; the cervix is immature, easily damaged, and vulnerable to infection), have chronic cervicitis, live where there are no sanitary facilities, and eat a diet lacking in vitamin C (less than 30mg a day increases risk sevenfold) or carotenes (under 5000IU daily triples risk). [79,80,81]

• Women whose cervical tissues are infected with HPV and inflamed – by herpes, gonorrhea, chlamydia, spermicides, or violent penetration – are twice as likely to be diagnosed with cervical cancer as women who have HPV but no inflammatory events.[82]

• Some procedures sound like diagnostic tests. A cone biopsy (page 203), despite its name, is major surgery, not a test.

★ Unusual vaginal bleeding – especially after intercourse or in postmenopausal women – abnormal pelvic pain, any out-of-the-ordinary discharge, especially a watery discharge, and deep discomfort in the belly are signs of cervical cancer.[83]

• If you have cervical cancer and have been exposed to HIV, get tested – twice! (Ten percent of positive HIV reports are false positives.) Cervical cancer is one indicator of HIV infection.[84]

• Women in Finland, Norway and Sweden who were infected with certain strains of chlamydia (page 156) were four times more likely to be diagnosed with cervical cancer.[85]

Step 2. *Engage the Energy*

★ Take back your power! Claim your cervix and your genitals as your own. Possess your cervix, your uterus, your vagina. Look at your cervix. Accept it; love it; cherish it. When we reject a part of ourselves, we can find ourselves "losing" that part to surgery.

• Women with cervical cancer are more likely to have been **sexually unhappy** than women with other types of cancer.[86] They may have disliked intercourse, but felt compelled to do it. They rarely have orgasms in the presence of a man. They're more likely to be divorced, separated, deserted, or "stuck" in a relationship with an unfaithful, undependable, or alcoholic man. [87] You can begin to change these patterns now, even if you have cervical cancer; even starting to change can help you beat the cancer.

> "Feelings of being used or raped are associated with chronic vaginitis, chronic vulvar pain, recurrent warts, herpes, cervical cancer, and abnormal Pap smears (dysplasia)."[88]

• **Reclaim your cervix**. How? One good way is to look at it; page 172 tells you how.

Another is **recapitulation**, a technique taught by Yaqui shamans. Sit quietly and vividly recall a situation where you felt sexually used or abused. It doesn't have to be dramatic or horrible. Perhaps you, like I, feel abused by ads showing a bikini-clad woman lying atop a car saying "Ride me!" Or perhaps the fact that millions of women have been sexually mutilated upsets you, as it does me. Feel your emotions as fully as you are able to.

Place your feelings into your right palm; let them have weight. Turn your head to the right; breathe in. Turn your head to the left and say out loud: "I reclaim my power." Say it again as you place your right hand on your left hand, palm to palm. Say it a third time as you withdraw your right hand and gently turn your left palm down, letting the feelings flow away. Repeat as often as needed. *Our emotions are an important part of our health.*

Help! Cervical Cancer

Expect results in 2–4 months.

• Try recapitulation (above).

• Take a dropperful of **astragalus, burdock**, and/or **dandelion root** tincture at least twice a day.

• Drink **red clover infusion.**

• Consider taking **poke root tincture**, cautiously.

★ Can **visualization** reverse cancer? Many healers and oncologists think so. If nothing else, visualization allows one to *do* something. One woman envisioned her ominous dark red *in situ* cervical cancer cells turning a bright healthy pink. Her follow-up Pap, three months later, found only normal cells.

Step 3. *Nourish and Tonify*

★ Women with cervical cancer often test low for selenium and for vitamins A, B_6, C, and folate/folic acid (a B vitamin).[89] To get more selenium eat mushrooms, garlic, and seaweeds. For vitamin A, eat orange, red, and green foods. Get vitamin B_6 from lentils, broccoli, and potatoes. Vitamin C-rich foods include sauerkraut, fresh whole fruits and salads, and potatoes baked in unpunctured skins. Folate (the natural form of folic acid) is abundant in leafy greens, lentils, and nettle infusion. Eating better doesn't "cure" cancer, but high-quality nutrition provides the basis for normal healthy cells to replace cancerous ones, and primes the immune system for "spontaneous remission."

• **Red clover infusion** – three quarts a week – is one of my favorite anticancer herbs. It is especially helpful against reproductive organ cancers (cervical, breast, uterine, ovarian, prostate).

Step 4. *Stimulate/Sedate*

• **Don't douche!** Women who douche weekly are nearly four times more likely to be diagnosed with cervical cancer.[90] Doesn't douching cleanse the vagina? Absolutely not. (*See* page 135.) The vagina harbors beneficial organisms (mostly bacteria) that prevent infection and may forestall cancer. Douching washes them away, leaving the cervix and vagina vulnerable to infection and inflammation.

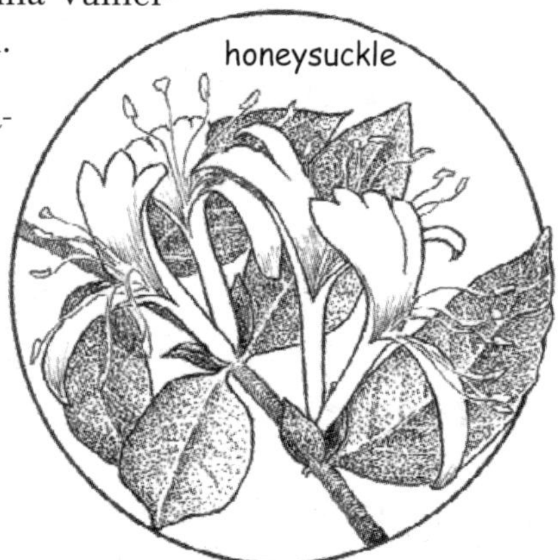

★ **Honeysuckle flower** is a traditional Chinese remedy for women with cervical distresses including ulcers, erosion, inflammation, and cancer. The tincture is applied directly to the cervix several times a day to disperse "heat" and move energy.[91] Recent research confirms its effectiveness.

★ **Castor oil** treatments against cancer were popularized by Edgar Cayce. In the case of cervical cancer, Cayce recommended daily castor oil packs over the uterine area, as well as five drops of castor oil orally at bedtime. Additional treatment options include Cayce's products Atomidine and Glyco-Thymol.[92]

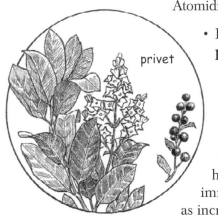

• Extract or tincture of common **privet berries** inhibits cervical cancers in mice.[93] A dropperful dose (or 5mg powder) taken 2–3 times a day may not directly eliminate cervical cancer in humans, but it may "tonify the yin," reduce cervical inflammation, enhance white blood cells, nourish the immune system and the liver, as well as increasing sexual responsiveness.

★ Because **milk thistle seed tincture** protects the liver without interfering with chemotherapy, it is *the* complementary medicine for those choosing chemo. It may be anticancer, too. Two of its alkaloids, silymarin and silibinin, reduce the growth of cervical, breast, and prostate cancer cells.[94]

Step 5a. *Use Supplements*

• Low levels of **folic acid** are associated with cervical cancer, perhaps because folate is needed for DNA repair. But supplements, even in very high doses, fail to reverse cervical cancer.[95]

• Low levels of carotenoids in the diet and blood increase the risk of invasive cervical cancer. **Caution**: Carotene **supplements** are not a cure, and may even prolong the presence of precancerous cells, helping them mature into cancers.[96] Studies have repeatedly found that beta-carotene supplements "decrease spontaneous healing." Women with CIN II who took beta-carotene supplements were more than twice as likely to progress to cancer as the control subjects.[97,98]

• **Caution**: High doses of supplemental vitamin C don't help those dancing with cancer, and may harm them.[99]

 DES Daughters & Sons 

"Yes, desPLEX prevents abortion, miscarriage and premature labor. Recommended for routine prophylaxis in ALL pregnancies."[100]

(Advertisement)

From 1938 until 1971, more than six million unborn children in the USA were exposed to the potent estrogen-like hormone diethylstilbestrol (DES or desPLEX). It was prescribed to their mothers in the mistaken belief that it could prevent miscarriage and create bigger, stronger babies. As early as 1954, studies found the opposite to be true – women who took DES were *more* likely to miscarry. Nonetheless, this dangerous drug continued to be given to pregnant women for seventeen more years.[101]

The daughters and sons of women who took DES often have malformed reproductive systems, malfunctioning immune systems, and a heightened sensitivity to carcinogens. DES-daughters and granddaughters are especially likely to be diagnosed with fast-growing clear-cell adenocarcinoma or intraepithelial neoplasia of the cervix or vagina.[102]

burdock

Though many DES-daughters are diagnosed when young, there is no age at which the danger disappears. All DES daughters need to remain vigilant their entire lives.[103]

The DES daughters and granddaughters can help themselves stay cancer-free by exercising regularly, meditating, and using **red clover** blossom infusion (1-3 quarts a week) and **burdock root** tincture (a dropperful a day, more when stressed).

Resources: www.descancer.org and www.desaction.org

Step 5b: *Use Drugs*

• One drop of lavender or rose essential oil added to a warm bath can help alleviate the stress of dealing with cervical cancer.[104]

• Smoking **tobacco** causes a tumor suppressor gene to lose its ability to kill cancer cells, says UCLA cervical-cancer researcher Dr. Christine Holschneider.[105] Perhaps that's why smokers are more likely to get, and die of, cervical cancer. Save your health, roll your own. Add coltsfoot or mullein leaves for a robust smoke; add cornsilk or mint for a lighter smoke. The semen of men who smoke tobacco contains carcinogenic chemicals, too.[106] And they increase the risk of cervical cancer. A condom or diaphragm can isolate your cervix from his ejaculate and reduce your exposure.

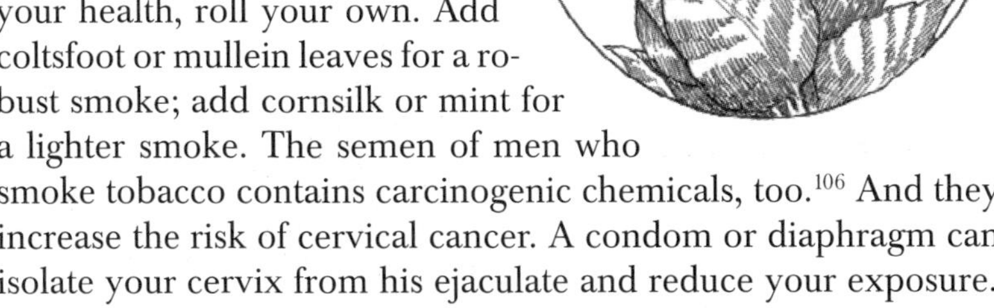

• **Chemoradiation** – chemotherapy plus radiation – improved four-year disease-free survival rates and reduced recurrences.[107] Women with early-stage cervical cancer (I or II) benefited more than those with late-stage disease (III and IV). Side effects were far more severe with the combined treatment.

Step 6: *Break and Enter*

> ". . . certain cancers, such as early-stage breast cancer, prostate cancer, cervical cancer and low-grade lymphomas, respond very well to herbal treatments, yet seem to be aggravated and sometimes worsened by surgical procedures or other conventional treatments." [108]

• The rates of cervical cancer are four times less among women whose partners have had a **vasectomy.**[109] Of course, once you already have cervical cancer, this intervention is too late.

• A **cone biopsy** is real surgery, not just a biopsy. It was originally conceived of as a uterus-sparing procedure for women with cervical cancer who, usually from a desire to have children, were reluctant to undergo hysterectomy. A cone biopsy requires anesthesia. It is not just a sample of cells, as are most biopsies, but surgery which aims to remove all possible cancerous tissues from the cervix along with a clean margin of unaffected tissue.

> "... a [1979] guideline for treatment of in situ cancer, stage 0: If the patient has completed her family and ... has no strong emotional reasons for preserving menstrual function, a hysterectomy can be done. There is no reason, however, to remove the ovaries."[110]

• Overtreatment of cervical carcinoma *in situ* is common. Except in the rare case of fast-growing microinvasive cancer, it is considered safe to explore alternative treatments for 3–12 months before resorting to surgery. A high percentage of *in situ* cervical cancers spontaneously disappear or can be reversed with appropriate dietary changes and adjunctive herbal remedies.

• Invasive cervical cancer has spread from the tissues of origin to the surrounding cells in stage I (only in the cervix) and stage II (in the upper vagina). A radical hysterectomy – which removes the uterus with its cervix, the tissues surrounding the cervix, and surrounding lymph nodes – is the safest treatment for women with invasive cervical cancer, says Lynda Roman, MD of the Anderson Cancer Center in Houston. "If less than that is done [such as a hysterectomy] half of all cases ... will recur."[111]

• When the cervical cancer spreads in stage III (to the pelvic wall) and stage IV (to the bladder and/or rectum), and when it metastasizes to other parts of the body such as the bones, the brain, the lungs, surgery will not be enough. The addition of radiation and chemotherapy is advised. A new technique – focused microwave heating coupled with radiation therapy – improves outcomes. Complementary medicines, like milk thistle seed tincture and carrot juice, can see to it that the quality of life is the best it can be.

Her Story

Lana is a DES daughter (page 202). She's had multiple chemical sensitivities and chronic fatigue immune dysfunction for ten years.

"I came out in my late twenties, and stuck strictly to women, but got my Pap smear every year. And every year they were normal.

"I don't know what made me suspect I had cancer. I was in my mid-forties, menopausal, menstruating for weeks on end, not just once, but over and over. My trusted experts, an acupuncturist and a lesbian gynecologist, said 'don't even think of cancer.' They told me not to worry, that heavy bleeding was normal during menopause. I did worry; I did think of cancer; I didn't seem right to me.

"I kept pressuring the gynecologist to do a biopsy, but then I refused to go through with it. She wanted to do it 'all at once,' that is, to do a cone biopsy. It seemed so invasive to have such a big piece cut out of my cervix.

"My bleeding slowed down, at last. Then I had a profuse watery discharge. My acupuncturist said: "Red changing to white means an improvement." It didn't feel that way to me.

"Fortunately, I followed my inner wisdom and sought other help. It wasn't easy: I was depressed, I didn't have much energy or any savings, and my health insurance was virtually nonexistent.

"At fifty-two, I was diagnosed with clear-cell adenocarcinoma. I never heard about DES (my mother took it) until my diagnosis.

"They operated on me for over five hours. My cancer was advanced; it was all over my bladder, uterus, and vagina. The surgeon said there was a 50 percent chance of cancer cells remaining. In the scan, it looked like there might be a metastasis to my lungs.

"Nonetheless, I refused chemotherapy and radiation, believing they would be the final blow to my already weakened immune system. Instead, I'm using remedies from Step 0 (serenity medicine), Step 1 (story medicine), Step 2 (mind medicine), Step 3 (life-style medicine), and Step 4 (herbal medicine).

"I don't expect these medicines to cure me. I chose them instead of chemotherapy because I want to be more in touch with myself and my life, and even with my approaching death."

Her Story

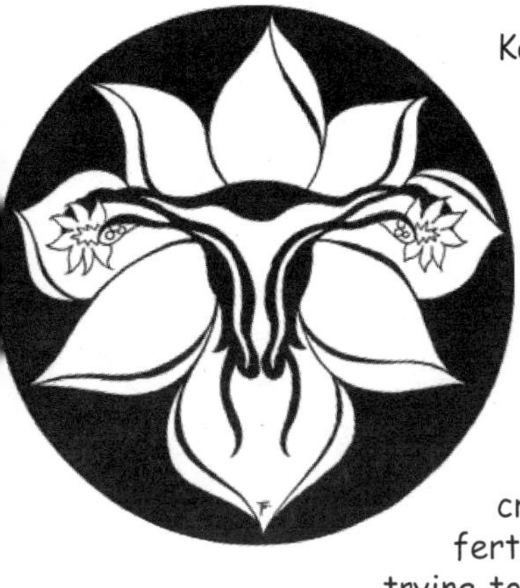

Kate is a menopausal suburban housewife.

"DES wasn't mentioned when I had a cervical polyp removed at the age of 19, by cryosurgery. I didn't find out that my mother took DES when she was carrying me until I was undergoing infertility treatment. I got the feeling she felt guilty for taking it. She never questioned her doctor, just as I never questioned mine thirty years later. I didn't find out the DES and cryosurgery were responsible for my infertility until years later. I finally gave up trying to have children. I don't have any reproductive cancers, yet. Herbs are my allies."

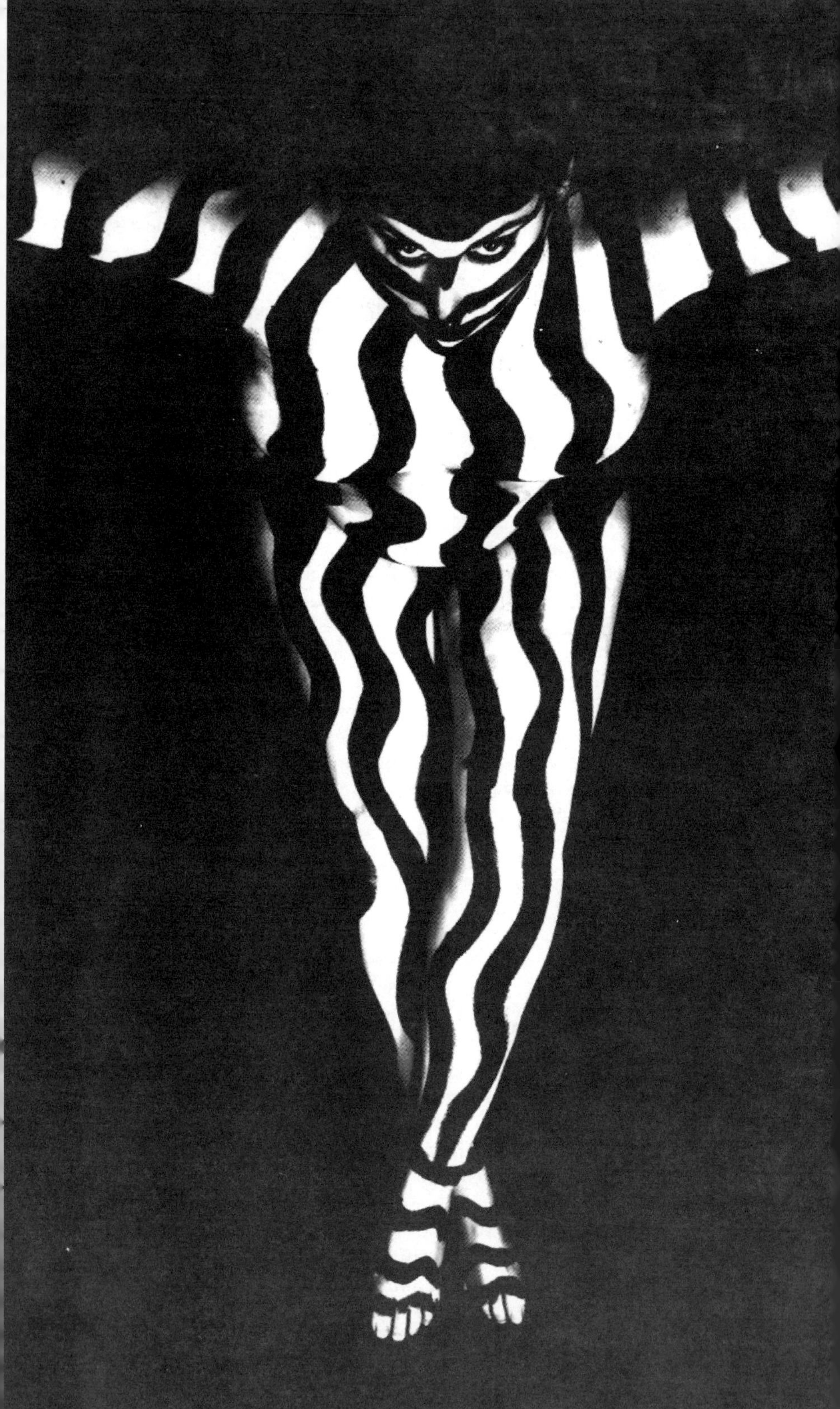

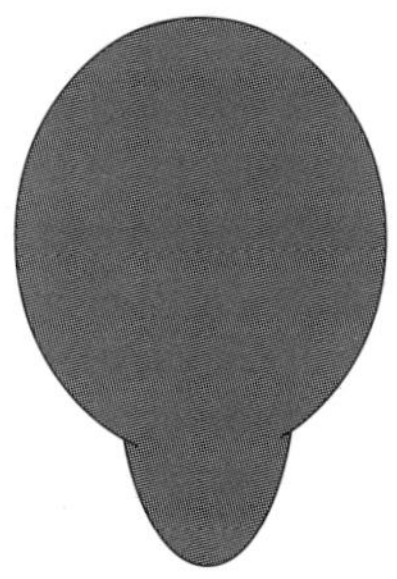

The Uterus

I am the center. I am the ballast. I am weighty. I am wise. I am a fist; I am a hand. I am muscular strength. I am spacious. I am whole.

I am spiraling power. I am the basin of chi. I am the palace of the child. I am the chamber of embodiment. I am your center.

I sway with the rhythms of your glandular orchestra. Sometimes my dance is slow and stately. Sometimes it is wild, pulsing with energy. At times I am loud; sometimes, you can barely hear my whisper.

In your childhood, I am less than a thought. In your cronehood, I hold the wisdom, I keep the wise blood inside. In between puberty and menopause, I go through changes.

Like the moon, I am tidal. During your fertile years, I wax and wane, fill and spill. The full moon wakes me to my tasks: start building a palace, begin the interior decorating. I grow as the moon wanes, swelling with potential. I thicken, I ripen, I prepare. New moon finds me at the height of expectancy. Will a fertilized egg snuggle into my velvety richness and compel me to grow large enough to hold and protect the future child? Or will I disassemble the palace and squeeze out the blood and chi, and dream for a while? Do I have more work to do, or is it time to let it go?

Like any hard worker, I may ache and cramp. Like a visit from your family, I may disturb and surprise. This is not to bother you, but to draw your attention.

I want you to love me. Honor me. Be proud of me. I want you to want me. Keep me. Fight for me. Know that you are safe in my magnificent strength. Remember that you can rely on my Ancient Wisdom.

I am your potential. I am your ground. I am your uterus.

Healthy Uterus

The uterus is an inverted-pear-shaped muscular organ, usually about three inches long and weighing about four ounces (about the size and weight of a lemon). It lies between the bladder and the rectum. Its neck, which is visible from the vagina, is the *cervix.* Its body is the *corpus,* the top of which is the *fundus.*

The uterus is attached to the lower back by the uterosacral ligaments, to the upper thighs via the round ligaments, and to the umbilical area by the urachus and obliterated umbilical arteries.

The uterus does not lie vertically but horizontally: the fundus points toward the belly and the cervix slants toward the spine.

The uterus consists of two layers of densely packed muscle fibers. The thicker outer layer is the *myometrium.* The thinner inner layer is the *endometrium.* The endometrium is sensitive to hormonal signals which direct it to grow, thicken, and become rich in blood when pregnancy has occurred or is possible – and to shed if pregnancy does not occur (menstruation).

The uterus is the strongest muscle in the body, surpassing both the tongue and the heart muscles. It can contract with enough force (150 pounds per square inch) to move a ten-pound baby through the birth canal. During pregnancy, the uterus builds two pounds of new muscle and gets twenty times larger.

The uterus moves during orgasm (page 108).

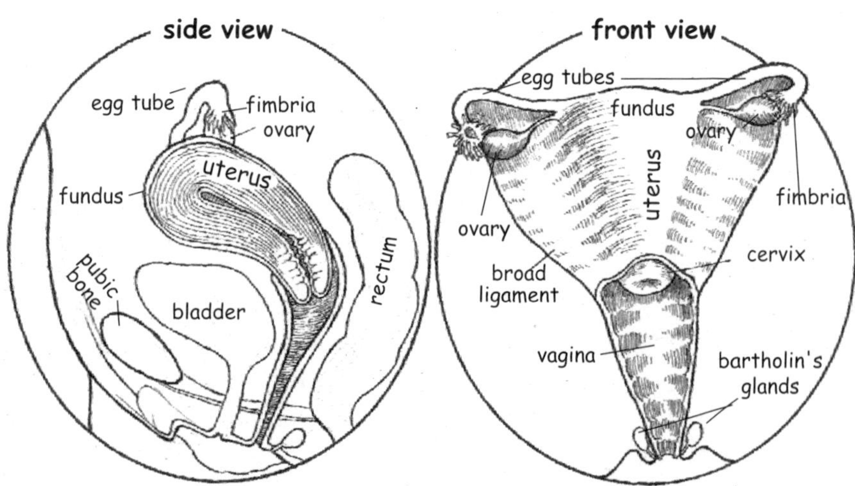

Uterine Distresses

"The uterus is the woman's center. If it is not in proper position and good health, nothing in her life will be right." Don Elijio Panti

The uterus is naturally healthy and resistant to disease, but menstruation (and pregnancy) put it through changes which can lead to pain and problems. Wise Woman ways are generally safer and more successful in dealing with uterine problems than drugs or surgery. **Hysterectomy** (page 235), the surgical removal of the uterus, is modern medicine's recommendation for most uterine problems. These remedies will help you keep your uterus if possble.

Herbs are wonderful helpers for women with menstrual distresses (page 210) such as **period pain** (page 211) and **flooding** (page 214).

Pain and heavy bleeding may also be due to **polyps** (page 251), **fibroids** (page 218), **adenomyosis** (page 227), or menopause.

A very, very few women will have **toxic shock syndrome** (page 211). Too many will experience chronic pelvic pain (page 15), which may be caused by **endometriosis** (page 229), **pelvic inflammatory disease/PID** (page 245), or trauma (page 79).

The endometrium of the uterus is vulnerable to growths including **polyps** (page 251), **hyperplasia** (page 241), and **endometrial cancer** (page 243). To **prevent endometrial cancer**, see page 238.

For help with uterine **prolapse**, see page 6.

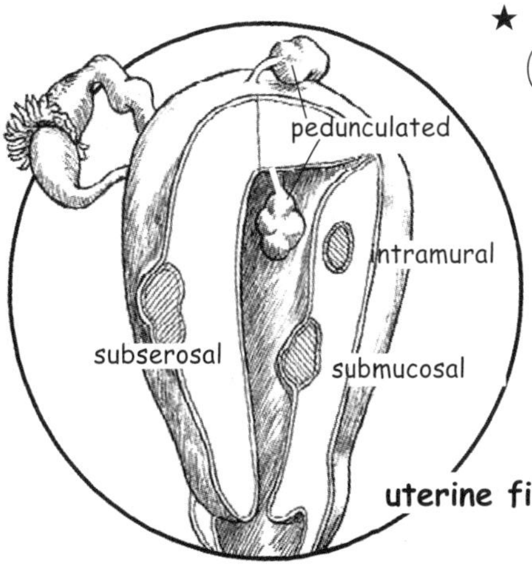

★ **Mayan Abdominal Massage** (MAM) is a "non-invasive, external massage which guides internal abdominal organs into their proper position for optimum health." This releases both physical and emotional congestion. MAM is effective for both men and women. More at www.arvigomassage.com

uterine fibroids

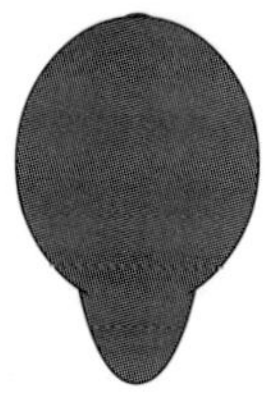

Menstruation

"Women are a mystery, are we not?" asks Grandmother Growth with the kind of gleam in her eye that makes you wonder what she'll say next. "Our wombs are the doorways of the next generation. We spin the umbilical cords that tie young to old.

"Times past, a woman's worth was the wealth of her womb. Not merely because she thought so, or because her culture believed so, but because her body told her so."

Menstruation is the shedding of the endometrium from the uterus. This blood-rich tissue grows during the last two weeks of the menstrual cycle, awaiting the implantation of a fertilized egg. If the endometrial nest is not needed, that is, if conception has not occurred, then it is released. The average blood loss during menstruation is usually only two tablespoons/one ounce/30ml.[1]

From the first menstruation (menarche) to the last (menopause), modern women prefer to manage their menstrual blood so it doesn't leave embarrasing stains on clothing and furniture. For most, that means buying manufactured "sanitary protection."

Feminists and ecologists question our reliance on "man-made" pads and tampons. Though convenient, they endanger the health of women and the earth. Instead, try pretty flannel rags, organic tampons, a menstrual sponge, or a keeper cup. Some women have more cramps with some of these; others feel liberated and great! Are the alternatives important? Read on and decide for yourself.

- ❖ Do tampons contain asbestos? No.
- ❖ Are tampons cancer-causing? Maybe.
- ❖ Can tampons cause endometriosis? Probably.
- ❖ Have women died from using tampons? Yes.

Are Tampons Safe?

• Most tampons and menstrual pads are bleached with chlorine, which leaves residues of the carcinogenic chemical dioxin.[2] In one startling study, 80 percent of the monkeys exposed to dioxin developed endometriosis. The higher the exposure, the more severe the endometriosis and the more likely death was.[3]

★ Dr. Philip Tierno Jr., of New York University Medical Center, a leading expert on the risks of tampons, believes that dioxin is a possible threat to women's health even at the trace levels (1 part in 3 trillion) that manufacturers acknowledge are present.[4] Tampons come in contact with highly-absorbent vaginal tissues. A woman will use about 11,000 tampons during her fertile years.[5]

• Toxic shock syndrome (TSS) is an uncommon, rarely fatal, blood infection linked to high-absorbency rayon tampons left in the vagina for extended periods.[6,7] For safety sake, use a low-absorbency, unbleached tampon, and change it at least twice a day.

Menstrual Pain/Cramps

Step 0. *Do Nothing*

★ Take a **"moon day,"** a day off from all responsibility, on the first or second day of your menses. Honoring your moontime (menses) "magically" cures PMS and chronic cramps, taps us into our creativity, and offers a respite from tending to loved ones.

Step 1. *Collect Information*

• The technical term for menstrual pain is *dysmenorrhea.* Clots in the blood are normal but may cause pain.

• The uterine muscle contracts to push the menstrual blood out. This contraction may be more or less painful, depending on the individual woman and the tone of her uterine muscle.

• Severe menstrual pain may signal a deeper problem such as endometriosis, fibroids, or pelvic inflammatory disease..

Step 2. *Engage the Energy*

★ Lie with your belly on the earth. Give yourself an orgasm. Take a nap. Take a toke. Sit in a hot bath. Tune into your uterus. Moan. Cry. Listen to soothing music. Read Jen Vaughn's comics: *Menstruation Station* or *Don't Hate, Menstruate!*

- **Homeopathic remedies** for women with menstrual cramps:
  - ~ *Chamomilla*: cramps like labor, birth.
  - ~ *Sepia*: intense, bearing-down cramps.
  - ~ *Sabina*: painful clots.

Step 3. *Nourish and Tonify*

• After "suffering for years," one woman freed herself from cramps in four days with four tablespoons of cod liver oil daily, generous amounts of organic raw-milk butter, and vitex tincture.[8]

Step 4. *Stimulate/Sedate*

★**Acupuncture** successfully reduces menstrual pain for more than 80 percent of women.[9] Pressing on the sacrum helps, too.

• Stop menstrual pain fast by smoking dried **catnip**. Roll it in a paper or smoke it in a pipe. One or two puffs usually does it. Smoke outside! It smells! Or go for a walk and breathe deeply; that reduces cramping fast.

★ **Motherwort** tincture (from fresh flowering tops) acts quickly to relieve cramps. Its tonic properties strengthen the uterine muscle, reversing cramps at the source. After taking motherwort tincture several times, many women find their menstrual cramps – and premenstrual symptoms – never return. I like a 5–25 drop dose, taken every five minutes for up to two hours, or until pain and cramping are eased.

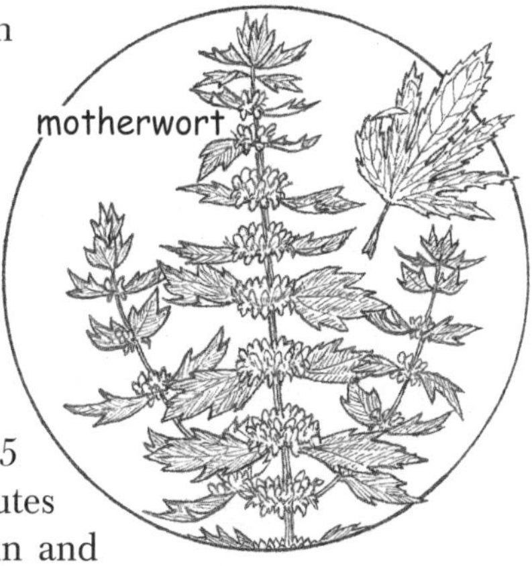

• All antispasmodic and pain-relieving herbs – such as **cramp bark** tincture (20–30 drops), **ginger** tea, or **willow bark** tincture (10–20 drops) – are allies against menstrual cramps.

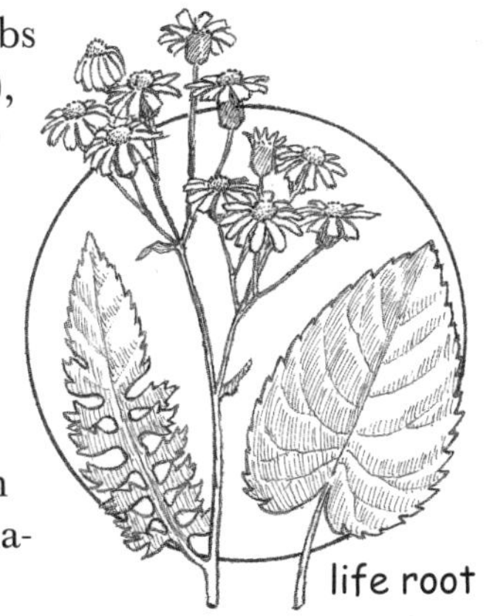

• Women with chronic menstrual pain plus nausea, headache/migraine, or sore muscles find relief with a little-known American herb, **life root** (*Senecio aureus*). A dose is 3–10 drops of the tincture of the fresh flowering plant, taken daily between ovulation and menstruation, for 4–12 months.

• For relief from intense menstrual pain, try **dong quai root**. It's "stronger than aspirin," according to Dr. Janet Zand.[10] A dose is a dropperful of the tincture taken daily from ovulation until menstruation. (Try it in miso soup.) Side effects – nausea, breast tenderness, digestive upset, and increased bleeding – are less likely when peony root, astragalus, and/or licorice are added to the dong quai.

Step 5. *Use Drugs*

• **Ibuprofen** relieves pelvic pain and slows bleeding. It is most effective if taken at the first sign of pain and repeated regularly.[11]

Step 6. *Break & Enter*

• Many women begin having painful menses after pelvic surgery, especially tubal ligation and diagnostic laparoscopic procedures.[12] Repeated use of **castor oil** compresses, **comfrey leaf** poultices, or **calendula flower** oil can dissolve (or prevent) adhesions and scar tissue, thus reducing menstrual pain.

Help!
Menstrual Pain

Expect results within 10–60 minutes

• Take 5–15 drops of **motherwort** or **dong quai tincture** as needed.

Expect results within 2–3 months

• Drink 3–6 quarts of **nourishing nettle** or **raspberry infusion** weekly.

• Take a **moon day.**

Heavy Bleeding/Flooding/Menorrhagia

Step 0. *Do Nothing*

• To calm chronic flooding, avoid raw foods and don't exercise (other than short walks) for 3–7 days before the menses begin.

Step 1. *Collect Information*

• *Menorrhagia*, from the Greek *meno* (menses) *rrhagia* (to burst forth), is heavy menstrual bleeding. Menses more often than every twenty-one days, periods that go on for more than a week, bleeding so heavy it soaks three pads in three hours, or loss of more than 80ml (three ounces) of blood altogether are all menorrhagia. *Metorrhagia* is bleeding or spotting *between* periods.

• Twenty percent of women with normal menses (30–40ml) call their period heavy. Forty percent of those with heavy menses (more than 80ml) consider their periods to be moderate or light.[13]

• Menorrhagia is common, and normal, during menarche and menopause, especially for women of color.[14] Other causes include fibroids, endometriosis, anovulatory cycles, PCOS, endometrial hyperplasia, polyps, vascular fragility, ectopic pregnancy, IUD, miscarriage, cancer, blood-thinning drugs, ERT, hypothyroidism, stress, and deficiencies of iron (anemia), copper, vitamins A or K. A third of those with fibroids flood frequently.[15]

Help! Flooding

Expect results within 5–15 minutes

• Take tincture of **shepherd's purse** or **cotton root bark**.

Expect results within 3–5 weeks

• Drink 3–6 quarts of nourishing **nettle** or **raspberry infusion** weekly.

• Try 4 tablespoons of **cod liver oil** daily for no more than two weeks.

• Endometrial polyps (page 251) cause about one-quarter of all cases of heavy bleeding.[16] Most polyps are benign and painless, but they can interfere with fertility. Polyps are rare after menopause. (Tamoxifen takers are less likely to have polyps.[17])

• Menorrhagia can exhaust you. Drink nettle!

• Thirteen to twenty percent of women with heavy menstrual periods have a bleeding disorder called von Willebrand disease.[18] Drugs (page 217) can control it; surgery is *not* necessary.

Flooding can worsen quickly. Use Step 4 remedies first!

Step 2. *Engage the Energy*

• Imagine something frightening, something that "chills your blood." Feel your belly and uterus tighten up, slowing bleeding.

• **Homeopathic remedies** for women with menorrhagia:

~ *Aconitum*: prolonged flow, very red; weakness, fear.
~ *Belladonna*: flow early, bright red, clotty, profuse.
~ *Calc-carb.*: profuse flow on exertion, at menopause.
~ *China*: flow early, dark, clotty; exhaustion.
~ *Cuprum met.*: flow late, prolonged, cramps; fearful, restless.
~ *Ipecac*: profuse red flow; pain, weakness, vomiting.
~ *Lachesis*: blood dark; pain intense.
~ *Phosphorus*: profuse bright red flow, intermittent.
~ *Secale*: blood dark, offensive, goes on and on; pain severe.

Step 3. *Nourish and Tonify*

★ **Raspberry leaf** infusion can stop menstrual flooding. Stinging **nettle** infusion helps prevent it by replacing iron, strengthening the blood vessels, and encouraging coagulation with its rich stores of vitamin K. Alternate, using 2–3 quarts of each per week.

• Low iron increases bleeding; bleeding robs **iron**. Compensate by eating iron-rich **red meat**, **organic liver**, or **salmon**. Iron from plants – **nettle infusion, yellow dock** tincture, **molasses**, **raisins**, or **beets** – is poorly absorbed. Eating vitamin C rich foods at the same time can double absorption of iron.[19]

> "Natural remedies can usually control menorrhagia . . . but may not take full effect for . . . months. You won't have the luxury of trying them if you . . . require immediate surgery or drugs."[20]

• Vegan and vegetarian women – as well as 40 percent of midlife women – are low in B_{12} or cannot absorb it well,[21] leading to flooding. Vitamin B_{12} is found only in meat, fish, eggs, and dairy products.

Step 4. *Stimulate/Sedate*

★ Apply an ice pack to the pelvis and elevate the feet.[22]

★ Try a dropperful of the tincture of fresh flowering **shepherd's purse** or of **cotton root bark** under the tongue to slow uterine bleeding quickly. Repeat the dose often to stop bleeding.

• **Witch hazel** bark is a hemostatic, astringent herb. A dropperful of **tincture** or several cups of strong tea stops bleeding fast.

• **Cinnamon** stops hemorrhage. It is specific against menorrhagia.[23] A large spoonful in a cup of hot water acts quickly.

Step 5a. *Use Supplements*

• Four tablespoonfuls of **cod liver oil**, or 60,000IU of vitamin A or beta-carotene, taken daily for no more than 2–5 weeks, counters even severe menorrhagia for 90 percent of women.[24,25] **Beware!** Vitamin A supplements weaken bones.[26]

★ Two doses of 500mg **vitamin C** daily reduces bleeding for 90 percent of women.[27] Dr. Susan Lark adds rutin.[28] Buffered ascorbic acid or mineral ascorbates are the preferred forms.

• **Iron deficiency** can cause flooding, shortness of breath, dizziness, weakness, fatigue, ringing in the ears, and headaches. Increase the effectiveness of supplements (ferrous gluconate, sulfate, or fumarate) – and reduce their side effects – by taking a dropperful of **yellow dock** root tincture at the same time.

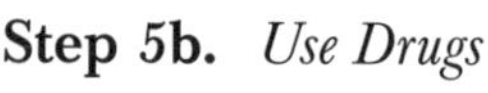

Step 5b. *Use Drugs*

• Using nonsteroidal anti-inflammatory drugs (NSAIDs) – such as 600mg **ibuprofen** every six hours each day of the menses – reduces blood loss by 20–50 percent in women with menorrhagia.[29] *Caution*: Long-term use of NSAIDs causes high blood pressure, gastrointestinal problems, and kidney distress.

• **Low-dose oral contraceptives** (birth control pills) reduce blood loss as well as NSAIDs or Danazol (by 30–50 percent).[30] Continuous use is best for those with fibroids. "The weight of the evidence suggests that taking birth control pills does not enlarge fibroids and *does* improve [that is, decrease] symptoms."[31]

• Half of women with heavy bleeding who use hormonal therapies (medroxyprogesterone acetate, or an intrauterine device containing levonorgestrel) get as much relief as those who have a hysterectomy.[32]

★ Two prescription drugs used against von Willebrand disease (a form of hemophilia) may help women who flood: DDAVP (page 52) and tranexamic acid. The later "significantly reduce[s] menstrual blood flow" in **all** women if taken during the days of the menses. It works better than NSAIDs or Provera, too.[33]

• **Gonadotropin-releasing hormone** (GnRH) **agonists** such as Lupron (leoprolide), Synarel (narfarelin, nasal spray), and Zoladex (goserelin), are powerful drugs with severe side effects. They relieve menstrual pain and flooding within 2–13 weeks, and can reduce the size of fibroids and endometrial implants.[34] How? By creating a chemical menopause – with hot flashes, mood swings, and bone loss – which may be permanent. Estrogen and progestin taken at the same time reduce side effects without reducing efficacy,[35] but cause other problems (page 233).

Step 6. *Break & Enter*

• Past the age of menopause? Experiencing spotting or bleeding? **Seek help**. Cancer could be brewing.

• Removal of the "offending organ"– especially in women over 40 – is the medical response to "dysfunctional, excessive" uterine bleeding. Women who have had a hysterectomy have four times more thromboembolic and cardiorespiratory events, and six times more postoperative infections than women who opt for ablation.

• **Endometrial ablation** (page 225) destroys the uterine lining while leaving the uterus intact. It is far safer than a hysterectomy, though not as "final" a solution to heavy bleeding.

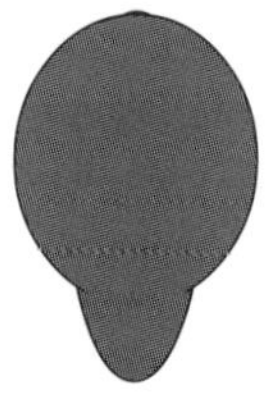

Uterine Fibroids

"Childbearing is still the goal of your body, dearest child. There are billions of children alive; you need not add to them. But your womb does not know that. It wants to swell with new life.

"Acknowledge that you are a womb-one. Hear the desires of your uterus: to create, to give birth. In time, menopause will end this dance of growth, and your womb will give you access to the Ancient Wisdom. For now, cease your struggle. You are gripped in the talons of creation. Create!"

Step 0. *Do Nothing*

> "Recent findings from over 850,000 counseling sessions conducted by the HERS Foundation. . . [suggest] almost all (98%) hysterectomies could be avoided with either conservative treatment or no treatment at all."[36]

• Every year in America a quarter of a million women undergo a hysterectomy due to fibroids.[37] Don't be one of them.

• About 80 percent of women with uterine fibroids have few or no symptoms.[38] They may simply wait until menopause brings an end to their fibroids; no need to do anything.

Step 1. *Collect Information*

> "Finding [help for fibroids] often leads her on a confusing journey in which she is likely to receive misleading information. . . ."[39]

> "It's appalling that so many women don't have access to good information; often the treatment you get [when you have fibroids] depends on which door you walk through."[40]

• Uterine fibroids are **benign** swellings. Despite the name fibroid *tumor*, cancer is extremely rare (0.1–0.5 percent).[41,42]

• Fibroids are also called leiomyomas (*leio* is smooth, *my* is muscle, *oma* is growth), myomas, myofibromas, fibromyomas, uterine leiomyomata, and fibroid tumors.

• Between the ages of 35–50, about 20 percent of white women, and nearly 60 percent of women of color, have uterine fibroids.[43,44] By age 50, more than 80 percent of black women and 70 percent of white women have fibroids.[45] Black women often have larger, more numerous, faster-growing fibroids at a younger age.[46]

• About one-third of reproductive-age women in the US have symptoms from fibroids: heavy, clotty, painful menses; abdominal and back pain; anemia from blood loss; a constant urge to urinate; constipation; pelvic pressure; pain on intercourse.[47]

• Uterine fibroids can grow rapidly or slowly. There is no way to predict if, or how fast, a fibroid will grow.[48] Surgery to remove a fibroid (or the uterus) "before it gets too big" is "bad advice."[49]

• Uterine fibroids can shrink spontaneously.[50]

• Uterine fibroids *do* run in families. A mutated gene that interferes with the production of fumarate hydratase may be the cause.[51]

• Fibroids have many estrogen receptors, but estrogen, even in birth control pills or ERT, does not cause fibroids, nor will a low-estrogen diet cure them.[52]

★ **Progesterone can increase fibroid size.**[53]

• "Women can relax about the big fibroids," says researcher Karen Hartmann. "Those are old and dormant. Small ones are the most active."[54]

• Women who have had four or more children, or who smoke, rarely have fibroids.[55]

Help!
Uterine Fibroids

Expect results within 6–18 months

• Take a dropperful of **vitex** or **saw palmetto tincture** 2–4 times a day.

• Investigate acupuncture.

• Listen to your uterus.

• Drink 2–3 quarts each of **nettle** and **raspberry infusion** weekly.

• Resist hysterectomy. Seek non-Western medical advice. Call HERS.

★ Fibroids usually go away after menopause.

• Women who began menstruating before they were twelve, who are obese, or who have not given birth are more likely to have problematic fibroids.[56]

• Most women have several types of uterine fibroids. Fibroids can also grow on the cervix or on the uterine ligaments.

~ *Subserosal fibroids* are the easiest to remove surgically.[57] They push into the outer uterine layer (*serosa*). They may put pressure on the bladder, rectum, or pelvic nerves, causing pelvic pain, leg pain, urinary frequency, and/or constipation, but rarely flooding.

~ *Intramural/interstitial fibroids* are most common.[58] They stay inside the uterine muscle where they can increase menstrual flow and pain, cause urinary urgency, and make the pelvis feel heavy, tender, or achy, especially during intercourse.

~ *Submucosal fibroids* are the least common. They begin in the uterine lining, but may protrude inward and cause heavy, painful menses. They interfere with fertility and sexual pleasure.

~ *Pedunculated fibroids* grow on stalks, like a mushroom or a ball on a string. If the stalk twists, severe abdominal pain results.

• Fibroids look like "white or pink potatoes."[59] Most are pea-sized; the largest ever reported weighed 140 pounds.[60] From one to dozens may occur at once. Large fibroids cause more symptoms. Small fibroids cause more miscarriages.[61]

• Doctors size fibroids by comparing the uterus (not the fibroid) to fruit or pregnancy. A uterus the size of a large grapefruit or a twenty-week pregnancy can contain a four-pound fibroid.[62]

• As fibroids grow, they create new blood vessels, thus increasing the blood flow to the uterus. If they hemorrage, blood loss can be so severe that a woman can become dizzy, suddenly faint, pass out, sometimes even bleed to death. Fibroids on the outside of the uterus bleed internally, invisibly, but with the same consequences.

• A fibroid that presses on the tubes connecting the kidneys and bladder can cause kidney damage.

> "The bottom line is that fibroids are not cancer, they don't cause cancer, and they do not even increase the risk of having cancer."[63]

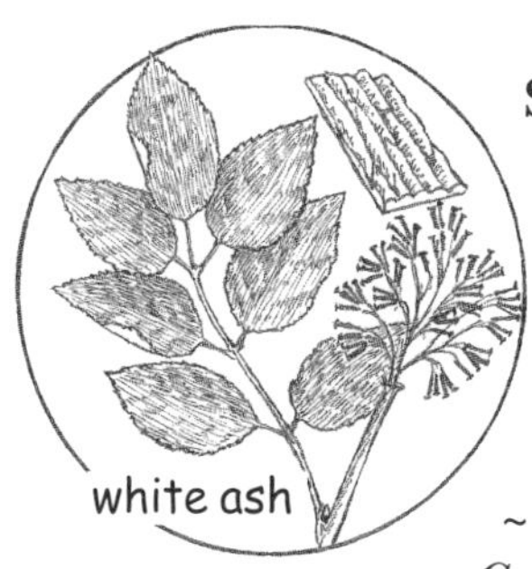

Step 2. *Engage the Energy*

• *Fraxinus americanus*, white ash, is the homeopathic specific for women with fibroids. Other homeopathic remedies include:

~ *Calc-carbonica*: pedunculated bleeding fibroids.

~ *Thlaspi*: continuous bleeding.

~ *Calc-fluorica*: large, hard fibroids, heavy bleeding.

~ *Calc-iodine*: with profuse yellow discharge.

★ Chinese herbalists say fibroids occur due to "stagnant Qi and Blood, which causes heat and dampness to accumulate in the pelvis."[64] In Ayurvedic tradition, fibroids are "an accumulation of emotions."[65] Christiane Northrup MD, says: "It's easy to see fibroids as hard, implacable anger."[66]

★ **Fibroids are a normal part of being a woman.** They are *not* caused by things stuck in your colon, though they may be linked to an unfulfilled desire to bear children, or a need to express bottled-up feelings. To shrink fibroids, naturally, persevere.

Step 3. *Nourish and Tonify*

> ". . . there are no studies that demonstrate that fibroid growth can be stopped by altering your diet."[67]

• Women who eat the most beef are 70 percent more likely to have fibroids than those who eat the least.[68] But a vegetarian or vegan diet won't cure fibroids. Reducing dietary estrogens has *not* been found to reduce fibroids.[69] Organic milk, meat, and cheese are nourishing foods, and don't make fibroids grow.[70] No association between eggs or dairy products and fibroids has been found.[71]

★ Women who consume the most fish and leafy greens (nourishing herbal infusions!) are the least likely to have fibroids.[72]

★ A dropperful of **vitex/chaste berry** tincture, taken 2–4 times a day, reduces uterine inflammation and changes the hormonal messages sent to fibroids, easing pain quickly and helping shrink the fibroid. In German medical practice, vitex is considered specific against uterine bleeding. Side effects – intestinal distress, rash, headache – are rare. Chaste berry works best when taken for a long time, so you will need a lot of tincture. It's easy to make your own; directions are on page 367.

★ There's a 3000-year-old Chinese remedy for women with fibroids that I call the "Triple Goddess Gift." It consists of equal parts of **maidenwort** (chickweed), **motherwort**, and **cronewort** (mugwort). I prefer to use tinctures of each, but a tea of dried leaves and flowers works well, too. (It tastes nasty though.)

• In Ayurveda, fibroids indicate "primarily a pitta [liver/manifestation] problem, and secondarily a kapha [emotion] imbalance."[73]

Unfortunately, Ayurvedic practitioners use cleanses and complicated herbal formulae (page 379) to treat fibroids. There is nothing wrong with taking a mixture of black cohosh, chasteberry, St. Joan's wort, wild yam, barberry, turmeric, dandelion, myrrh, valerian, fenugreek, cumin, ginger, yellow dock, fennel, and cinnamon. Except, only **chasteberry** has been shown to reduce fibroids.

When I take an Ayurvedic view of fibroids, a simpler solution comes to mind: **motherwort**. Its bitterness eases pitta/liver problems. It's also full of acceptance and self-love to ally kapha/emotional issues. I'd use 5–25 drops of tincture, once or twice a day.

• Neither exercise nor weight loss will get rid of fibroids.[74] Both moderate symptoms, however. Exercise increases the level of pain-reducing endorphins in the blood, but it increases flooding.

Fibroids and Pregnancy

♥ Babies born to women with fibroids are *not* more likely to die or have birth defects.[75]

♥ "For the vast majority [70–75 percent] of women, fibroids sit quietly during pregnancy."[76]

♥ Fibroids present at the beginning of a pregnancy may, or may not, grow as pregnancy progresses. This is a problem only 10 percent of the time.[77] They shrink after the birth.[78]

♥ Subserosal fibroids are least likely to create problems.[79]

♥ Women with small fibroids are more likely to miscarry.[80]

♥ Women with fibroids are at increased risk of preterm labor during pregnancy, but 90 percent deliver at full term.[81]

Step 4. *Stimulate/Sedate*

• As with any hard-to-solve problem, many herbs have been tried – with some success, sometimes, for some women – to relieve pain (P), check bleeding (B), and/or shrink fibroids (F).

~ **Chasteberry**: P, B, F, tincture (2–4 dropperfuls daily).
~ **Comfrey leaf**: P, F, sitz bath (warm) or compress.
~ **Lady's mantle**: B, F, tincture (10–25 drops 3 times a day).
~ **Poke root**: P, F, tincture (1–3 drops daily); rub oil on belly.
~ **Reishi mushroom**: P, tincture/tea, reduces inflammation.[82]
~ **Raspberry leaf**: P, B (iron), F, infusion, (2–4 quarts weekly).[83]
~ **Shepherd's purse**: P, B, F, tincture (1 dropperful daily, from ovulation to menstruation only).
~ **Yarrow** (*use only white-flowered*): P, B, sitz bath (warm).

★ **Acupuncture** can relieve the "stuck energy" of fibroids.[84] **Moxibustion** and/or **acupressure** work, too. Do-it-yourself directions are in Dr. Susan Lark's *Fibroid Self Help Book*.[85]

Step 5a. *Use Supplements*

• **Lipotrophic factors** – vitamin B_6, inositol, choline, and magnesium – are suggested for women with fibroids. Instead of supplements, I eat lipotrophic foods like **beets**, **garlic**, and **lentils**.

★ **Avoid** progesterone cream. It is promoted for women with fibroids, but the evidence suggests progesterone feeds fibroids.[86]

Step 5b. *Use Drugs*

• Menopause usually ends fibroids, so drugs that induce it are used to treat fibroids. Three months of a GnRH agonist can halve the size of a fibroid. Beware! There are "formidable" side effects (page 233). And once the drug is stopped, fibroids recur.[87]

• Women who took a daily oral dose of the hormone ulipristal acetate (**Ella**) for three months had less bleeding and smaller fibroids with fewer side effects than those taking other drugs.[88]

• **Asoprisnil**, a selective progesterone receptor modulator, inhibits fibroid formation and suppresses bleeding. There may be unanticipated, unforeseen, or unexpected side effects. Be cautious.

• The morning-after pill, RU-486 (mifepristone) in 10mg doses – 600mg induces abortion – shrinks fibroids and reduces pain, but causes uterine abnormalities in one-third of the women treated.[89] When the drug is stopped, the fibroids recur.

• The anti-osteoporosis drug **raloxifene** (60mg daily) reduces uterine size and shrinks fibroids for 83 percent of the women who take it.[90] Side effects include joint aches and serious blood clots.

• If you have your uterus and take hormone replacement (HRT), you may encourage fibroids. Stop HRT, lose the fibroids.

Step 6. *Break and Enter*

> "Fortunately, most uterine fibroids . . . are comfortably diagnosed with history, a bi-manual exam, and a pelvic ultrasound."[91]

• Not sure it's fibroids? A lighted telescope-like device (a *hysteroscope*) inserted into the uterus under general anesthesia allows a visual check for the causes of uterine pain and bleeding.

• Needle biopsies that are done to rule out leiomyosarcomas (cancer) are "expensive, invasive, and impractical."[92]

• Are you considering surgery now . . . before your fibroid enlarges? Don't. Women with large fibroids have no more surgical complications than women with small fibroids.[93] Fibroids usually disappear after menopause. Wait it out if possible.

These surgical treatments are listed in order of least invasive and dangerous, to most invasive and dangerous.[94,95] **All pelvic surgeries, even laparoscopic ones, can cause painful adhesions.**

• Ask about the risks, side effects, benefits, and advantages of any treatment. How long does it take to recover? Will your fertility be impaired? What is the recurrence rate? How will it affect your sexuality? Your bowels? Your bladder? Get it in writing!

• Most new, less-invasive treatments for fibroids rely on heat. Heating a fibroid to 150–180°F will cause it to die, be sloughed off, and passed from the body. But high heat injures the endometrium to the extent that infertility is likely. Heat can injure adjacent organs like the uterus, the bladder, or the rectum. Other side effects may include burns, back/leg pain, cramping, urinary tract infection, premature menopause, blood poisoning.

• **Balloon ablation**: A balloon, inserted through the cervix and into the uterus, is filled with fluid, and heated to 200°F to destroy fibroids. Infertility is the primary side effect; pregnancy can be "life-threatening." Not suitable for submucosal fibroids.

• **MRI-guided focused high-intensity ultrasound**: This incision-free, but radiation-rich procedure requires a woman (under mild sedation) to be in an MRI scanner for 3–4 hours, lying on a focused ultrasound transducer encased in a sealed water bath. Like a magnifying glass focusing light into a fiery hot spot, the transducer focuses ultrasound energy into a hot spot that kills the fibroid. Recovery is one day. At the six-month follow-up, 80 percent of women report major improvement in their quality of life.[96] About 25 percent are likely to need further procedures, either to treat new fibroids or to finish off the original one.[97]

• **Endometrial ablation**: A hysteroscope is inserted through the opened cervix; an electrical current destroys the endometrium and fibroids. Perforation of the uterus or bladder, and burns to adjacent organs can occur. Orgasm may be permanently disrupted. It stops excessive bleeding 80 percent of the time.[98]

• **Laser ablation**: Thin hollow needles, guided by MRI into the fibroid, allow laser fibers to be inserted and heated to over 140°F to coagulate the fibroid. The procedure takes two hours under light sedation; women are free to go home four hours later. After six months, fibroids were 37 percent smaller.[99]

• **Radio frequency ablation**: This laparoscopic surgery uses radio waves to heat up and eliminate fibroids as large as four inches. Most women are able to resume normal activities within three days. At the 11-month follow-up, most women reported freedom from bleeding, pain, and no regrowth of fibroids.[100]

• **Uterine-artery embolization** (UAE): Small polyvinyl plastic particles are injected into the arteries which supply the uterus and the fibroid with blood. (Polyvinyl can be carcinogenic.[101])

Women can return home the next day. (A five-day stay is usual after a hysterectomy.) During the next two weeks there is usually intense pelvic pain – often requiring morphine – while the fibroid dies and is absorbed by the body.[102,103]

This surgery induces menopause about 5 percent of the time. More than 90 percent of women choosing it are relieved of heavy bleeding and pelvic pressure; 10 percent need another procedure.[104] After one year, most fibroids are half as big. The five-year success rate for UAE is 73 percent.[105]

Less than one percent of women who have UAE develop an infection.[106] About 3 percent develop complications that require a hysterectomy.[107] Occasionally a massive blood infection develops, and despite immediate hysterectomy, death may ensue.[108]

- These types of surgery require general anesthesia:
  - ~ **Laparoscopic** surgery (for subserosal fibroids)
  - ~ **Hysteroscopic** surgery (for small submucosal fibroids)
  - ~ **Myomectomy** (for larger fibroids). Myomectomy is done with a laparoscope or via a vaginal or abdominal incision. It is "extremely difficult" and bloody; fibroids are likely to recur.[109] About 20 percent of women need a transfusion.[110] From 20 to 50 percent need repeat/multiple surgeries.[111, 112] Painful adhesions are common.[113] Recovery time is 3–4 weeks. Myomectomy weakens the uterine wall, so delivery by C-section is necessary.[114]

Pregnancy is possible after any of these interventions. No woman older than 35 who had a myomectomy got pregnant in the next 18 months, but 83 percent of those younger than 35 did.[115]

★ **About 40 percent of hysterectomies are done as a response to uterine fibroids.**[116] A quarter of a million American women a year lose their uterus because they have fibroids.[117] Most of these hysterectomies are unnecessary! Keep your uterus!

Her Story

Chris is a self-employed woman.

"I always felt 'cowed' by OB/GYNs — and they're so expensive. A friend suggested Planned Parenthood. Wow! They're thorough, cautious, respectful, and open to alternatives. Best yet, neither the questions I ask nor the diagnosis they make end up on my permanent health insurance file."

Her Story

Irene is a massage therapist with two grown children.

"Lying in bed one night, just as I was falling asleep, I suddenly felt as if I'd peed myself. The bed was full of blood. The gynecologist confirmed my fear that the hard canteloupe-sized protuberance in my abdomen was a fibroid. The size of a 10-week pregnancy, it pressed on both my bladder and my colon, causing pain during bowel movements and frequent urination. Determined to avoid surgery, I took chaste berry tincture three times a day, had acupuncture and moxibustion treatments, used castor oil packs regularly, and (to replace lost blood) drank nourishing nettle infusion. It took six months for me to shrink the fibroid. It hasn't returned."

> "Using different words [not tumor, but mass; not disease but distress] to describe fibroids will not stop a woman's bleeding or banish her pain, but it can impact the way she feels about the situation, and how she addresses [her] symptoms."[118]

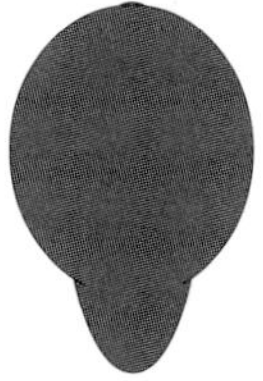

Adenomyosis

"Like a spring too tightly wound, you are turning in on yourself, growing into yourself rather than out, beloved one," says Grandmother Growth. Are those tears glistening on her cheeks . . . or rain? Lightning flashes.

Step 0. *Do Nothing*

• Unless you have symptoms, let it be, leave it alone.

Step 1. *Collect Information*

• Adenomyosis is a benign condition. It occurs when endometrial tissue grows *within* the uterine muscle, instead of lining it. It usually spreads throughout the uterus, and is not lumpy, like fibroids.

Adenomyosis can be symptomless, or can cause significant pelvic pain (page 15), heavy bleeding (page 214), pain with urination or intercourse, and cramping.

• Diagnosis is difficult. Symptoms of adenomyosis, fibroids, and endometriosis are very similar. "The only way to diagnose adenomyosis with certainty is to remove the uterus."[119] Don't!

• Adenomyosis often occurs in women in their forties and fifties who *have* had children.

• Cytokines – inflammatory substances – create the pain of adenomyosis, and may initiate premature labor.[120] **Linden** flower infusion is a great-tasting anti-inflammatory ally.

Step 2. *Engage the Energy*

• Put yourself out. Get out. Sing out. Speak up. Let it out.

Step 3. *Nourish and Tonify*

★ **Raspberry** leaf infusion – a quart a week or more – tones the uterine muscle, reduces menstrual pain, decreases bleeding, counters inflammation, and shrinks swelling. Ahhh.

Step 4. *Stimulate/Sedate*

• Tori Hudson ND says women have successfully countered adenomyosis using a protocol including tinctures of licorice, partridge berry, blue cohosh, and wild geranium.[121] (Make it: page 371).

• Curanderas, grandmothers, and midwives use a strong tea of **oregano** leaf to counter bleeding and ease uterine pain.

Step 6. *Break and Enter*

• Magnetic resonance imaging (MRI) is "one of the few tests that can differentiate fibroids from adenomyosis."[122]

• The usual orthodox treatment for adenomyosis is hysterectomy (page 235). No matter what your age, *it is important to keep your ovaries* if you elect to have your uterus removed.

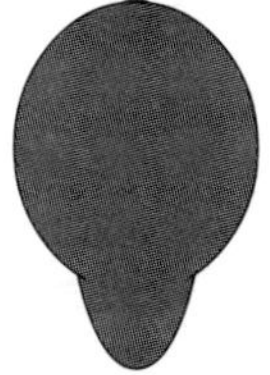

Endometriosis

"Contain yourself, my pride, my joy. Activate your human craving for order and order your organs, they are getting out of bounds," complains Grandmother Growth.

"You are making a mess of your insides, you know. A bloody mess, in fact. Tighten up your act. Draw the line. Oh, and get rid of those tampons, too," she commands with a frown.

Step 0. *Do Nothing*

> "Because endometriosis can cause so many different symptoms, doctors refer to it as 'the chameleon disease of the pelvis.'"[123]

• One in ten women with pain from endometriosis endures ten or more years of misdiagnosis.[124]

• Menopause usually, but not always, eliminates endometriosis. Postmenopausal women do continue to produce non-ovarian estrogens, and their ovaries are still slightly active. For some, this is enough to keep endometriosis going.

> "I think of endometriosis as a chronic disease that often—but not always—improves after natural or surgical menopause."[125]

Step 1. *Collect Information*

• Endometriosis is the growth of endometrial tissue in places other than the uterus, such as on the egg tubes, the ovaries, or the intestines. It may occur on the arms and thighs, or in the lungs or nose, too.[126]

• Women with endometriosis may be free of symptoms, or they may deal with severe, chronic, sometimes disabling, pain.

• Non-uterine endometrial tissues develop into nodules or "implants" of invasive cells which are described as "dark black powder burn lesions." (But see entry about Dr. Redwine, below.) These are endometrial cells, and just like the endometrial cells lining the uterus, they bleed monthly. This internal bleeding causes inflammation, scar tissue, adhesions, and severe pain.

• Endometriosis primarily affects women in their fertile years, with 75 percent of all cases occurring between the ages of 25 and 45. But it may begin at menarche and linger after menopause.

• Sixty percent of infertile women have endometriosis.[127]

• It is uncertain how many American women have endometriosis. Those without symptoms are undiagnosed. Those who do have symptoms often suffer for years before being correctly diagnosed. Estimates range from "as many as 10 percent of women of reproductive age"[128] to five million women.[129]

• Women with endometriosis are 100 times more likely to have chronic fatigue syndrome, 7 times more likely to have hypothyroidism, and twice as likely to have fibromyalgia as other women. Lupus, multiple sclerosis, rheumatoid arthritis, and immune system problems are also more likely among women with endometriosis.[130]

• Endometriosis has become more common since the middle of the twentieth century. Dioxin, a potent carcinogen that causes birth defects, liver diseases, and a variety of cancers, may be to blame.[131] Monkeys who ate dioxin in their food for four years developed endometriosis.[132] "The severity of endometriosis directly correlated with the dose of dioxin administered."[133]

• Dioxin is produced during the manufacture of some plastics, chemical herbicides and pesticides, when garbage is incinerated, when diesel fuel is burned, and from the bleaching of paper products, including sanitary napkins, tampons, toilet paper, tissues, and cigarette paper. When dioxin blows or falls onto plants that animals eat, the dioxin accumulates in their meat and milk.

• Dr. David Redwine studies women with endometriosis. His startling conclusions: One, endometriosis exists at birth. It is triggered by hormonal events, not by "retrograde menstruation." Two, while symptoms may become worse over time, the disease itself does not spread. Three, more than 60 percent of lesions are clear, red, white, gray, and/or blue. If only black lesions are removed during surgery, there will be recurrence.[134]

Step 2. *Engage the Energy*

• **Homeopathic remedies** useful for women with endometriosis: *Aconitum*, *Bryonia*, and *Xantoxylum fraxineum*.

Step 3. *Nourish and Tonify*

★ Use only organic menstrual supplies; consider a sponge.

• Can your diet influence your risk of having endometriosis?
~ Red meat daily doubles risk.[135]
~ Two servings of fruit a day reduces risk by 40 percent.[136]
~ Two servings of greens daily reduces risk by 70 percent.[137]
~ Trans-fats in the diet increase risk.[138]
~ Two grams of omega-3 fats (from oils and fish) daily reduces risk by 22 percent.[139]

• If you're concerned about chemicals (especially traces of dioxin) in your food, **buy organic meat, milk, cheese, yogurt, eggs**, and **butter**. For optimum health, a whole-grain, vegetable-rich diet of well-cooked food which includes gifts from the animals and the oceans is superior.

• Restricted diets – which shun the supposed estrogenic effects of meat, milk, eggs, wine, beer, wheat germ, and yeast – create a fearful, restricted attitude that is contrary to healing. Keep red meat in your diet, but eat it less often. Eating meat *helps* the liver remove estrogens from the blood.

Help!
Endometriosis

Expect results within 3 months

• Eat **shiitake** several times a week.
• Stop using tampons; **let it flow**.
• **Exercise** daily. • Try acupuncture.
• Get **pregnant**. • Try **dong quai**.
• Love your liver.

Plant foods are estrogenic, too.[140] Focus on quality. **Eat a wide variety of whole foods lovingly prepared at home.**

★ **Shiitake** are mushrooms that inhibit endometrial cell growth and may inhibit endometriosis too.

★ The only known "cure" for endometriosis is **pregnancy** and lactation. The hormones of gestation and breast feeding counter the hormones that promote endometriosis. One-third of women with endometriosis have difficulty conceiving, are more likely to miscarry, and are at a higher risk of ectopic pregnancy.

★ Women with endometriosis who can't, or don't desire to, get pregnant, can reduce their symptoms by **exercising heavily**.

Step 4. *Stimulate/Sedate*

★ **Dong quai** is a treasured Chinese herbal medicine for all uterine problems. Three months of daily doses of 10–20 drops of the tincture of this smoky-tasting root in combination with the same amount of white peony or astragalus root tincture relieves endometriosis pain as well as drugs, with fewer side effects.[141, 142]

• Herbalist Rosemary Gladstar uses liver-strengthening, hormone-supportive herbs like dandelion, burdock, vitex, and dong quai for women with endometriosis. (Her formula: page 371.)

• Naturopaths and heroic herbalists favor combinations of herbs like vitex, motherwort, poke, and dandelion to help reverse endometriosis. (Make it: page 372.)

★ **Acupuncture** can reduce the pain of endometriosis for most women, and may cure some.

• **Castor oil** packs, popularized by Edgar Cayce, soothe pain and may reduce the extent of endometriosis. (Make it: page 259.)

Step 5a. *Use Supplements*

• **Fukepenkayen Pills**, available at Chinese pharmacies, warm and decongest the uterus, which is considered critical for those with endometriosis. The list of ingredients is on page 371.

Step 5b. *Use Drugs*

> ". . . endometriosis may be the first human disease definitely linked to hormonal and immunological disruption due to pollutants."[143]

★ Using prescription pain killers? A dropperful of **skullcap** tincture every 4 hours helps you decrease or eliminate your need for pharmaceuticals, but may make you sleepy.

• Hormones that may help women with endometriosis include:

~ The **progesterone-only mini-pill** (birth control pill), taken continuously, controls symptoms in 60 percent of women. It also reduces the risk of ovarian cancer, which may be more common in women with endometriosis.

~ **Danazol**, a testosterone derivative, is highly effective but can cause facial hair growth, loss of head hair, and other problems.

~ **Gonadotropin-releasing hormone** (GnRH) **agonists** can relieve pain and flooding, and reduce the size of endometrial implants, but with severe side effects.[144] They "shut down the pituitary," reducing testosterone and estrogen. This chemical menopause is permanent for some women.[145] Taking estrogen and progestin concurrently can reduce side effects without reducing efficacy,[146] but causes other problems.

• The National Women's Health Network **warns** that some women have a severe reaction to Lupron (a GnRH), and there is no way to predict who will experience "frightening and debilitating side-effects." Of the 4228 women who reported adverse reactions to Lupron, 325 required hospitalization and 25 died.[147] The others had a variety of symptoms including hot flashes, migraines, severe joint pain, loss of bone mass, difficulty breathing, hypertension, chest pain, vomiting, depression, dimness of vision, fainting, dizziness, weakness, amnesia, muscle pain, insomnia, chronic enlargement of the thyroid, and liver function abnormalities.[148]

Step 6. *Break and Enter*

• Laparoscopic surgery under general anesthesia is required for a definitive diagnosis of endometriosis. Best to schedule removal of lesions at the same time. Fight to keep your ovaries!

• The intrauterine device (IUD) **Mirena** can be left in the uterus for up to five years. It releases the progestin levonorgestrel, mimicking pregnancy, and gradually eliminates ovulation, menstruation, and the pain and distress of endometriosis.

• **Hysterectomy** doesn't help women with endometriosis. Even with the uterus gone, ovarian production of estrogen continues, endometrial implants continue to grow, and pain may increase.

• Laser surgery and **electrocautery** can remove errant endometrial tissues. This usually restores fertility and reduces pain without removal of the uterus or ovaries.

• In extreme instances, the sacral nerves in the lower back are severed in an attempt to resolve pain.

Her Story

Barbara is a writer.

"After years of pain before, during, and after my menses, I was finally diagnosed with endometriosis. From puberty on, I always had at least a week of PMS followed by a long, heavy, painful period.

"Surgery relieved some, but not all, of my pain. I was offered hormone treatments; but no one could tell me what the long-term effects would be. I didn't want to be a guinea pig, so I decided to trust myself and to find a way for my body to heal itself.

"With much skepticism, I went to a homeopath.[149] The remedy I took (*Sepia 6x*) not only relieved my physical symptoms, it showed me what led to my disease. I changed my diet, took 25,000IU of vitamin A daily, exercised, meditated, did yoga, and went for emotional/spiritual counseling. Today I am proudly pain-free!"

Her Story

Kate is a lawyer in a small town.

"After taking Lupron [for endometriosis] I now have bone loss, severe bone and joint pain requiring heavy painkillers, chest pain, tachycardia, fibromyalgia, and horrible memory loss, hair loss, and weight gain. Prior to Lupron I ran and boxed every day. I was healthy even though endometriosis caused significant pain. It has now been a year since my Lupron treatments and my life is in medical shambles."[150]

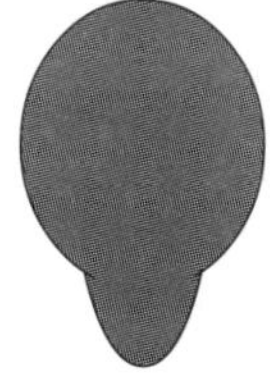

Hysterectomy

Grandmother Growth is sitting by your bed. You hear her words with your heart as well as your ears. "Beloved, I am with you. I will be with you if you remove your uterus. I love you. Your choices are your own to make. You are whole whether you have a uterus or not. Your brain registers only wholeness, never loss. Choose well, my love.

"Consider carefully, my dear. Look at all your options. Are your expectations of the aftermath of surgery grounded in fact? Or fantasy? Sit here and talk to me, my dearest. Pour out your misery. Let us see if we can use it to grow joy for you."

Step 0. *Do Nothing*

• Ask yourself: "What would happen if I did nothing right now?" Many uterine problems resolve as we age. Is surgery really needed?

Step 1. *Collect Information*

> "Hysterectomy involves removing the uterus and severing the ligaments that support . . . the entire pelvic structure. As a result, the pelvis broadens and becomes wider and the individual's blood supply can be disrupted. Women who have had a hysterectomy may lose sensation to the vagina, clitoris, and/or nipples, experience chronic pain, or have inflammation of the nerve endings."[151]

★ Six hundred thousand (600,000) hysterectomies are done every year in the US.[152] That's a little more than one every minute of every day. This rate stayed constant from 1998 to 2008.[153]

• More than one-third of US women have had a hysterectomy by age 65, one of the highest rates in the world.[154] About 70–98 percent of the time the operation is "inappropriate."[155] Ninety percent of hysterectomies are done for reasons other than cancer.[156]

• Excessive bleeding, fibroids, and pelvic pain are the most common reasons for hysterectomy. But 14 percent of those operated on have no symptoms at all.[157]

Step 2. *Engage the Energy*

> "The 20 million women who have had hysterectomies indoctrinate their daughters, sisters and friends: Just do it. You'll feel so much better once the pain is over."[158]

★ If you are agreeing to a hysterectomy because you don't want to argue with your doctor or hurt their feelings, stop! Ask for some time to think it over. Investigate options other than hysterectomy. Go in for monitoring, if you wish, but be wary of invasive diagnostic tests.

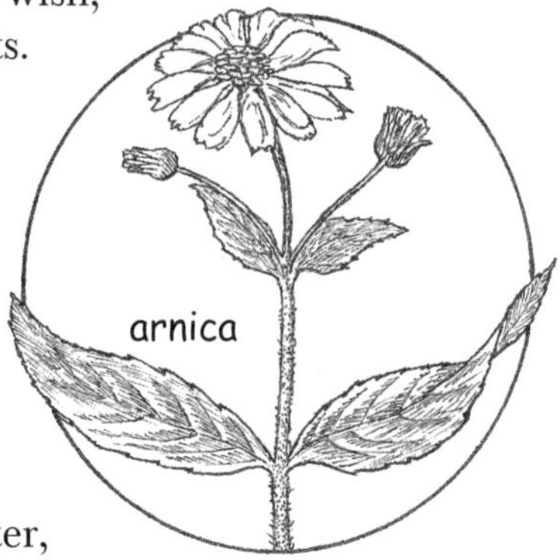

★ If you choose to have a hysterectomy, consider taking homeopathic *Arnica* before and after surgery to counter swelling and bruising. After surgery, I use arnica gel on the soles of the feet, where it is absorbed and carried to the traumatized areas.

arnica

• Get the feelings, before and after, straight from women who've been there, done that, in *Women Talk About Gynecological Surgery.*[159]

Step 3. *Nourish and Tonify*

• Taking 2–3 dropperfuls of **echinacea** tincture 3–4 times a day for the week before surgery can help you protect yourself against the nasty infections found in hospitals.

• Drinking 2–4 cups of nourishing **nettle infusion** a day in the week or two before surgery helps to protect against blood loss and fosters faster recovery.

Step 4. *Stimulate/Sedate*

> "I'm wary of such studies [that claim improvement in sex]."[160]

• One study of over 1000 women, average age 43, found they "wanted and had sex more often, were more likely to reach orgasm, experienced less vaginal dryness, and were less likely to have pain during sex [after a hysterectomy]. . . ."[161] Many other studies find hysterectomy to have the opposite effect on sexuality.

Step 5. *Use Drugs*

• Taking birth control pills or having an IUD inserted can resolve heavy uterine bleeding and pelvic pain. . . or worsen them.

Step 6. *Break and Enter*

> "Removing [the uterus] is like pulling out the cork from an upside-down wine bottle. Unless the woman has strong muscles, her bladder or her bowels can descend into her vagina [prolapse]."[162]

• Should you keep your **cervix**? A review of 700 women found no difference in urinary incontinence or bowel problems. Vaginal bleeding was twelve times greater in those who kept their cervix.[163]

• Women who have a hysterectomy are 60 percent more likely to be **incontinent** after age 60 than those who refuse surgery.[164]

• Fifteen percent of women who have a hysterectomy and keep their **ovaries** experience "postoperative ovarian failure."[165]

• Women who have had a hysterectomy are more vulnerable to heart disease, stroke, and other cardiovascular problems.[166]

• Women who are **sterilized** are four to five times more likely to have a hysterectomy. (Other biological factors were ruled out.)[167]

Her Story

Jan is a successful professional woman in her sixties.

"I had a hysterectomy because I thought it would be an easy solution to my problems. I really underestimated the amount of physical, emotional, and psychic pain it would trigger. My feeling of loss is enormous. Time has not lessened it, but made it worse. I'm still depressed when I think about what I did. I warn women against choosing a hysterectomy for any reason except cancer. Now I do everything I can to support the uterus that I no longer have. Sad, isn't it?"

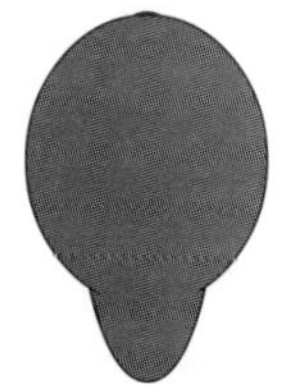

Preventing Endometrial/Uterine Cancer

"I am the Ancient Wisdom encoded in every cell of your body. I am the Ancient Children of your womb. I am the Ancient Stories of your eggs. Listen, listen, listen, dear granddaughter. Listen . . . ."

Step 0. *Do Nothing*

• Endometrial cancer is slow-growing and rarely diagnosed in women younger than 35.[168]

Step 1. *Collect Information*

• There are many risk factors for uterine cancer including excess weight in young adulthood and a low level of physical activity.[169]

• Although 40,000 American women are diagnosed with uterine cancer yearly, 83 percent survive five years or more.[170]

Step 2. *Engage the Energy*

• Envision your uterus glowing in health. Bathe it in loving kindness, compassion, and forgiveness. Imagine it smiling back at you. Listen to the Ancient Ones.

 Risk Factors for Uterine Cancer 

- ❖ Use/d ERT
- ❖ DES daughter
- ❖ No births
- ❖ Obese
- ❖ Have PCOS
- ❖ Hypertensive
- ❖ Aged 55–70
- ❖ Diabetic
- ❖ Early menarche
- ❖ Late menopause
- ❖ Daily use of soy or alcohol

Step 3. *Nourish and Tonify*

★ Uterine cancer has a hard time getting started in the body of a woman who drinks a cup or more of **tea** daily, eats **leafy greens** and other foods rich in carotenes daily, consumes four servings of **cabbage family** plants a week, and includes **seaweed** and **mushrooms** such as shiitake and maitake in her diet.[171]

• **Fiber** from **whole grains** not only lowers the risk of stroke, type-2 diabetes, and heart disease, it protects against uterine cancer, too. Uterine cancer rates drop as women's fiber intake increases.[172] For every five grams of fiber per 100 calories consumed, risk falls by 18 percent. Those who consume the most fiber are 29 percent less likely to be diagnosed with uterine cancer than those who consume the least.[173]

> "There's laboratory evidence that the plant estrogens in soy actually promote the growth of breast and endometrial tumors."[174]

• Eat **lentils** and **beans** (but not soy) often to reduce endometrial cancer risk. Women whose diets are high in fiber and beans lower their risk by 54 percent.[175]

★ Women who consume the most **phytoestrogenic foods** (such as legumes and red clover) reduce risk by 41 percent.[176]

• Those who eat the most foods rich in **lignans** (found in whole grains, beans, and flax) reduce uterine cancer risk by 32 percent.[177]

• The risk of uterine cancer doubles in postmenopausal women who have gained 11 to 44 pounds since the age of 18.[178] Counter risk with exercise, diet, and **nourishing herbal infusions**.

Step 4. *Stimulate/Sedate*

★ A study which followed 6000 pairs of female twins for 25 years found that women who exercise hard are 80 percent less likely to develop uterine cancer than those who don't exercise at all.[179] Even light exercise lowers risk considerably.[180] Women who exercise 20 minutes five times a week reduce their risk by 30 percent.[180A]

• Postmenopausal women who are lean and who drink two or more alcoholic beverages per day double their risk of endometrial cancer.[181] Obese and overweight women who drink at least two cups of coffee a day reduce their risk.[182]

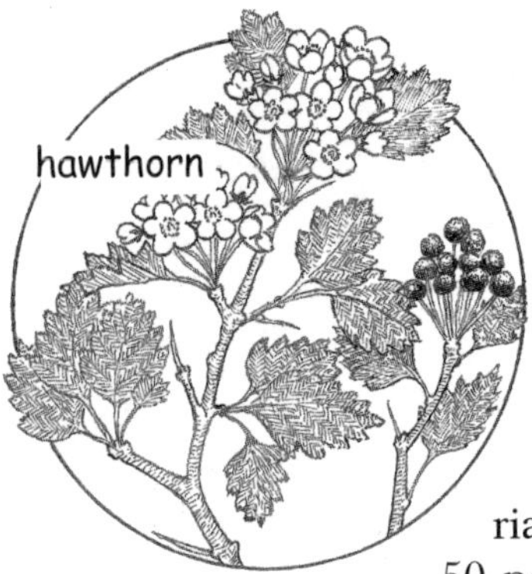

hawthorn

• Reduce hypertension, a risk factor for uterine cancer, with dropperful doses of **hawthorn** or **motherwort** tincture taken 2–3 times daily. Motherwort is an especially fierce protector of uterine health.

Step 5a. *Use Supplements*

★ **Vitamin D** reduces the risk of breast, ovarian, endometrial, and bladder cancer by 30–50 percent.[183] Best: get 20–30 minutes of direct sun exposure daily; try supplements of D_3.

Step 5b. *Use Drugs*

• Taking **birth control pills** for as little as one year cuts risk of uterine cancer by 50 percent.[184,185] The risk reduction continues for at least ten years.[186]

• A primary cause of endometrial cancer is ERT (estrogen replacement therapy). When the craze for ERT was at its highest, MDs advised healthy women to have their uterus removed so it would be "safe to take estrogen." Taking progestin concurrently (like Prempro) protects the uterus, but doubles breast cancer risk.

• Six or more uses of the (in)fertility drug clomiphene citrate – a selective estrogen receptor modulator that induces ovulation – puts a woman in the highest risk category for uterine cancer. Instead, try Wise Woman ways: 2–3 quarts of red clover infusion weekly, animal fat at every meal (butter, eggs, cheese, yogurt, fish, meat), and a joyous call to the spirit of your child every day.

• Taking tamoxifen increases the risk of endometrial cancer, and the risk of it being hard to find and resistant to treatment. The longer one takes this drug, the higher the risk.[187] Taking it for up to five years doubles the usual risk. Taking it for five or more years increases risk by a factor of seven.[188]

Step 6. *Break and Enter*

★ Women with an intrauterine device (IUD) are 40 percent less likely to get uterine cancer according to recent studies.[189]

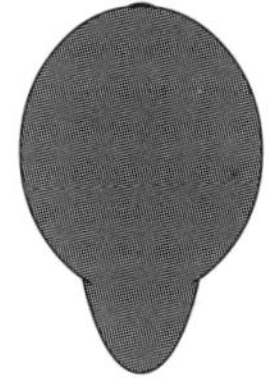

Endometrial Hyperplasia

"Something is ready to grow. What have you planted, dear granddaughter? Your womb prepares the soil.

"I say, let your garden be fallow. The days are shorter; winter is on the way. Throw out your old seeds of pain and anger, confusion and regret, unmet love and unwanted love. Open your belly. Give your belly full of feelings to the Earth. Belly ache to her. Open the space of your uterus to Ancient Wisdom. Abandon your personal projects.

"Nothing new grows here now. Walk with me, hold my hand."

Step 0. *Do Nothing*

> "When properly treated, endometrial hyperplasia rarely progresses to cancer."[190]

Step 1. *Collect Information*

• Uterine hyperplasia means the number of endometrial cells has increased. They are usually benign, but may presage uterine cancer, so a biopsy is in order, along with consistent follow-up.

• Hysterectomy is usually recommended as the best treatment because it "prevents cancer in the future." This is overkill. Stop!

• Hyperplasia is triggered by strong estrogens. Women who take any form of estrogen – ERT, tamoxifen, or bio-identicals – are at the highest risk. Red clover infusion counters strong estrongens.

• Hyperplasia usually causes flooding and/or spotting.

Step 2. *Engage the Energy*

• Homeopaths use the nosode for DES to counter hyperplasia.

Step 3. *Nourish and Tonify*

• Hyperplasia and uterine cancer are fed by strong estrogens. The liver degrades strong estrogens into weak ones, which don't feed cancer. **Liver-helper herbal tinctures** like milk thistle seeds or the roots of dandelion, burdock, or yellow dock can ease hyperplasia. The dose is a dropperful, 1–3 times a day.

★ **Red clover** infusion (2 quarts a week), **miso** (a tablespoon a day), and ground, cooked **flax seeds** (3 tablespoons a day) are powerful allies for women who want to reverse atypical cells. Their weak estrogens counter cancer-promoting strong estrogens.

Step 4. *Stimulate/Sedate*

★ **Avoid** the strong estrogens in black cohosh and hops (beer!).

Step 5a. *Use Supplements*

• **Evening primrose oil** can help reverse hyperplasia.

Step 5b. *Use Drugs*

> "Treatment for both hyperplasia and early endometrial cancer involves either taking hormones to counter estrogen's effects, or hysterectomy."[191]

• Progestin counters mild hyperplasia. Prescription Provera or Prometrium are more effective than progesterone creams.[192]

• Megace (megestrol acetate), a potent oral hormone, reverses atypical hyperplasia, but with severe side effects.

Step 6. *Break and Enter*

• An **endometrial biopsy** is required to differentiate between hyperplasia and cancer. This is best done in the doctor's office with a thin straw inserted through the cervix (a vacuum draws cells into it). It is rare that a D&C (dilatation and curettage) is justified for diagnosis. Resist pressure to have one.

• A Mirena IUD, which delivers progesterone directly to the uterus, can stop the progression to cancer. (More, page 234.)

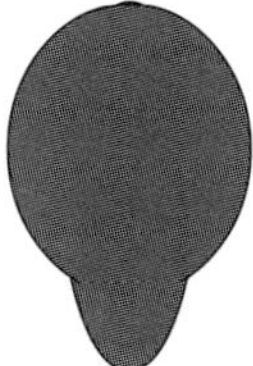

Uterine/Endometrial Cancer

Step 0. *Do Nothing*

• The **symptoms** of uterine/endometrial cancer – unexpected bleeding, vaginal discharge, pelvic pain, dyspareunia, bloating, painful urination, bladder and bowel changes – mimic those of fibroids, endometriosis, PID, and ovarian cancer. If your symptoms are not relieved quickly with the Wise Woman remedies in this book, get help. Do not delay.

Step 1. *Collect Information*

• Most cancer of the uterus occurs in the endometrium, hence uterine cancer and endometrial cancer are the same.

• While it is important to seek medical advice for abnormal uterine bleeding, only 3 to 10 percent of women with postmenopausal bleeding actually have uterine cancer.[193]

• Uterine cancer is the most common gynecological cancer in America, with 40,000 new cases a year, and 7000 deaths annually.[194,195] The number of new cases has been rising since 1987.

• The number of women who die from endometrial cancer has increased by 128 percent in the fifteen years between 1987 and 2002.[196] Nearly a third of women with endometrial cancer have a variant type.[197] Half of these women will have a fatal recurrence within five years despite undergoing "standard treatment: radiation therapy following hysterectomy, removal of the Fallopian tubes, ovaries, and lymph nodes."[198]

• An inherited mutation – Lynch syndrome – increases risk for uterine cancer, primarily in younger women. This syndrome has recently been found in women over 50 as well.[199]

Step 2. *Engage the Energy*

• **Homeopath** Suzy Meszoly uses Dr. A. U. Ramakrishnan's[200] approach – *Carsinosin* one week and one of these remedies at 200C every other week – with "great results." She cautions: "All cancers require consititutional treatment by an experienced homeopath."

~ *Aurum muriaticum natronatum*: cancer of the uterus, ovaries, or cervix, with ulceration and induration, cold abdomen.

~ *Lilium tigrinum*: cancer of the uterus or cervix, with a weighty, bearing-down sensation; especially for those who are hurried, impulsive, high-strung and overly sensitive.

~ *Pulsatilla pratensis*: reproductive cancers; especially for those who are gentle, soft spoken, and weep easily.

~ *Sepia officinalis*: cancer of the uterus/cervix; for strong-willed, hard-working women who avoid sex and get depressed.

Step 3. *Nourish and Tonify*

> "Endometrial cancer and hyperplasia both result from an excess of circulating estrogen."[201]

• To counter excess strong estrogen, strengthen the liver and increase dietary intake of weak estrogens from leaves and seeds.

Step 4. *Stimulate/Sedate*

• Alcohol, soda pop, and fast food are out. Herbal infusions are in.

Step 5. *Use Drugs*

• Women who have taken **clomiphene citrate**, a fertility drug, have the "highest risk of developing uterine cancer, as do women who used the drug 20 or more years ago (which is consistent with the fact that uterine carcinomas are slow-growing tumors)."[202] All ovulation-stimulating drugs pose a similar risk.[203]

• Chemotherapy and radiation after surgery are adjunct treatments that delay relapses and metastasis, but they do not prevent them, nor do they lengthen life.[204] Taking milk thistle seed tincture before chemo and carrot juice (or a baked sweet potato) before radiation can moderate side effects.

Step 6. *Break and Enter*

• The standard diagnostic for uterine cancer is a D&C biopsy, an invasive operation. Instead, ask for a vaginal ultrasound, or, if needed, a biopsy done with a thin hollow tube that can be inserted through the cervix without the need for dilation or anesthesia (page 242).[205]

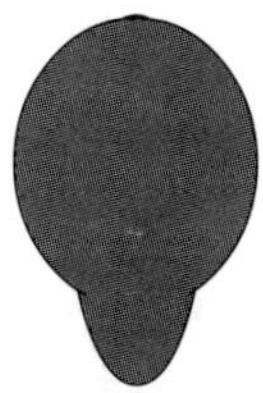

Pelvic Inflammatory Disease

"Give me your hands, my sweet. Put them here," encourages Grandmother Growth as she clasps your hands and puts them firmly against her belly, low, near her notch.

"Yes, put your hands here on my womb. Close your eyes and feel the throb, the pulse, the Earth drum beating there."

"Now, put your hands on your womb." Suiting action to words, she moves your hands to your belly and presses them, leaving her hands on yours.

"There is heat in your belly. It paces. It is dissatisfied. It has stopped yearning and has turned in on itself in bitterness and vengeance, fear and frustration.

"It has gone too far for kindness. You must strike swiftly and deep. You must kill the cells of doubt, eliminate the infections that are eating your core. Consume them before they consume you, my precious, my beloved granddaughter."

Step 0. *Do Nothing*

• Untreated, pelvic inflammatory disease (PID) can lead to infertility, ectopic pregnancy, chronic pelvic pain, and even death. *Start taking echinacea as soon as you think there may be a problem.* (Dosage on page 248). It could save your life.

Step 1. *Collect Information*

• Pelvic inflammatory disease is a general term that covers a range of infections. Symptoms vary widely, from unnoticeable to unbearable. About 170,000 US women, 15–44 years of age, are diagnosed with PID in emergency rooms yearly.[206]

• A woman with PID may have an infection in her endometrium (endometritis), egg tubes (salpingitis), ovaries, and/or uterus.

• PID is "polymicrobial"; it has more than one causative agent.[207] Infective agents include gonorrhea, chlamydia, *Mycoplasma*, hemophilus, *Streptococcus aureus,* and *Ureaplasma urealyticum.*

• Chlamydia is the cause of 50 percent of the PID in Europe and 20-30 percent of the PID in the USA.[208]

• More than one million American women deal with PID on a yearly basis.[209] One-quarter of them will require hospitalization.[210]

• Those at highest risk for PID are active heterosexuals, aged 14–24, with new or multiple partners, with a current (or previous) STD (95 percent of cases),[211] who douche, have an IUD, have had recent pelvic surgery (including miscarriage or abortion), and/or are HIV positive. PID may be acute or chronic, silent or loud.

• Symptoms of PID – tenderness, tightness, pain – often begin during or after menstruation. PID pain is usually on both sides; it may be achy or sharp. There may be low grade fever with a heavy tiredness, lymph node swelling, smelly vaginal discharge, nausea, spotting between periods, and/or a heavy flow/flooding.

★ If you have a **fever** and **severe pain,** you could have a life-threatening infection. Take echinacea and **seek help** immediately.

 Prevent PID 

♥ Be monogamous (one partner only) or always use a barrier.

♥ If you have an IUD or are at high risk, treat yourself promptly with anti-infective herbs if you have pelvic pain – no matter how slight.

♥ Don't drink, take recreational drugs, smoke, or eat processed food.

♥ Love yourself.

• Partner(s) are infected too, even if they don't have symptoms. Take antibiotic herbs/drugs together, please, and refrain from sex until the treatment is done. If not, you could get chronic PID.

• PID can linger for years with symptoms that come and go. Diagnosis is difficult. Hard-to culture organisms slip past the tests. Infections of the tubes and uterus don't show up on a cervical culture. Blood tests are not reliable. Abscesses form and create scar tissue. Some women endure years of mis(sed)diagnosis.

Step 2. *Engage the Energy*

• Combine prayer, visualizations, or dreamwork with your antibiotic therapy for enhanced health.

• **Homeopathic remedies** for acute PID (use *with* antibiotics):

~ *Aconite*: abrupt onset, fever, anxiety, cold worsens.
~ *Apis*: burning pains mainly on the right side, no thirst.
~ *Belladonna*: severe pain, abrupt onset, face red and hot.
~ *Colocynth*: intense cramping pains
~ *Mercurius corr.*: alternate chills and sweats, rest helps.

Step 3. *Nourish and Tonify*

• If you are running a fever or feel achy, be sure to hydrate. Plain water is fine, but nourishing herbal infusions are better.

• The arguments are endless: To eat probiotic ferments during, or after, taking antibiotic drugs is the question. The current answer is "during." Eat 1/2 cup of plain yogurt, kefir, or unheated sauerkraut daily to feed your gut flora. You can take probiotics in capsules, too, but they're more expensive and less effective.

Help!
PID

Expect results within 36 hours

• At the first sign of pelvic pain take 3 dropperfuls of **echinacea** tincture 3–4 times a day for 4–6 days.

• If pain continues or worsens, use twice as much echinacea twice as often, plus one drop of **poke** tincture.

• If symptoms continue or worsen, seek help, take **antibiotics**.

Step 4. *Stimulate/Sedate*

★ **Echinacea** is the herbal antibiotic. It increases production of T-cells, promotes natural killer cell activity, and increases the growth and amount of bacteria-munching white blood cells.[212] A dose of the tincture is one drop per two pounds of body weight, taken at least every two hours initially. (More on page 342.) **Hint**: Look carefully at the label – front and back – be certain it contains *only* echinacea root, no golden seal, no leaves.

• If echinacea does not lessen or remove symptoms within 6–12 hours, I add one drop of **poke root** tincture to each full dose. If there's no response within 24 hours, it's time for antibiotics.

★ **Usnea**, a lichen common throughout the temperate forests and orchards of both northern and southern hemispheres, is another powerful anti-infective. Look for the white cord in every branch. A dose is a dropperful taken each hour.

Usnea is very tough, making it difficult to tincture. Some herbalists freeze and pulverize it before making a tincture. Others boil it and add the softened herb plus the tiny bit of cooking water to the alcohol.

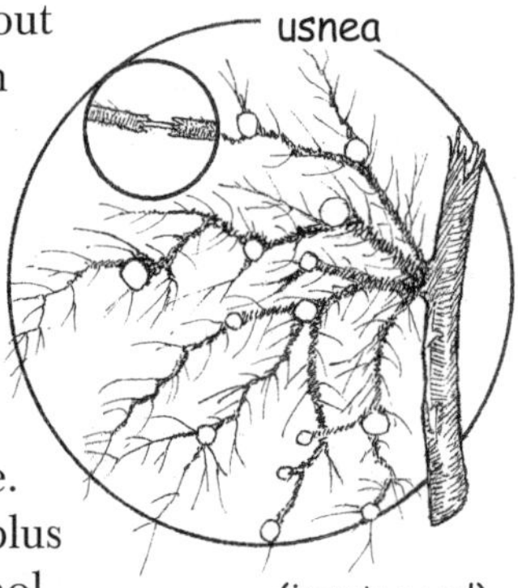

(inset: cord)

★ Experts recommend that any woman with suspected PID go to the hospital immediately.

Advantages of Using Herbs to Treat Suspected PID

- ❖ Non-prescription
- ❖ Safe to take with drugs
- ❖ Available by mail
- ❖ No harm done if PID is not present
- ❖ Long shelf-life, can be kept on hand
- ❖ Can be taken at first signs of infection
- ❖ Counters infection while waiting (for doctor appointments, results of tests/cultures)
- ❖ Few/no side effects
- ❖ Aids antibiotic drugs
- ❖ Can be made at home

★ Counter pain and inflammation (and strengthen the immune system) with ice packs on the belly and alternating hot–cold sitz baths. Sitz in hot water (or a hot herbal soak) for three minutes, then in icy cold water for one minute. Alternate three times to make one treatment. Repeat twice a day.

Step 5. *Use Drugs*

> "Women who suffer from PID and have strong opinions about not being treated with antibiotics should be fully educated and informed, so their decision . . . is not naive. A short course of antibiotic therapy is rarely detrimental to one's health."[213]

★ Do you have to take all of your antibiotics? Yes. PID is tricky and can linger without symptoms. If you take antibiotics, the minimum treatment length is 14 days. More than one antibiotic, or more than one course of antibiotics, may be needed to eliminate your PID completely. Take herbal antibiotics like usnea, echinacea, or yarrow too, if you wish. And be sure your partner doses up!

• Young women who come to emergency rooms with PID are usually admitted and put on intravenous antibiotics to guarantee compliance. The consequences of missing a dose are not immediately obvious, but can cause lifelong problems.

• Taking birth control pills may reduce the risk of PID.[214,215] Using condoms, or being mutually monogamous, definitely will.

Step 6. *Break and Enter*

> "Hysterectomy is rarely necessary for PID."[216]

• Women are most likely to contract STDs/PID during ovulation and menstruation. The cervix is slightly open then, allowing infected sperm to move more easily into, and beyond, the uterus.

• Untreated PID can cause death or necessitate a hysterectomy.

• Uterine biopsy "if not performed carefully, can further spread [PID-causing] organisms . . . to the uterus."[217]

• Women cured of PID have a high risk of ectopic pregnancy. Be prepared; see page 269.

☆ Uterus Star: Sea Sponge Tampons ☆

Sea sponge tampons have been used safely by hundreds of thousands of women since the mid-1970s. Cleopatra used one too.

Sea sponges are small, soft, absorbent, and reusable. They are sustainably harvested and ecologically sound. More than 20 million chlorine-bleached menstrual pads and tampons are sold yearly in the USA. That adds up to a lot of trash. When you use a sea sponge, there is nothing, not even a wrapper, to discard.

Sea sponges are free of dyes and dioxin. They help prevent endometriosis, ovarian and cervical cancers, PID, and toxic shock.

They can be soaked in herbal teas, yogurt, colloidal silver, or other agents for healing applications to the cervix and vagina. Or soak in ascorbic acid and use as a contraceptive barrier.

There is a magic to letting your blood flow. I highly recommend it! But if you can't let it flow, try a sea sponge.

Her Story

Angela is a devout Catholic and mother of three.

"They say I have fibroids. I've always had big clots when I bleed. After switching to cloth pads my periods were shorter and less heavy. The pelvic relaxation exercise I learned from *Luna Yoga* reduced my two weeks of agonizing pre-period pain by 60 percent.

"I'm listening to what my womb is telling me, rather than letting the doctors torture me. They want to cram a tube through my poor cervix and fill my womb with dye!!! My very soul recoils. I prefer prayer to these violations. I will keep my womb!!"

Her Story

Margaret is an unemployed single mother.

"I am *so* frustrated with women doctors. One screamed at me that herbs were more dangerous than ERT! The male doctors acknowledge that I understand my body better than they do. All three women doctors I consulted recommended a hysterectomy because I had fibroids, ovarian cysts, PMS, and a history of uterine problems. 'It will be easier in the long run,' they said. I resisted, and finally found a male OB/GYN who said 'You're almost 40, let's wait and see.' Then I found someone who took seriously the lump in my thyroid. It was thyroid cancer! Since my surgery (to remove the tumor), I am feeling much, much better. My menstrual problems are gone; my uterus isn't."

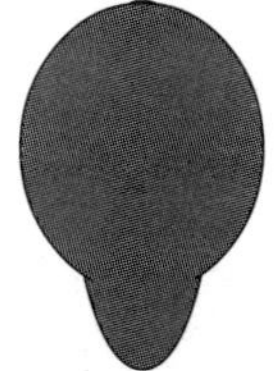

Endometrial Polyps

Step 0. *Do Nothing*

★ Unless you are bleeding heavily, there is no reason to treat or remove endometrial (or cervical) polyps.[218]

Step 1. *Collect Information*

• Polyps may cause bleeding or spotting between menses. For remedies, see page 214.

Step 2. *Engage the Energy*

• **Homeopathic remedies** for women with uterine polyps:
- ~ *Belladonna*: menses early, profuse, painful.
- ~ *Calc-carb.*: staining, worse in cold and wet; menses profuse.
- ~ *Sanguinaria*: with profuse bleeding/hemorrhage.
- ~ *Thuja*: with terrible pain; woman feels thin and fragile.
- ~ *Phos.*: bleeding heavy, sexual desire increased.

Step 3. *Nourish and Tonify*

★ **Oak bark** sitz baths shrink the blood vessels that serve the polyp as well as diminishing the polyp itself. Make it: page 368.

Step 4. *Stimulate/Sedate*

• Uterine and cervical polyps are said to arise from "pelvic stagnation." Counter with castor oil packs. Make it: page 259.

Step 6. *Break and Enter*

• Though rarely needed, both D&Cs and hysterectomies are offered as a (too invasive!) "solution" to uterine polyps.

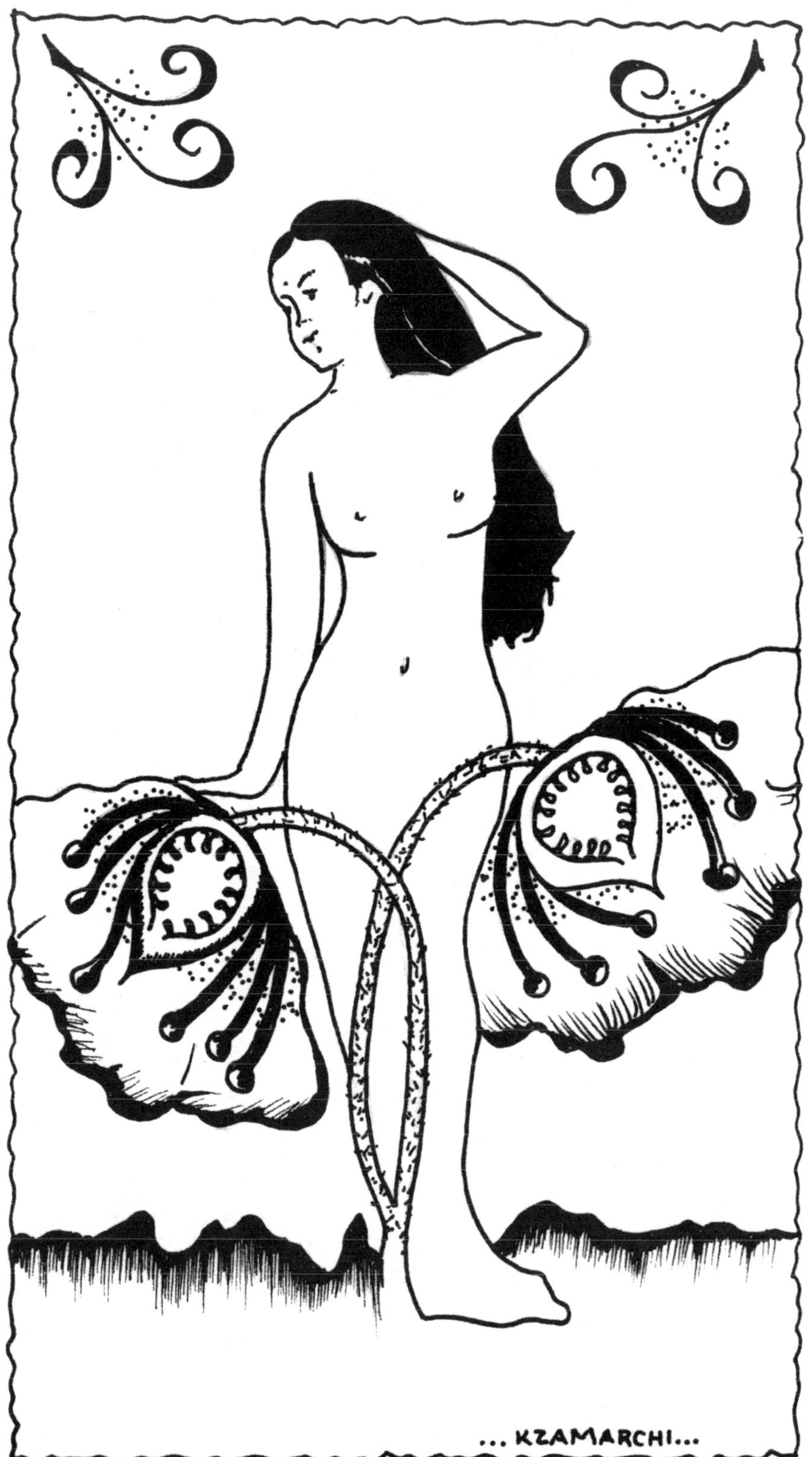
... KZAMARCHI ...

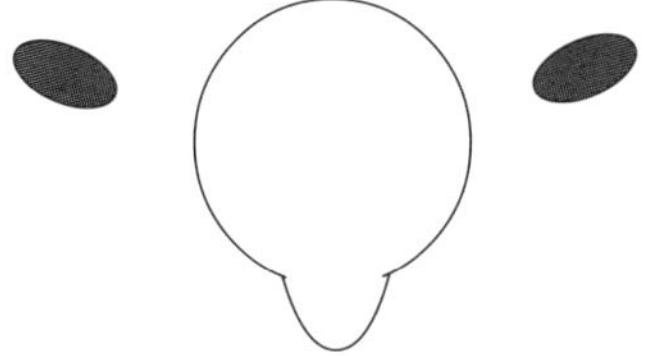

The Ovaries

We are baskets of potential. We are treasure chests of stories. We are passionate and protective; we are profligate and problematic. We are the innermost turning of the spiral. We are the mainspring of existence; we contain the irresistible forces of creation.

We are your gyroscopes; we are your inner guidance system. We are a giveaway blanket strewn with gifts. We are the vault where the most precious and valuable things are kept. We are the library of DNA; we are your high-speed inner*net access. We are the eternal flame. We are star stuff vibrating in you, weaving the patterns of heredity.*

We are a team; we work independently. One per side, one at a time, exploding with joy, exploding with life, we burgeon, we burst. We stir the magical cauldron, adding carefully-crafted hormones, adjusting the heat so it boils over at just the right moment to spew forth an egg, ripe and ready.

One egg is blasted forth. She leaves her yellow coat behind, and that mystical coat now conducts the hormonal orchestra for her alone. The eggs that lost are supposed to shrivel up and die. But every once in a while, there's a sore loser. An egg that won't quit, that makes a pain of itself, or gets uppity and tries to make a baby on its own. We call it a cyst.

Frankly, the more eggs we release, the worse it is for us. We appreciate some time off, if you please. Without the constant pressure to ovulate, we can do some housekeeping, nourish ourselves, get some rest.

We are always with you – even if you cut us away. We send you healing dreams. We awaken the wisdom of the Ancient Ones within you. We hold the grandmothers' memories. We are your ovaries.

Healthy Ovaries

The ovaries are two almond-shaped, plum- to almond-sized endocrine glands that sit in the lower pelvis, one on each side of the uterus. They contain immature, unripe eggs: Graafian follicles.

The ovaries "float" near the *fimbria*, the fluttering fringed openings of the egg tubes. They are held in place by ligaments.

The ovaries produce many hormones, the most important being estradiol, the strongest of the many human estrogens, and the one that is required for ovulation.

The ovaries grow at puberty and contract a little after menopause, but postmenopausal ovaries are no more "shriveled" or inactive than an older man's testes. Our ovaries continue to secrete estrogens and other hormones for as long as we live. No matter how old we are, ovaries are important for optimum health.

Proto-ovaries are present in the four-week-old fetus. By the fifth month of gestation, they are filled with millions of follicles, which die off as we age. By puberty, only 300,000 remain in the ovaries. Even after menopause, hormonally-active follicles are present.

During the years between puberty and menopause, the ovaries take turns, one each month, ripening follicles and ovulating. The ripe, mature follicle tears itself out of the ovary, wounding it. Women who are neither pregnant nor using horomonal birth control are wounded most often because they ovulate most often.

When a mature follicle releases a ripened egg, it becomes the *corpus luteum* (yellow body) and secretes progesterone, which readies the uterus for the fertilized egg and encourages rapid cellular growth in the breasts. If the egg is not fertilized, the corpus luteum dissolves, progesterone levels fall, and menstruation occurs.

Normal menstruation and conception can occur with as little as five percent of the ovary remaining.

Psychic healers see the ovaries as collected wisdom or creative potential (including, but not limited to, childbearing).

In Traditional Chinese Medicine, the ovaries and eggs are viewed as a manifestation of life force energy or *chi*, specifically, Ancestral Chi. Ovarian problems are seen as disruptions in the flow of energy/chi; the cure lies in improving the flow of chi, with special attention to liver chi and spleen chi.

Ovarian Distresses

Ovarian problems – cysts, pain, cancer – may be seen as blockages or impediments to the release or manifestation of creativity.

Ovarian cysts (page 257) are a natural, normal part of the ripening of a follicle into a fertile egg. Most (94 percent) ovarian cysts are small and cause no pain except occasionally at ovulation (*mittelschmerz*). Cysts that form in the ovaries before puberty or after menopause are generally benign.[1] Larger, persistent cysts, especially in postmenopausal women, bring up fears of ovarian cancer. Alternative remedies can successfully eliminate ovarian cysts and help **prevent ovarian cancer**, too (page 275).

Polycystic ovarian syndrome – PCOS (page 264) – is a body-wide problem that can cause ovarian pain and menstrual distress. Alternative treatments are as effective as modern medicines.

Ovarian pain (page 261) may range from mild discomfort to acute agony. Sudden, severe abdominal pain warrants emergency care. Ovarian pain can be caused by a large cyst pressing on tender tissues, a twisted cyst, an ectopic pregnancy (page 269), pelvic inflammatory disease (PID, page 245), endometriosis (page 229), or (rarely) a ruptured cyst. *Ruptures in the pelvic cavity can be fatal.* Visualization and meditative breathing, along with herbs such as skullcap or passionflower tincture, can help ease the pain while you await surgery.

Ovarian cancer (page 281) is "silent but deadly." Fear of this rather rare cancer exaggerates the risk, leading to potentially harmful biopsies, exploratory surgeries, even oophorectomy.

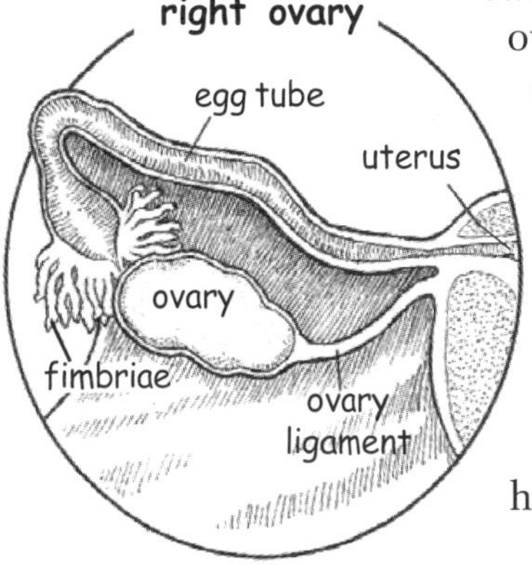

Read this! Surgical removal of healthy ovaries, for any reason, does not reduce mortality from ovarian cancer.[2] It does increase a woman's risk of developing severe problems later in life, including osteoporosis, heart disease, and Parkinsonism (tremors, stiffness, and poor balance).[3] Removal of both ovaries doubles the risk.[4] The younger a women, the higher her risk.[5]

Ovarian Cysts 

There are numerous types of ovarian cysts; these are the most common. A functional cyst arises from a follicle.

Cyst larger than 4 inches? There for 3 months? Take action!

Cysts are, by definition, benign.

Normal functional follicular cysts rarely produce symptoms and require no treatment. They occur in all women who ovulate. Fertility drugs may increase risk. Small follicular cysts generally go away on their own within three months. Homeopathic and herbal remedies can support their remission.

Luteal cysts are functional cysts filled with blood. They can persist for many months, becoming large and painful. Aspiration of the blood with a fine needle eases pain, but the recurrence rate is 30 percent. A dropperful of shepherd's purse tincture every four hours helps stop luteal cyst bleeding/swelling. Daily use of lady's mantle tea helps prevent it.

Dermoid cysts, or *teratoma*, are functional cysts that contain an oily fluid and hard tissues, such as cartilage, teeth, or hair. Orthodox treatment is removal of the ovary. But preservation of the ovary by removing only the cyst is possible. Faithful, persistent use of chickweed or Triple Goddess tincture can resolve these cysts, but it may take a year or more.

Chocolate cysts, or *endometrioma*, form when endometrial tissue clumps on the ovary. They can be very painful. Orthodox treatment is removal of the ovary or, at least, drainage done with a laparoscopic procedure. Herbal remedies and patience are effective alternatives.

Tumors are swellings; they may be benign or malignant.

Borderline tumors, including *mucinous cysts* and others with "low malignant potential" are often overtreated with aggressive removal of uterus, tubes, and ovaries. Herbal remedies are highly effective – usually within 3–9 months – with or without surgical removal of the tumor.

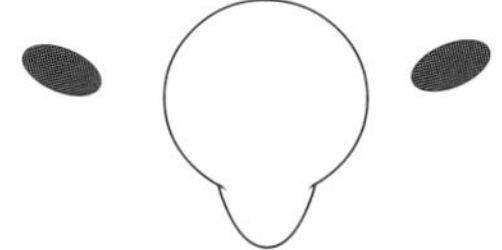

Ovarian Cysts

"Listen closely to the soft, old, wise voice of your ovaries," counsels Grandmother Growth. "Your ovaries embody the Ancient Mother of All, the First Mother. She lives within you, as she lives in every woman.

"Each follicle in your ovary is one of Her stories. Each egg in your ovary is one of Her tales. She wants you to bring them to life, to let your creativity, your "baby," in any form, out to play. Listen, listen, listen. Your ovaries have much to tell you. The Ancient Ones urge you to act, act, act. Come from your ovaries; put it out, let it show, make it real.

"Cherish your creative power, daughter. If you stifle it, you will harm your ovaries. Their energy will become frantic and desperate; they will bother you. Ignore your need to create too long and your ovaries will become depressed, their energy congested, dragging, heavy. Their lightness will become a burden, a weight far too heavy to bear. Their stories will be stories of loss and grief. And you may lose them. Be assured, though, you can never lose your connection to me and to the Ancient Mother of All. We live in every cell of your being, my dearest child, in every cell."

Step 0. *Do Nothing*

★ The vast majority of ovarian cysts dissolve on their own, with no treatment, within three months.

• Watchful waiting is appropriate for women with *nonsolid* ovarian cysts smaller than ten centimeters (four inches). There is a "virtually nonexistent" chance of these tumors being malignant.[6] In premenopausal, asymptomatic women, 70 percent of such masses resolve without any therapy.[7]

Step 1. *Collect Information*

> ". . . every month women develop ovarian cysts as part of their normal menstrual cycle."[8]

• Ovarian (*adnexal*) cysts are fluid-filled sacs. Rarely malignant, they may be quite painful, or cause no symptoms at all.

• Ovarian cysts are normal during the fertile years. The maturing egg is a cyst, which breaks out of the ovary. If it doesn't, it's a *follicular cyst.* If it creates hair and bones, it's a *dermoid cyst.* When the corpus luteum bleeds, it's a *luteal cyst.*

• Ovarian cysts can interfere with fertility. They can burst or twist, causing intense pain and sudden weakness.

• Beware! Transvaginal ultrasound (TVU) shows masses on the ovary, but can't distinguish between benign cysts and cancerous growths. Doctors, fearing cancer, remove healthy ovaries.

• Smooth ovarian masses smaller than two centimeters (an inch) in premenopausal women rarely trigger medical panic. However, if you have a large mass or are postmenopausal, expect to be urged to have a total hysterectomy or "at least" exploratory surgery "for peace of mind."[9] Peace of mind?! Abdominal surgery is life-disrupting and can be life-threatening; it is *not* a safe diagnostic.

• Older women *are* more likely to have ovarian cancer, but at least 15 percent of their ovarian masses are simply benign cysts.[10] Surgery can ruin your life, not save it. Proceed with caution.

Step 2. *Engage the Energy*

• **Homeopathic remedies** for women with ovarian cysts:
~ *Apis*: burning pain on the right, worse with heat.
~ *Aurum muriaticum nat.*: ovarian pain extends up to scapula.
~ *Baryta-carb.*: timid woman with a large single cyst.
~ *Calc-carb.*: corpulent, slow, passive, cold cystic woman.
~ *Colocynth*: small round cysts, violent, cramping pain.
~ *Graphites*: cysts cause pain on intercourse.
~ *Kali-br.*: left-sided pain, especially during intercourse.
~ *Lachesis*: pressing, stitching pain on left; highly emotional.
~ *Lycopodium*: boring pain on the right; craves sweets.

• **Visualize** the cyst dissolving. Pretend there is a river flowing through it, washing it away. Bathe it in a healing color. Let go. . . .

• Dr. Mona Lisa Schultz, neuroscientist and medical intuitive, says ovarian cysts are stored energy. To release it, she suggests "giving birth" by creative expenditure of pelvic energy.[11]

Step 3. *Nourish and Tonify*

• Either a cup of **burdock** root infusion 4–8 times a week, or a dropperful of **wild yam** root tincture, 1–3 times a day, can help tonify the ovaries.

Step 4. *Stimulate/Sedate*

★ **Chickweed** is a reliable dissolver of ovarian cysts. I prefer tincture of the fresh plant in flower, though infusion of the dried herb may be used with good results. The key is consistency: a dropperful of tincture, or a cup of infusion, taken 3-4 times a day until the cyst is gone. Very large cysts and dermoid cysts *will* dissolve eventually, but it may require more than a year's effort.

★ Herbalists around the world recommend **castor oil packs** to reduce ovarian cysts. A flannel cloth is soaked in castor oil and applied to the abdomen, or the oil is rubbed right into the skin over the ovary. For deeper, more penetrating heat, wrap the castor-oil soaked flannel in foil (seal well) and warm in the oven; remove foil before applying. Or cover oiled skin with a towel and a heating pad. Success follows repetition (yes, you can use the same flannel over and over) and patience (yes, you must do it over and over). Several applications a day is most effective. If your skin gets irritated, stop for a while.

• Other poultices used to eliminate ovarian cysts/cancers include fresh mashed **tofu**; fresh

Help!
Ovarian Cysts

Expect results in 2–4 months

• Take a dropperful of **chickweed tincture** 1–3 times a day.

• Or take a dropperful of chickweed, motherwort, cronewort (mugwort) tincture 1–3 times a day.

• Commit to a **creative project** that delights you.

• Experiment with **poultices**.

or dried **comfrey leaves** boiled until soft and applied, cold or hot, as desired; and fresh **chickweed**.

★ Improving the flow of blood and lymphatic fluid to the pelvis helps eliminate ovarian cysts. A dropperful of the tincture of fresh flowering **cleavers**, taken 2–3 times a day, does it best. It also relieves ovarian pain. Cleavers and chickweed are good friends who work well, and grow well, together.

★ **Triple Goddess tincture** is a Chinese formula for women that goes back several thousand years. It is made from equal parts **maidenwort** (*Stellaria media*), **motherwort** (*Leonurus cardiaca*), and **cronewort** (*Artemisia vulgaris*). Each herb is harvested, and tinctured fresh, when it blooms: the maiden in the spring, the mother in the summer, and the crone in the fall. To dissolve cysts, I use 1–2 dropperfuls of mixed tincture 3–4 times a day.

Step 5. *Use Drugs*

• Although birth control pills are frequently prescribed as a means to prevent ovarian cysts, they are no more effective than a placebo.[12] Neither is progesterone cream, nor Norplant (tiny progestin-bearing silicone rods implanted in the upper arm).[13]

Her Story

Sarah is a healthy postmenopausal woman.

"I was so distressed. My doctor wanted to do immediate surgery to check out a large, possibly cancerous, mass he found on my ovary.

"I asked for some time to think about it. I was certain I didn't have ovarian cancer, but I was shaken by the doctor's fervor.

"The first thing I did was make some red clover infusion. Then I took some motherwort tincture, to calm down. I went to Susun's website and read about chickweed tincture. I bought some and started taking 2-4 dropperfuls a day the very next day.

"Six weeks later, another sonogram showed the same mass, no bigger, no smaller. I knew the cyst was dissolving. My abdomen felt softer than it had in months. I refused surgery again, to my doctor's dismay, and continued with my chickweed tincture.

"A month later, another sonogram. The doctor was speechless. The mass on my ovary was nowhere to be seen."

Step 6. *Break and Enter*

> "If the ovaries can be felt in a postmenopausal woman, that in itself indicates the necessity of a complete hysterectomy."[14]

• Do cysts larger than two inches require surgery?[15] **Laparoscopic** diagnosis or treatment of ovarian cysts can cause infertility, chronic pain, bleeding disturbances, and pelvic adhesions which may occasionally be lethal.[16] *Try other remedies first.*

> "Not only is abdominal surgery unnecessary [for ovarian cysts], it can be downright dangerous, with repercussions that can impair fertility and eventually lead to tremendous pain."[17]

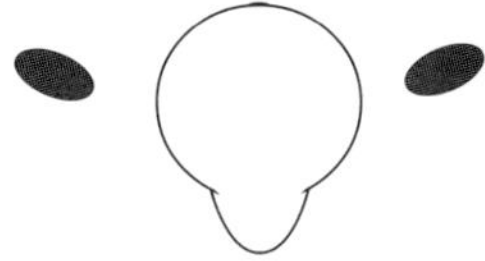

Ovarian Pain

"Some of the stories held in your ovaries are painful," Grandmother Growth whispers. "Your mothers and their mothers' mothers' mothers' lost their babies, died in childbirth, were raped or married to men they feared. Their memories hurt. You have the power to soothe the pain of the generations. Let me help you, with love."

Step 0. *Do Nothing* / **Step 1.** *Collect Information*

• Is your acute pelvic pain gas? It is if it lessens with rest, time, and some slippery elm. Do nothing. If not, it could be: an ectopic pregnancy (page 269), PID (page 245), appendicitis, or a cyst (page 257). If it keeps getting worse, seek help. For help with chronic pelvic pain, turn to page 15.

Step 2. *Engage the Energy*

★ The best **homeopathic** remedy for women with *mittelschmerz* (pain with ovulation) is *Atropine.*

- Other **homeopathic** remedies for ovarian pain:
  - ~ *Arg-met.*: pain on left.
  - ~ *Colocynth*: severe pain, eased by warmth.
  - ~ *Belladonna* or *Lycopodium*: pain on right.
  - ~ *Mag-phos.*: ovarian neuralgia, mostly on right.
  - ~ *Naja*: violent cramping pain, worse on left.
  - ~ *Nux vomica*: pain with loss of appetite.
  - ~ *Sabina*: pain worse with heat.
  - ~ *Staphizagria*: ovaries very tender, pain worse on sitting.
  - ~ *Zincum met.*: pain worse with touch.

Step 3. *Nourish and Tonify*

★American folk herbalists use **wild yam root** to relieve ovarian pain. Chinese herbalists say it tonifies chi. A daily dose is a cup of dried root infusion, or 2–4 dropperfuls of fresh root tincture. Wild yam is especially effective in relieving nerve pain after pelvic surgery.

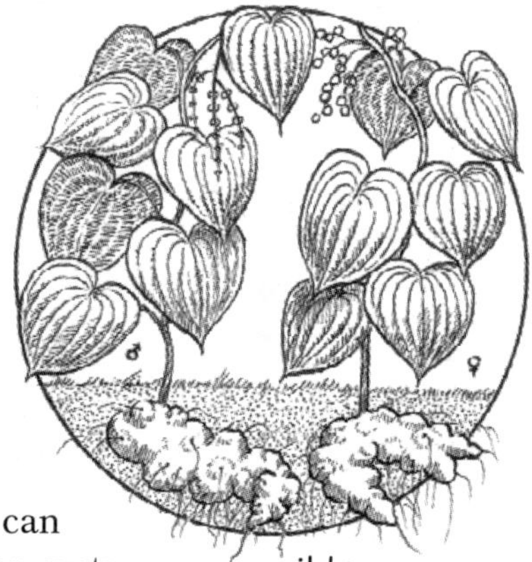

wild yam

- **Saw palmetto berry** tincture can relieve ovarian pain, eliminate ovarian cysts, and address PCOS.

Your Story?

Colleen was still contemplating having children. During her annual exam, her gynecologist found a large mass on her ovary. She was frightened by what the doctor said, and agreed to have it surgically removed, "just in case there's cancer."

With tears in her eyes, she recounts awakening after the surgery. Her surgeon was beaming at her. He said: "The mass was benign. And you won't ever have to worry again. We went ahead and removed your ovaries and your uterus. Aren't you happy?"

This story is true. And I've heard it from more than one woman.

(One reader wrote in the margin of my manuscript: "I can't imagine a doctor would remove the uterus of a woman of childbearing age without good reason." Another reader penned this reply: "Believe it! It happened to my sister, too.")

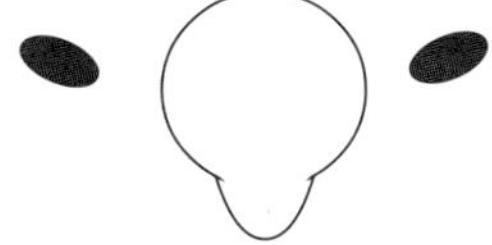

Polycystic Ovarian Syndrome (PCOS)

"What are your ancestors saying?" asks Grandmother Growth. Tears streak her wrinkled cheeks and hang in the folds. Her smile is so compassionate, your heart breaks open. You step into her embrace and feel your own tears flowing.

"Their voices are faint. Their faces are faded. They have no hands. They are destitute; they have nothing to give you. They are sad, so sad. But there was nothing left for you. They love you, but cannot change what is.

"To compensate, your ovaries compulsively create possibility after possibility. But without the energy of your ancestors, none of those possibilities can be born. You are stuck with them.

"You are special. You start a new story. A story that has never been told before. Yes, doors are closed to you that are open for others. Knocking on them will not avail you. Come , let us find your gift. It is hidden, but it is within you. Follow me. . . ."

Step 0. *Do Nothing*

• Stress causes an increase in cortisol production, and cortisol exacerbates the symptoms of PCOS. Ommmm . . . . Mindfulness meditation, yoga, and tai chi are easy ways to lower cortisol.

• PCOS affects different women differently. Take some quiet time – alone in nature if possible – to feel into what you want before embarking on any treatment. Do you want to get pregnant? Get rid of unwanted body hair? Improve the appearance of your skin? Have regular periods with normal bleeding? Protect yourself against heart disease and diabetes? You can! Read on.

Step 1. *Collect Information*

• PCOS is also known as chronic oligoanovulation. It was formerly called Stein-Leventhal syndrome.

• PCOS affects between 5–10 percent of women of reproductive age in the USA – that's about five million women.[18]

• Women with PCOS have a variety of symptoms: sudden weight gain, facial hair, infertility, and irregular menses are the classic ones. Others include: growth of body hair, dandruff, sleep apnea, snoring, acne, chronic pelvic pain, high blood pressure, high cholesterol, and insulin resistance. Numerous cysts on the ovaries frequently occur.[19] The type and severity of symptoms varies widely. Not all women have all symptoms; about one-third have severe symptoms, such as uncontrollable bleeding, baldness, and *acanthosis nigricans*, a condition in which dark velvety patches appear on the skin. Symptoms may begin at puberty, or not until the woman is in her thirties.[20]

• Hormone levels are skewed in women with PCOS. They usually have *twice as much testosterone* and androstenedione as other women,[21] higher levels of luteinizing hormone (LH), and virtually no progesterone.[22] Their base estrogen levels are generally normal, but there's little or no estradiol, thus, no ovulation.[23]

• Women with PCOS are frequently insulin-resistant.[24] Up to 40 percent of women with PCOS develop insulin resistance or diabetes by the age of forty.[25]

• The causes of PCOS are unknown at this time. *There may be a genetic component.*[26] Women with PCOS are often daughters of men who have gone bald early in life. A defect in a single gene is responsible for both conditions. If a women inherits that one gene from either her father or mother, her chances of developing PCOS are high; if from both, very high.

Help!
Polycystic Ovarian Syndrome

Expect results within 2–4 months

• **Remove** vegetable/seed oils from your diet. **Eat more** animal fats.

• Take 2–4 droppersful of **vitex** or **saw palmetto** tincture daily.

• Take dandelion tincture as needed.

• Control bleeding with frequent doses of shepherd's purse tincture.

• Drink 3–6 quarts of **nourishing herbal infusion** weekly.

• Why do women with PCOS have too much testosterone? It can be due to abnormalities in the hypothalamus, abnormalities in the ovaries, or **too much insulin**. A genetic defect in an enzyme pivotal to the manufacture of ovarian androgens (testosterone) allows insulin to overstimulate production.[27]

• Women with PCOS who ally with **motherwort** tincture lessen their increased risks of diabetes, endometrial cancer, heart disease,[28] coronary artery blockages, and calcifications.[29]

Step 2. *Engage the Energy*

• To counter an abundance of testosterone: Claim your Wise Woman within. Welcome her, nurture her, embrace her.

• **Affirmations** for women with PCOS:
I surrender to the sweetness of life.
I burst out of my bounds and venture all.
I manifest my own inner Wise Woman.

Step 3. *Nourish and Tonify*

★ Regular **exercise** equals less depression, a reduction in breast and reproductive cancers, fewer heart attacks, better blood pressure, less diabetes, and a reduction in the symptoms of PCOS.[30]

• Women with PCOS do better with **high-fat**, **whole-grain** diets.[31,32] Since hormones are essentially fats, essential fatty acids are critical to reproductive health. **Omega-3 fatty acids** – found in **olive oil**, **butter**, full-fat yogurt and cheese, nuts, fatty fish, **purslane** and flax seeds – help. Omega-6 fatty acids – in vegetable oils, especially soy, canola, corn, and cottonseed – inflame.

★ **Avoid** trans fatty acids, preservatives, and processed foods. They disrupt healthy hypothalamus functioning and distort hormonal messages, according to lipid chemist Sally Fallon.[33]

• Herbalist David Winston offers **self-heal** (Xia Ku Kao) as a tea (1–2 cups) or tincture (1–2 dropperfuls) to women with PCOS.

• A diet low in processed carbohydrates is the best for all women, and critical for women with PCOS. Replace white flour and white sugar with whole grains and honey. Eliminate all high-fructose corn syrup and artificial sweeteners, too.

★ Instead of soda pop, **drink nourishing herbal infusions**. A quart a week of nettle, oatstraw, raspberry, or linden (use one at a time and rotate) will give you results within a month.

• **Linden** flowers are one of the nicest anti-inflammatory herbs around. Put one-half ounce of the dried herb in a quart of cold water, bring it to a boil, turn off the heat, cover the pot, and let it steep for at least four hours. Try it warm with a spoonful of honey.

• Women with PCOS often have high levels of insulin in their blood.[34] A diet that includes yogurt and salmon, but no other animal products, reduces insulin and the need for drugs.[35]

• Don't substitute soy for meat or dairy; it is contraindicated for PCOS. Nutritionist Dr. Mary Enig says PCOS is strongly related to consumption of commercially-processed soy products, especially soy-based infant formula.[36] Dr. Naomi Baumslag, president of the Women's International Public Health Network, reminds us: "The amount of phytoestrogens in soy [products] varies as much as tenfold. . . . The soy used today . . . has more isoflavones. . . ."[37]

Step 4. *Stimulate/Sedate*

> ". . . weight loss alone may correct hyperinsulinemia, and reverse other characteristics of PCOS — even infertility."[38]

• Many "healthy" protein bars, promoted to help weight loss, are soy-based and not healthy at all for PCOS women.

• For women with PCOS, herbalist Terry Willard offers **Female Restorative Roots**.[39] (Make it: page 375.)

★ **Saw palmetto** has androgen-modulating effects. Herbalists David Winston and Karta Khalsa consider it the perfect ally for women with PCOS. In high doses (4–6 dropperfuls or more a day) saw palmetto tincture can reduce hair growth, reverse weight gain, eliminate acne, and even stimulate suppressed ovulation. David Winston suggests combining it with moderate doses (1–4 dropperfuls daily) of **vitex** and **dandelion** tinctures.

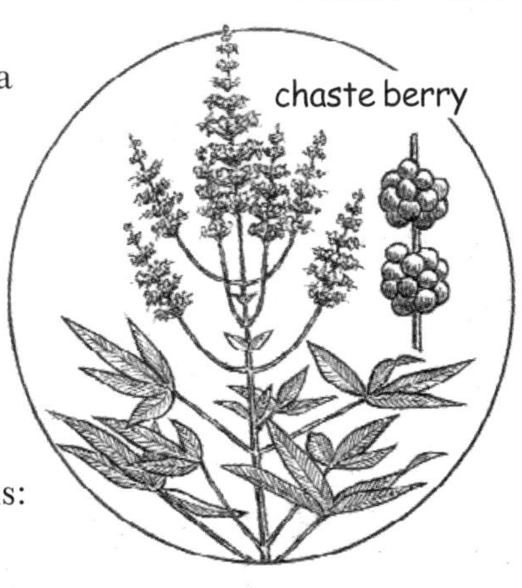

★ **Chasteberry** (**vitex**) has a strong effect on the entire hormonal system. It's especially helpful for women who have trouble conceiving, as regular use can trigger ovulation, even in older women. A dose is a dropperful of tincture, 1–3 times a day for 12–36 months. It's more effective, and a lot less expensive, to make your own. (Directions: page 367.)

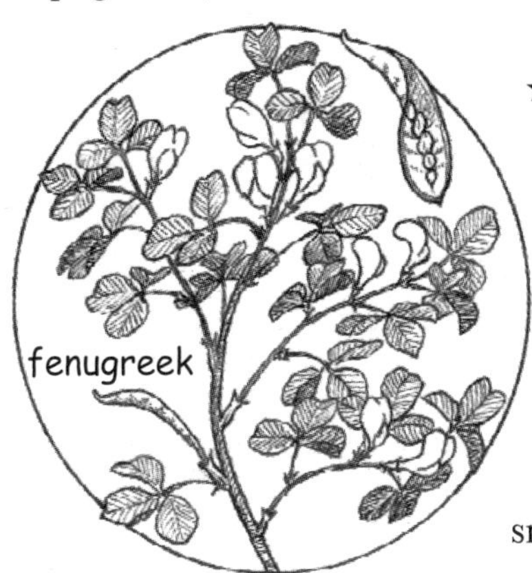

★ A cup a day of great-tasting **fenugreek seed** tea helps your cells accept insulin. Make it: Put 6–8 teaspoonfuls into a quart jar or a big teapot, add one quart of boiling water, cover, and brew for 5–20 minutes. Strain and refrigerate. Keeps for up to a week. Added benefit: It makes one's perspiration smell like maple syrup.

Step 5a. *Use Supplements*

• Women with PCOS are often low in vitamin A.[40] Get more by eating more well-cooked green, red and orange foods. If you must supplement, cod liver oil is best.

Step 5b. *Use Drugs*

• Instead of fertility drugs, try **chasteberry** tincture.

• Drugs that increase the body's sensitivity to insulin can help women with PCOS. After a month on **Metformin** (glucophage), 90 percent of women with PCOS ovulated.[41] (Some took Clomid too.) Use of Metformin increases the chances of getting pregnant. It is known to cause severe diarrhea; perhaps that's why it is said to mitigate weight gain in women with PCOS.

★ Oral contraceptives (birth control pills), prescription progesterone, and/or spironolactone are used to block the action of androgens. These drugs may alleviate symptoms and can help decrease the risks of endometrial hyperplasia and cancer.[42]

• Despite the known connection between high cortisol and PCOS, naturopaths "always give cortisol (cortef) for PCOS. It stops the syndrome and rests the ovaries."[43]

• The **essential oils** of clary sage (2 drops), fennel (2 drops) geranium (2 drops) and rose (1 drop), diluted in two tablespoons of olive oil – and a little rubbed on the belly – may ease PCOS pain. Essential oils are strong medicine. Carefully consider your ability to withstand their concentrated energies before using them, even externally.

Step 6. *Break and Enter*

> "I can remember it clearly, as if it were just yesterday. Throughout my medical training I was told that when performing a hysterectomy for *any* reason on *any* woman 40 or older, it was my responsibility to persuade her to have her ovaries removed. . . ."[44]

• Exploratory surgery is not simple, safe, pain free, or "noninvasive." Consider carefully, then consider again, then reevaluate and reconsider, before you agree to removal of your ovaries for any reason except cancer – not the fear of it, not the threat of it, but actual cancer.

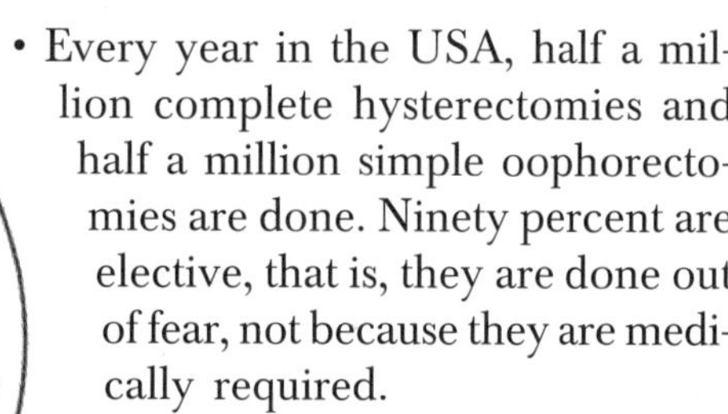

• Every year in the USA, half a million complete hysterectomies and half a million simple oophorectomies are done. Ninety percent are elective, that is, they are done out of fear, not because they are medically required.

• **Keep your ovaries!**

★ Women who keep their ovaries live longer and are less likely to die of heart disease or lung cancer.[45]

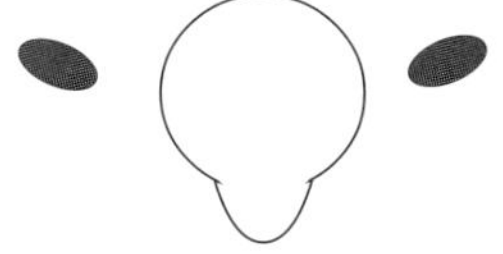

Ectopic Pregnancy

"Come here and rest your head in my lap," says Grandmother Growth with a sigh and a small grimace of pain. "What I have to tell you is difficult to say. It is even more difficult to do.

"The spirit life within you must leave. It is time to give death to that growing light. Give death with love. Give death with compassion. Give death with peace in your heart. Withdraw your support. Cut the thread.

"This creation cannot live. Let it go. Now."

Step 0. *Do Nothing*

★ This is a potentially fatal condition. **Seek help now.**

Step 1. *Collect Information*

• A fertilized egg ought to implant in the uterus. If it grows somewhere else – usually in the egg tube, but occasionally in the ovary, cervix, or abdominal cavity – it is an ectopic pregnancy.

• During our fertile years, once each month, a ripe follicle (mature egg) tears its way out of the ovary and is enticed intothe egg tube by the fimbria (fingers). Rhythmic pulsations carry the egg to the uterus. If the egg tube is scarred or narrowed, or unable to pulsate, a fertilized egg may get stuck and grow there.

• Symptoms of ectopic pregnancy usually begin about six weeks after conception. They include spotting or staining, abdominal or shoulder pain. Some women bleed heavily.

• A growing fertilized egg can rupture the egg tube, creating excruciating pelvic pain – some women pass out – and life-threatening internal bleeding.

• Pelvic pain can be caused by a great many things, from appendicitis to gas. Some can be fatal; others, just embarrassing.

Some require emergency surgery; others will resolve themselves. Diagnosis can be difficult. Ultrasound and blood tests make it a bit easier. Sometimes laparoscopic surgery is necessary, however, to diagnose – and treat – ovarian/pelvic pain.

• A radio-immunoassay, or -receptorassay test can reveal beta human chorionic gonadotrophin, a hormone produced by the dividing cells of the embryo even before it is implanted in the uterus.

• The rate of ectopic pregnancies has more than doubled in the past ten years. Formerly, about 0.5 percent of all pregnancies were ectopic. The rate is now between 1 and 2 percent.[46] This is most likely due to increases in PID and chlamydia infections, not to increases in the use of IUDs or the rates of tubal ligation.

• Previously, ectopic pregnancy was one of the three leading causes of maternal mortality in the USA.[47] Today, modern diagnostic techniques allow time to act to prevent hemorrhage and death.

• Ectopic pregnancies are more common in women who were exposed to DES (page 202) in utero.[48]

> "Before we had these drugs, women who had pelvic infections [PID] would often become totally infertile. With antibiotic treatment, they can become pregnant, but their tubes may be scarred . . . and damaged, so the fertilized egg [sticks] in the tube."[49]

Step 2. *Engage the Energy*

• While awaiting help – in the emergency room or before surgery – visualize those who love you. They are comforting you, easing you, holding you, crying with you, lending you strength.

Risk Factors for Ectopic Pregnancy

- Present or previous chlamydia infection
- Present or previous PID
- Present or previous endometriosis
- Previous ectopic pregnancy
- Previous abdominal surgery of any kind, including C-section, tubal ligation, appendectomy, laparoscopic diagnosis

Step 3. *Nourish and Tonify*

★ If you go to a hospital, **take an advocate** with you. Really!

• Help yourself heal after the surgery by drinking comfrey leaf infusion. I like mine with a hint of mint. Make it: page 367.

Step 4. *Stimulate/Sedate*

★ If you are at risk for ectopic pregnancy, keep powdered **tumeric** and **ginger** on hand. Herbalist Sarah Elisabeth says repeated doses (taken in capsules or mixed with yogurt, honey, or tea) can prevent an ectopic pregnancy from bursting.

★ Tincture of mature, ripe **wild carrot seed** – a dropperful taken every 15–20 minutes – helps prevent rupture of the tube and may help you pass the conceptus. (Make it, page 367.)

• "Mad dog" **skullcap** relieves pain. A dose is 10–20 drops of tincture of the fresh plant in flower, repeated as needed. Skullcap is sleep-inducing, so several doses may put you out.

• Tincture of fresh **shepherd's purse** stops internal bleeding – fast. A dropperful dose may be repeated every 15 minutes, or as needed, until effective.

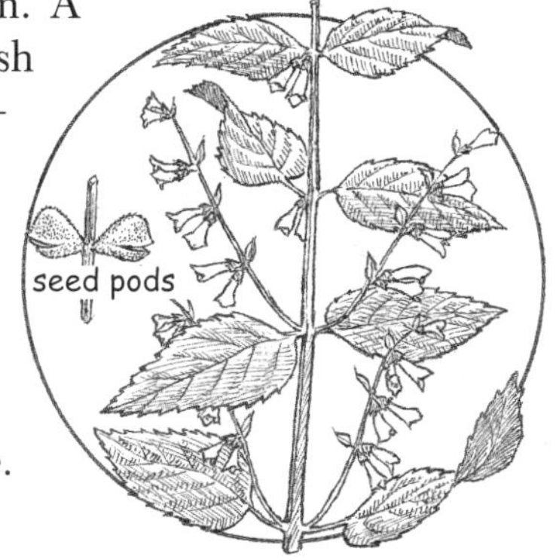

skullcap

Step 5. *Use Drugs*

• Ectopic pregnancies can be ended with the chemotherapeutic agent methotrexate. Methotrexate kills all rapidly-dividing cells, including the embryo. Since it takes time to work, it is not suitable for women who are already in severe pain or at a point in their tubal pregnancy where rupture seems likely.

Step 6. *Break and Enter*

• Many hospitals routinely remove the entire egg tube when there is an ectopic pregnancy. This impairs fertility and is not necessary. Take an advocate with you to insure that your egg tubes are saved. Surgeons can almost always cut open the tube, remove the ectopic pregnancy, and leave it to heal naturally.[50] Don't just ask for a **salpingostomy**; insist on it!

Her Story

Martina is 24, single, and vastly enjoying her life. She is the only woman in her family who doesn't deal with PCOS.

"My mother was told that surgery was the only way to take care of the numerous cysts on her ovaries and the horrible pain she was experiencing. Before she was 30, they had removed one whole ovary and half of the other one. She continued to get cysts and pain despite the surgery. At last, she discovered that taking birth control pills eased the pain and shrunk the cysts! She is now in menopause and still suffering. When the pain gets too bad, the Pill still helps. Her father was bald by the age of fifteen."

Her Story

Windsong is the devoted mother of two.

"Last night, after drinking sage tea, was the first night in years I didn't awaken in a puddle of sweat. I'm in menopause at age 30.

"A few months after my second son was born I got my tubes tied. My doctor never explained any possible side effects. I developed post-tubal-ligation syndrome, and wham, slam, I was menopausal. The problem didn't stop there. The post-tubal-ligation syndrome kicked my *adenomyosis* into overdrive. My uterus grew at an alarming rate. In the end, at the age of 28, I agreed to have it removed (a hysterectomy), but they removed my ovaries too.

"I have no trust in doctors. I won't take their hormones. I'm learning about herbs; the ones I've tried are already helping me feel better."

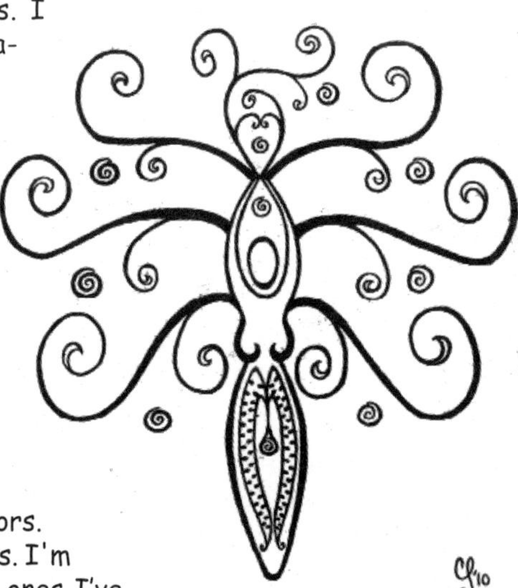

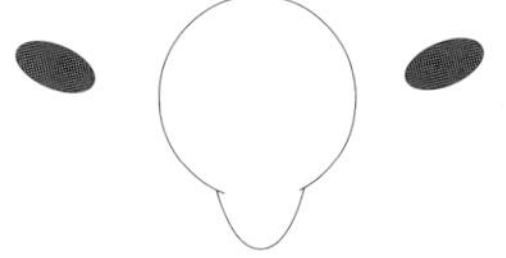

Screening for Ovarian Cancer?

Screening for ovarian cancer seems like a good idea. For early-stage cancer, the five-year survival rate is over 90 percent; at later stages, less than 30 percent.[51] But there are severe problems with the methods currently available for screening.

The available tests – CA-125 and transvaginal ultrasound (TVU) – used alone, find only 25 percent of the women who actually have cancer,[52] and vastly increase the number of women frightened into unnecessary abdominal surgeries and oophorectomies.

Calcium-125 has a very high false positive rate. *Any individual positive CA-125 test has less than a one percent chance of being correct.*[54] Only half of women with early ovarian cancer will have elevated CA-125.[55] Menstruation, pelvic inflammatory disease, endometriosis, hepatitis, liver disease, cirrhosis, poorly-controlled diabetes, pneumonia, and systemic lupus increase CA-125 levels, too.[56]

In 100,000 symptomless women screened for ovarian cancer with TVU, 40 cases of ovarian cancer will be found, but 5398 women will be subjected to unnecessary surgery.[57]

> ". . . the minimum bar for an acceptiable screening test is, at most 10 surgeries to find one ovarian cancer."[53]

Used together – letting rising CA-125 levels trigger a TVU – twice the number of early cancers are found (50 percent rather than 25 percent) and only 1.5 women out of 100,000 will undergo surgery to find the one with ovarian cancer.[58]

New tests, such as PreOvar, look for abnormal genes or protein fragments from the cancer in the blood or urine.[59,60,61,62,63]

Even monitoring of CA-125 levels in women known to have ovarian cancer is questionable. It increases the amount of chemotherapy given (which decreases quality of life) without increasing the life span.[64]

Ovarian Cancer Risk Factors[65] 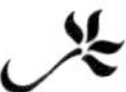

- Age over 55 (the median for onset is 63)
- Lives in an industrialized country
- Douches frequently
- Unchecked ovulation for thirty or more years
- Never pregnant; never lactated/nursed
- Never used birth control pills (oral contraceptives)
- Uses/used estrogen or hormone replacement
- Uses/used dusting powders with talc[66,67]
- Took fertility drugs for three cycles or more[68]
- High consumption of industrial dairy products[69]
- High consumption of domesticated-animal fats[70]
- Eastern European Jewish descent; BRCA mutations
- Family history of ovarian, breast, uterine, or colon cancer*

* 90 percent of women with ovarian cancer have no family history.[71]

To Lower Risk of Ovarian Cancer 

- Eat a soy-free, semi-vegetarian diet.
- Eat 5 servings of fruits/vegetables daily.[72]
- Eat red/cured/processed meat less than 4 times a week.[73]
- Drink freshly-brewed (not bottled) green or black tea.
- Drink nourishing herbal infusions, especially red clover.
- Maintain a normal weight.
- Take birth control pills for five years or more.
- Be pregnant, at least once, even if you don't give birth.
- Never have a diagnosis of breast, uterine, or colon cancer.
- Start your menses after age 12; end them before age 52.
- Have no family member with ovarian cancer.

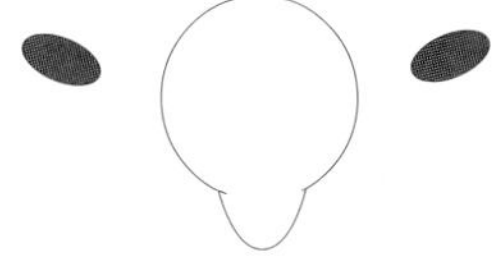

Preventing Ovarian Cancer

"Did you like stories when you were young? Do you still enjoy them? Remember that your ovaries are story baskets," confides Grandmother Growth, as she takes your hand in hers.

"This is a talking stick," she says, placing a small beaded rod with two feathers hanging from it into your open palm. "Hold it. Let it gently lift the cover of your ovary basket so the stories can flow. Let it loosen your tongue so the emotions can flow. Let it act as a needle to weave you into the healing cloak of the Ancients.

"Grasp the stick. Grasp your strength. You are deserving of respect and honor. You are precious, worthy. Stand up now, here, beside me, and put your feet on the path to power."

Step 0. *Do Nothing*

• Gynecologists in America and Europe are trained to "prevent" ovarian cancer by removing the ovaries of any woman older than forty who is having pelvic surgery of any kind. Avoid pelvic surgery . . . or avoid gynecologists. . . or be prepared to fight.

> " . . . thousands of women's ovaries are . . . sacrificed to save one or two from getting ovarian cancer."[74]

Step 1. *Collect Information*

• An American woman's lifetime risk of ovarian cancer is less than one in eighty.[75]

★ Any **pregnancy** reduces the risk of ovarian cancer, and the later in life the last pregnancy happens, the greater the risk reduction. A woman who has a child before age 25 reduces her risk by 20 percent; after the age of 35, by 50 percent. Women who have four or more full-term babies reduce their risk by nearly 70 percent. Even incomplete pregnancies confer "significant protection."[76]

Step 2. *Engage the Energy*

• Christiane Northrup, holistic medical doctor, suggests that unexpressed rage and resentment can build up in the ovaries, setting the stage for ovarian cancer. She reflects that many women feel "paralyzed by their [unacknowledged] rage."[77]

★ To **unstick your rage** from your ovaries, you need to believe that you have hidden anger, and that it can be expressed in a healthy, non-injurious way. This exercise will help you do both. You'll need a rolled-up newspaper and a cushion, or (the choice of my mentor Elisabeth Kubler Ross) a large phone book and a piece of rubber hose. Sit or kneel on the floor with the cushion or phone book in front of you, about three feet/a meter away. Hold your newspaper or rubber hose above your head, at arm's length. Groan aloud, or say "Nnnn." Continue the groan, adding "Ooooh" to your "Nnnn," as you bring your paper (or hose) down on the cushion (or phone book). Use your voice. Be loud. Repeat at least ten times for one session.

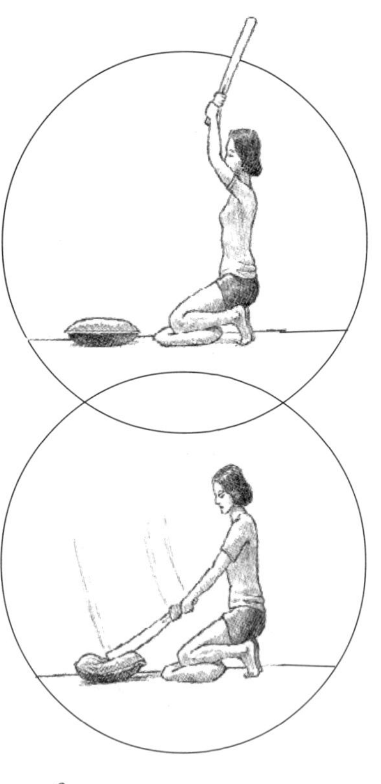

This exercise is about feelings, not reasons. *Why* you are angry is not the point.

You, like all women, like all people of every age, have hidden some of your anger in your body, usually in the large muscles. Exercise of any kind can reveal and move that anger. This type of exercise concentrates the anger and allows us to access it in a reasonably safe and fairly easy way.

Concentrate on your sensations; abandon words. Let your tears flow. Let your rage show. Be kind to yourself afterwards, too.

Step 3. *Nourish and Tonify*

> "Antioxidant polyphenols [found in tea], including flavonols, catechins, theaflavins and thearubigins, have been shown to inhibit cancer formation in both laboratory and animal studies."[78]

• Many tasty foods can significantly reduce one's risk of being diagnosed with ovarian cancer: black tea, onions, garlic, tomatoes, carrots, spinach, nettles, citrus, and organic dairy products.

★ Of 61,000 women aged 40–76, those who drank two or more cups of black or green tea a day lowered their risk of ovarian cancer by 46 percent.[79,80] **Black tea** provided the most benefit. Additional cups of tea, up to four a day, reduced risk even further. In lab studies, gallocatechin-gallate – a polyphenol abundant in green tea – killed ovarian cancer cells. Neither bottled nor decaffeinated teas contain significant amounts of polyphenols.

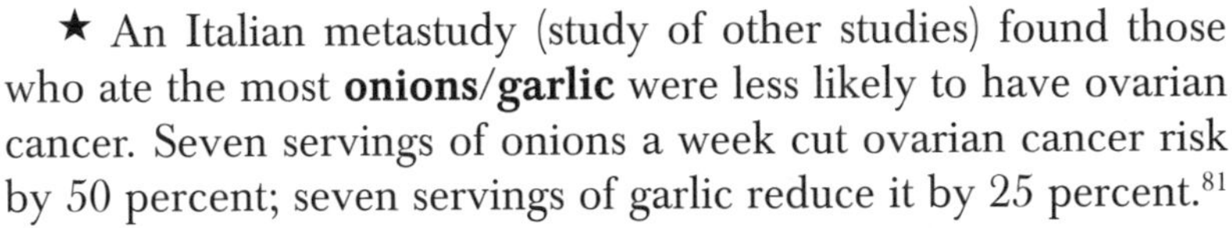

★ An Italian metastudy (study of other studies) found those who ate the most **onions/garlic** were less likely to have ovarian cancer. Seven servings of onions a week cut ovarian cancer risk by 50 percent; seven servings of garlic reduce it by 25 percent.[81]

★ Vegetables generally, **cooked tomatoes** and **carrots** particularly, lower ovarian cancer risk. Women who eat one cup of tomato sauce weekly lower risk by 40 percent. Twenty carrots a week decreases risk by 54 percent.[82] Women who eat three or more daily servings of any vegetable reduce their risk by 46 percent.[83] Two servings of vegetables a day lowers risk by 34 percent.[84]

★ Women with the highest intake of *kaempferol* – an antioxidant flavonoid found in leafy greens such as **spinach**, **nettles**, cabbage, broccoli, and green tea – are 40 percent less likely to be diagnosed with ovarian cancer than women with the lowest intake.[85]

• Another antioxidant flavonoid, *luteolin*, found in citrus, is also protective. Of the 67,000 women in the Nurses' Health Study, those who consumed the most were 34 percent less likely to be diagnosed with ovarian cancer than those who consumed the least.[86]

• **Milk** consumption does not increase ovarian cancer risk, say Japanese researchers who looked at 22 prior studies. Milk fat raises risk slightly, but lactose and other milk components don't.[87] A study of more than 550,000 women also failed to find an adverse connection.[88] "Three glasses of milk a day may slightly raise risk."[89]

• Other researchers found that women with high intakes of dairy products are 54 percent *less* likely to be diagnosed with ovarian cancer.[90] Lactose (milk sugar) helps promote the growth of bacteria that reduce cancer-causing compounds in the reproductive tract. One glass of milk a day can reduce risk by 41 percent.[91]

• An Australian study found women with the highest intake of red meat were 2.5 times more likely to develop ovarian cancer than those with the lowest intake. Consuming wine with the meat moderated the risk, but eating more vegetables didn't.[92]

• Does the **fat** you eat influence your risk of ovarian cancer? A dietary modification trial with nearly 50,000 American women, aged 50–79, found a 40 percent difference in ovarian cancer rates between those eating a low-fat diet (24–29 percent of calories) as compared to those eating a high-fat diet (more than 35 percent of calories).[93] For each 10 grams of *saturated fat* eaten daily, ovarian cancer risk can increase 20 percent. Ten fewer grams of saturated fat a day can lower risk 20 percent.[94] Women with the worst diets benefit the most from reducing the amount of fat they eat.[95]

• Perhaps it's not fat itself, or saturated fat, or animal fat that raises cancer risk. Perhaps it's the fat in *commercial* meat and dairy, from animals kept inside and fed lots of corn. So when I eat dairy or meat, it's always organic or pasture-raised and often local, too.

• Hyperthyroidism, and to a lesser extent, hypothyroidism, may protect against ovarian cancer.[96] Perhaps the thyroid "malfunctions" common to menopausal women actually improve health!

Step 4. *Stimulate/Sedate*

• Maintain a **healthy weight**. Women who were overweight when young and who've never given birth are more than twice as likely to be diagnosed with ovarian cancer.[97]

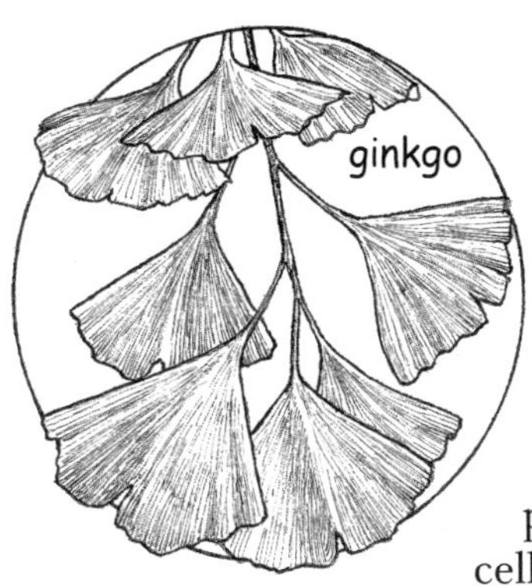

★ Six hours of **exercise** a week reduces ovarian cancer risk 30 percent.[98]

★ Women who took *Ginkgo biloba* tincture or capsules once or twice a day for six months or longer were 60 percent less likely to have ovarian cancer than women who never took it.[99] Ginkgolides – special compounds found in **ginkgo** – kill cancer cells in the ovaries.

• Ovarian cancer is encouraged by genistein, a phytoestrogen abundant in non-fermented soy products. Genistein is more carcinogenic than DES *when exposure occurs during infancy.*[100] Avoid tofu, soy milk, and all processed soy foods.

Step 5. *Use Drugs*

• Women who take **acetaminophen** – an over-the-counter pain and fever reliever – as few as five times a month, or as frequently as once a day, are 30 percent less likely to develop ovarian cancer than those who rarely or never do so. This common painkiller seems to shrink the ovaries.[101]

Caution: Seventy percent of healthy volunteers (aged 18–45) who took 4 grams (8 doses) of acetaminophen (Tylenol) daily for two weeks showed signs of liver damage including itchy skin, jaundice, dark urine, abdominal tenderness on the upper right side, flu-like symptoms, and elevations of alanine aminotransferase.[102] Long-term use of acetaminophen has caused kidney and liver failure. Hives, facial swelling, and breathing difficulties may also occur. Large doses are lethal.

★ Women who take second-generation **birth-control pills** have less ovarian (and uterine) cancer – even if they have hereditary risk factors.[103] After 3–6 months on the Pill, ovarian cancer risk decreases by 40 percent.[104] After 3 years, by 50 percent (20 percent if you inherited BRCA).[105,106] After six years, it's 60 percent less for everyone. The longer you take the Pill, the lower your risk. Newer, third-generation, pills also lessen risk, so far.

• If you must dye your hair, please use henna, rosemary, lemon juice, or anything other than commercial dye. One study found women who dyed their hair one to four times a year were 70 percent more likely to get ovarian cancer, while women who used hair dye five times a year increased their risk by 100 percent.[107] Other studies find little or no risk increase with use of hair dyes.

• Taking supplemental DHEA increases risk for ovarian cancer in both pre- and post-menopausal women.[108]

Step 6. *Break and Enter*

• Only 20 percent of the women who have surgery (which can be fatal) for suspected ovarian cancer actually have it.[109]

★ For women with BRCA mutations, a tubal ligation reduces ovarian cancer risk by 60 percent.[110] A bilateral salpingo-oophorectomy reduces risk by 80 percent.[111] Those with BRCA1 mutations are helped far more than those with BRCA2.[112]

★ Removing any woman's uterus will reduce her risk of ovarian cancer by 30 percent.[113] **If you are having a hysterectomy and don't have cancer, insist on keeping your ovaries**. If you are under 65 years of age, the removal of your ovaries will increase your risk of dying from coronary heart disease more than it will reduce your risk of dying from ovarian cancer.[114]

Her Story

Serena is "just an ordinary married woman."

"Menopause freaked me out. First I lost my interest in sex and was sure my husband would leave me. Then I started to flood.

"Shepherd's purse stopped the bleeding, but someone told me it meant that I could have, gasp, cancer, so I went to my doctor. He recommended a D&C, but said a hysterectomy would be the safest option to prevent cancer. So I agreed. I was so afraid of my body.

"I wanted to keep my ovaries, but they said I could die of ovarian cancer, so out they came too. Slam! Like hitting a brick wall at full speed, I was plunged into a menopause nightmare.

"That was three years ago. I finally feel better. I drink nourishing herbal infusion daily and listen to what my body wants. Why didn't I just do that in the first place? Fear!"

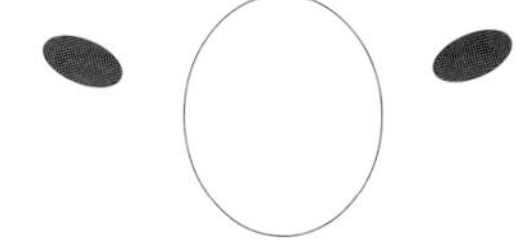

Ovarian Cancer

"I love you, dear granddaughter," croons Grandmother Growth as she rocks you in her arms. "Lay your head down on me and let me accompany you on your journey.

"Hold my hand as we dive deep within and swim in the sea of your pelvis. Use your inner sight and your inner knowing. Pay no attention to the voices of fear. Is this cancer a challenge? Does it ask you to stand up for yourself and do whatever it takes to overcome, to conquer, to survive?

"Or does it suggest that you let go and turn your face toward your death? Those who love you will want you to stay and do battle. If this is not the time for struggle, find a way to leave in love. Compassion for them need not require you to abandon what is truly best for you.

"If you choose to go on, give it all you've got. Be fierce. Be adamant. Be more than you've ever been before. Lean on me. Complain to me when the going gets rough and you wonder if you made the right choice. Throw yourself into my lap and sob whenever you have the need. I am here for you.

"If you choose to let go, do so with a smile. My friend Morpheus will come to ease your pain. He and I will stand guard and cheer as you step over the final finish line."

Step 0. *Do Nothing*

• **Avoid CA-125 screening**. Only one out of 126 women with elevated levels of CA-125 actually have cancer.[115]

Step 1. *Collect Information*

• **Speak up** if you think you have ovarian cancer. Half of diagnosed women have had at least one target symptom for three months prior; many have had symptoms for a year or more.[116]

• Ovarian cancer is rare. A woman's lifetime risk is only 1 percent. If her mother, sister, or aunt have been diagnosed, then it's 5 percent. If found in a distant relative, it's 7 percent.[117] Ovarian cancer accounts for 1 percent of deaths in women.[118]

• Average age at diagnosis for an American women is 65.[119]

• Women with BRCA1 or BRCA2 genes (often Ashkenazi Jews) have a very high risk – 45 to 80 percent – of getting ovarian cancer. Taking birth control pills for six or more years, or having a tubal ligation, can lower that to a 25 percent risk.[120]

• After increasing 30 percent between 1985 and 1995,[121] the rate of invasive ovarian cancer has fallen significantly, due to women's greater awareness of early symptoms. Nonetheless, in 2006, more than 20,000 American women were diagnosed with ovarian cancer; that's 1 out of 57 women.[122] More than 15,000 will die. The survival rate has not changed in the past fifty years.[123]

★ **Abdominal swelling**, **pain**, **bloating**, **constipation**, and **urinary problems** are symptoms of ovarian cancer.[124] All women have some of these symptoms sometimes. What distinguishes the woman with ovarian cancer is the **severity**, **frequency**, and **persistence** of her symptoms. She has daily symptoms, while a healthy woman experiences pelvic discomfort only a few times a month. Of women with ovarian cancer, 74 percent are constipated,[125] 64 percent have abdominal swelling, difficulty eating and feelings of fullness, 70 percent have bloating, and 55 percent have frequent, urgent urination or other urinary problems.[126]

• Other symptoms of ovarian cancer include: indigestion, gas, back pain, diarrhea, abnormal menstrual bleeding, fatigue, and painful intercourse.

• Most (90 percent of) ovarian cancers are thought to

Help!
Ovarian Cancer

Use complementary medicines alone or with other treatments.

• Drink 3–4 quarts of **red clover** infusion weekly.

• Try 1–4 drop doses of **poke root tincture** *carefully*.

• **Visualizations** create miracles.

• Connect with your anger.

• **Love your vagina**. No douching, no soap. **Exercise it.**

begin in the outer layer of the ovary (*epithelial).* The deadliest forms may be those that start on the fimbria. The connective tissue of the ovaries can host *stromal cell cancers.*

• When ovarian cancer is confined to the ovary and treated aggressively, 92 percent of women survive for five years. When it has spread to the lymph nodes, the five-year survival rate is 71 percent; if it is in other areas, 28 percent.[127,128] Ovarian cancer causes more deaths than all other reproductive cancers combined.[129]

★ What causes ovarian cancer? Nitrates in drinking water increase both bladder and ovarian cancer in older women says the World Health Organization.[130] In young women, ovulation may be to blame. When the egg pushes its way out of the ovary, it causes mutations on a gene that prevents damaged cells from multiplying; this sets the stage for ovarian cancer.[131] Limit or eliminate ovulation to limit ovarian cancer. How? By becoming pregnant, breast feeding, or by taking the Pill (oral contraceptives).

> "Ovarian cancer is not one disease; it's a spectrum of diseases. There's a large group of chronic survivors."[132]

> ". . . speculate that early-stage and late-stage ovarian cancer are actually two distinct diseases . . . fimbrial-end ovarian cancer may account for the 75 percent of cases that turn deadly."[133]

Step 2. *Engage the Energy*

• When Elisabeth Kubler Ross asked a Quaker woman to envision her immune system destroying her cancer, she said, "I don't make war." She sent her cancer cells to a happy, loving, far-away place.

• Move anger out of the ovaries with the exercise on page 276.

• Integrate **homeopathic** remedies such as: *Carcinosin, Aurum muriaticum nat., Viburnum prunifolium, Thuja, Sepia, Lilium tigrinum.*

Step 3. *Nourish and Tonify*

• Women with a Body Mass Index under 25 at the time of their ovarian cancer diagnosis survive one-third longer than those with a higher BMI, and their cancers recur less quickly after treatment.[134]

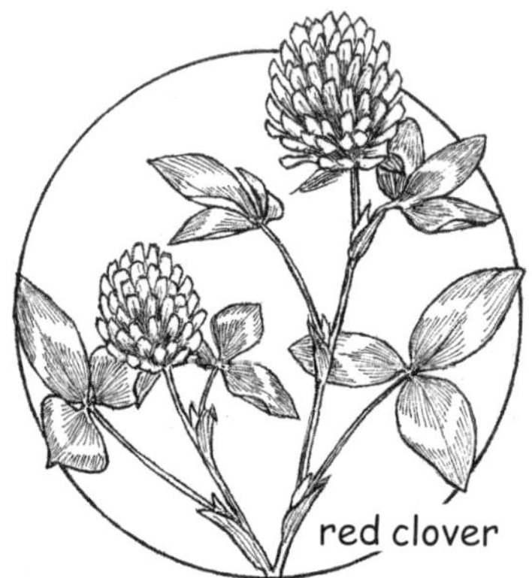

★ **Red clover infusion** is the world's safest and most respected anti-cancer herb. The dose is 2–4 quarts a week. I don't consider capsules or tincture effective. (Make it: page 367.)

Step 5. *Use Drugs*

★ The "Million Women Study" in England found those who took estrogen/progestin (hormone replacement) were 63 pervent more likely to be diagnosed with ovarian cancer and 20 percent more likely to die of it than non-users.[135] Among a quarter of a million American women, those who took estrogens were twice as likely to die from ovarian cancer as those who did not.[136] Dietary phytoestrogens – except isolated isoflavone from soy (which is often added to health foods) – do not appear to increase risk.

• **Timing chemotherapy** – administering cisplatin in the evening and doxorubicin in the morning – improves efficacy from 11 percent to 44 percent.[137,138]

★ If ovarian cancer recurs, consider hospice. **Hospice** care is available in the USA to anyone with a life expectancy of six months or less. Hospice offers emotional support as well as pain and symptom management, often in the "residence of choice." Hospice workers are generally accepting of alternative medicines such as massage, prayer, visualization, and herbal remedies.

Step 6. *Break and Enter*

> "Surgery is critical to diagnosis and appropriate treatment of ovarian cancer. . . ."[139]

• Women with ovarian cancer treated by gynecological oncologists live longer than women treated by general surgeons.[140]

• Orthodox treatment against ovarian cancer includes surgical removal of the ovaries, uterus, egg tubes, and omentum. This eliminates 60 percent of stage I cancers. Additionally, all women are prescribed paclitaxel (Taxol) and carboplatin or cisplatin. This significantly increases the risk of developing leukemia.[141]

★ Removal of both ovaries (oophorectomy) causes instantaneous, intense, **menopause**. Many women say sex is adversely affected, too.[142] Hormone "replacement" therapies do counter the severe and rapid bone loss that follows oophorectomy,[143] but cannot replicate the natural, nuanced, intricate, and responsive flow of hormones that the ovaries provide. Nourishing herbal infusions – like nettle or oatstraw – can. They counter bone loss, ease symptoms, and restore sexual functioning. Make it: page 367.

> "[Natural ovarian hormones] give her a subtle sense of well-being which is not easily replaced with pills."[144]

Twenty-first Century Treatments

• **Monoclonal antibodies** can find and bind to cancer cells and deliver tumor-killing agents. **Avastin** (bevacizumab) is a monoclonal antibody that interferes with blood supply, starving cancers.

• **Vaccines** against ovarian cancer are under study. One triggers the immune system to attack cells producing CA-125.

• **Intraperitoneal chemotherapy**, a fifty-year-old technique, delivers chemotherapeutic agents directly into the space between the abdominal wall and the vital organs. It increases survival among women with advanced ovarian cancer by an average of 16 months.[145] A combination of intravenous and intraperitoneal chemotherapy confers a 25 percent overall survival advantage.[146] The side effects – infection, fatigue, severe pain – are so debilitating that few women are able to endure all six treatments.

• Catheter-delivered drugs plus **hyperthermia** (intense heating) is **intraperitoneal hyperthermic chemotherapy**, a new treatment used against advanced ovarian cancer.[147]

• **Genetic techniques**: Herceptin, to counter over-expression of the cancer-receptor gene HER2/neu. Injections of working copies of gene p53, a tumor-suppressor, to stop cancer growth.

★ A single session of **high frequency electric current** (radiofrequency ablation) killed targeted metastatic cancer cells completely in five of six patients with advanced ovarian cancer; four of those five tumors did not recur over a three-year follow-up.[148]

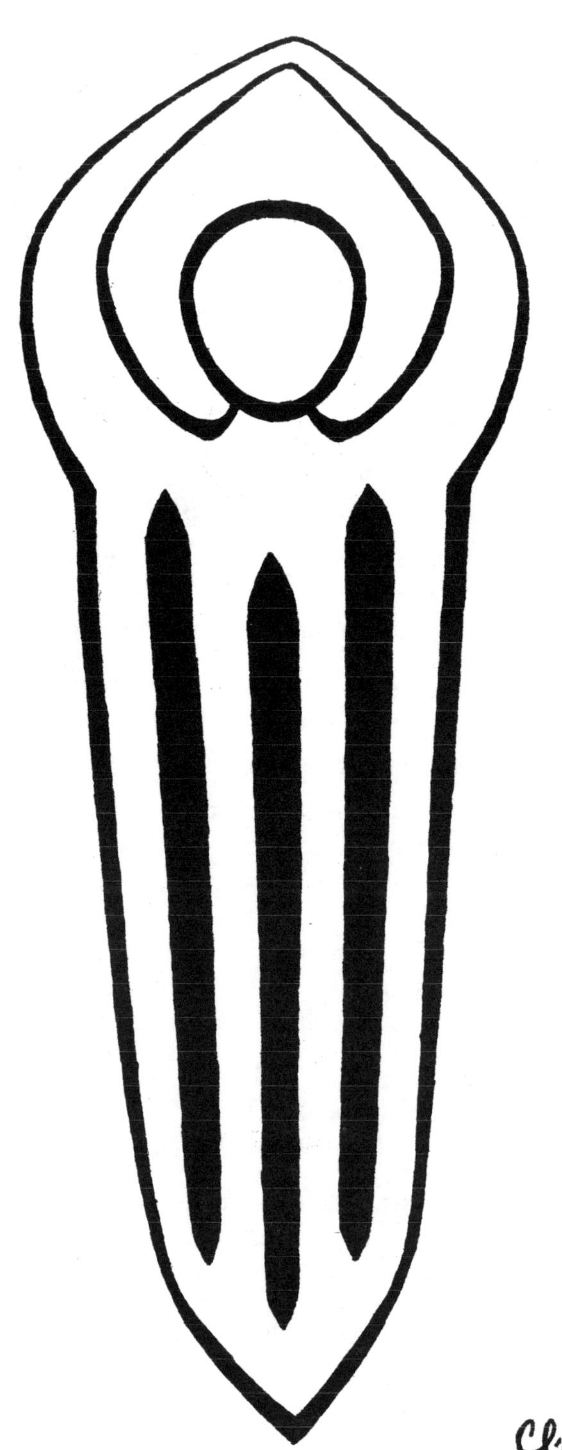

Part Three

Especially for Men

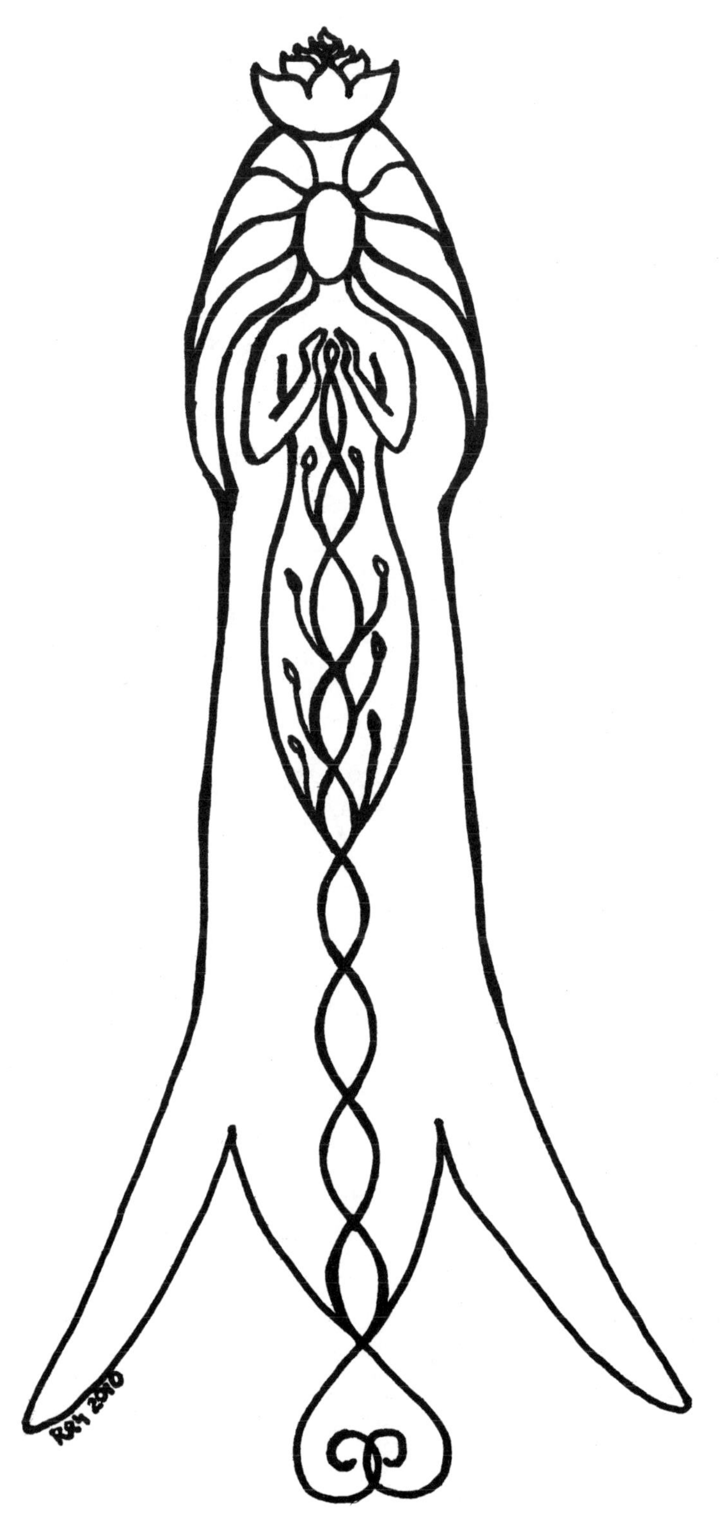
2010

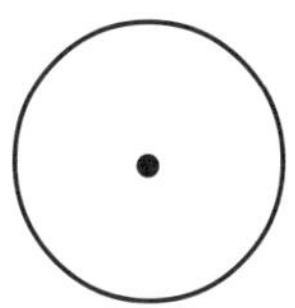

The Penis

Man is a toolmaker; I am his tool. Man is a thinker; I am his thought.

As a tool, I am an extension of the hand. But I am stronger than the hand that uses me. And more clever. Tools are dangerous. To use a tool well requires training and attention, skill and thoughtfulness.

As a thought, I am an extension of mind. Still, I am more powerful than mind. Thoughts are the seeds. But thoughts limit and define the mind. To think well requires care and diligence, rigor and flexibility.

Pound, hammer, drill, and screw. I am a tool of creation; I am the thought of something new. I am not the creation; I am the delivery system.

I prefer to act first and think later. My task is not the specific but the general. I am not fussy. In fact, I crave variety.

My names are legion, diverse, and unlimited. Although I am only your tool, merely your thought, simply the means to the end, you so identify yourself with me that you call us by the same names: peter, dick, jack, john, peterson, dickson, jackson, johnson.

If I seem to have a life of my own, unconcerned with your life and needs, it is because I view you as my *tool, my access to what I want. I seek to control your thoughts and turn them to my wishes. You owe your existence to me – how can you refuse?*

If I seem simple-minded, single-minded, close-minded, and proud, it is because I know you are enthralled with me and will indulge me. I can control your actions and turn them to my desires. Without me, your line ends. Without me, you are alone. How can you thwart me? How can you resist?

I will never stop demanding your participation in my vision of eternity. If you allow me to, I will make you a god. Together we will manifest multiplicity, discharge responsibility, and get the precious burden deposited safely, where it may thrive and grow.

I will not be ignored. I am your penis.

The Healthy Penis

"A notorious organ that no one trusts."[1]

The penis consists of a shaft, with a head, the *glans*, and an opening, the *meatus*, covered by a foreskin, the *prepuce*.

The meatus is the opening of the urethra, through which urine and semen are passed out of the body. The urethra starts at the bladder, goes through the prostate, then down into the seminal vesicles, and up between the corpus cavernosa to the meatus.

The shaft is not one but three cylindrical bodies of erectile tissues interwoven with many nerves and covered with a loose skin devoid of fat. Two of the bodies of erectile tissue – the *corpus cavernosa* – lie next to each other on the top of the shaft, and a smaller one – the *corpus spongiosum* – lies under and between them.

The bodies of erectile tissue are spongy tissues packed with tiny blood vessels. As blood flows into these blood vessels, little valves trap it, causing engorgement, tightening of the penile skin, and hardening the shaft: an erection.

At orgasm, all the valves open at once, ejaculation occurs, and the penis becomes flaccid. It takes some time before another erection can be achieved. (Woman's erectile tissues, which are, ounce for ounce as large as a penis, though spread out over a larger area, are unvalved. This gives women the ability to have orgasm after orgasm without pause.)

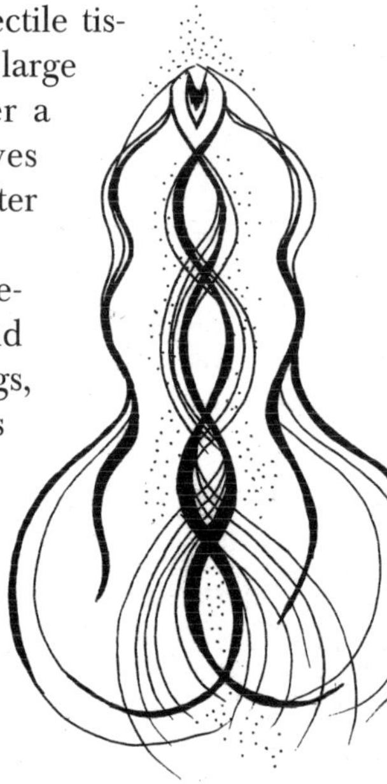

Foreskins are protective, like eyelids. The foreskins of both men and women contain many nerve endings, blood vessels, and sebaceous glands that produce antibacterial and antiviral proteins known as *smegma*. (Latin for "soap.") Smegma moisturizes the glans penis and the clitoris and protects against inflammation and infection.

Penile Distresses

The penis is vulnerable to **irritation** (below), infections (**STDs**, page 292), and, occasionally, cancer.[2] It is also vulnerable to **circumcision**, a hotly debated topic (page 294).

As the ads for, and sales of, Viagra testify, the primary problem with the penis lies in its in/ability to become erect and stay that way long enough. Instead of drugs, try herbal, homeopathic, and lifestyle remedies for **erectile dysfunction** (page 296).

Natural treatments for **Peyronie's disease** and **priapism** (inability to lose an erection) are in *The Sexual Herbal*.[3] **Phimosis** is treated in *The Male Herbal*.[4] (*See* glossary for more information.)

 A Word About Condoms 

One of the best ways for a man to protect himself and his lovers from STDs and unwanted pregnancy is to use a condom, a thin, flexible covering for the shaft and head of the penis. Condoms made from skin have been used for thousands of years and are still available, although at least twice as expensive as others.

Modern condoms are made of latex or synthetics. They release chemicals that are **carcinogenic** in humans.[5] Most of the chemicals are released "soon after contact," and are magnified by sweat and saliva. Nitrosatable compounds, which can turn into carcinogenic nitrosamines in the body, are very high in condoms.[6]

Some wo/men find that lubricants and spermicides on condoms cause rashes, redness, irritation, vaginal rawness, urethral pain, and herpes outbreaks. Avoid these additives whenever possible.

 Penile Redness/Irritation 

• Homeopathic **calendula** gel is soothing. Calendula oil is too.

• **Aloe vera** gel, especially from the fresh leaf, is highly effective in relieving all skin irritations.

Sexually Transmitted Diseases (STDs)

Men with sexually transmitted diseases may have few or no symptoms. Symptomless men can still pass STDs to any partner. Uncircumsized men are more likely to carry STDs,[7] and more likely to have symptoms, such as small red spots on the foreskin.

Remedies for women with STDs begin on page143. Men can **use the same remedies** with good results, but there are a few special things only they can do.

Foremost among them is the **penis soak**, originated by herbalist Cascade Anderson-Geller. (Make it: page 374.)

• **Candida** is a yeast that lives on men's pubic hairs and skin, and in the anus and urethra as well. To avoid passing your yeast on to your lover, **soak your penis in plain yogurt or vinegar** mixed half and half with water for five minutes. *Candida* shrivels up in acidic environments. Acidifying the urine with unsweetened cranberry juice or high doses of ascorbic acid (vitamin C) can kill *Candida* in the urinary tract so you can avoid antifungal drugs.

• **Chlamydia** is the exception to the rule: Men are more likely than women to develop symptoms, only one-third will remain symptomless. Chlamydia burrows into the lining of the penile urethra, inflaming it (*urethritis*), causing pain or burning on urination, and sometimes giving rise to a mild discharge. Chlamydia can also burrow into, inflame, and ultimately scar the epididymis, the fine tubing that carries sperm out of the testicles; this is a primary cause of male infertility. Men without symptoms can pass chlamydia to women. Men who have sex with men: Chlamydia thrives in the rectum if it is introduced there.

It is vitally important for any man who suspects a chlamydia infection to **alert all his partners**. Untreated chlamydia in women can cause severe, life-threatening problems. Over 9 percent of all adults between the ages of 18 and 35 have undiagnosed and untreated chlamydia and/or gonorrhea infections: 6.4 percent of men of color, and 2.8 percent of other men.[8] **Herbal anti-infectives** (page 159) **used in conjunction with prescription antibiotics** offer the best results.

Chlamydia can lead to **Reiter's syndrome** in young men. This syndrome involves eye infections, urethritis, and arthritis. One in three men who develop it become permanently disabled.[9]

• **Trich** is a single-celled organism that can live in a man's urethra. If any partner has trich, you do too. Eliminate it in **ten days** by doing these three things: A daily **penis soak.** (Make it: page 374). **Avoid ejaculation.**[10] Take **antimicrobial herbs**, such as garlic, goldenseal, or yarrow. (Continue for 3–4 weeks to avoid the possibility of trich surviving in your prostate and seminal vesicles.)

• **BV**, or bacterial vaginosis, is a chronic vaginal irritation or infection. **Your urethra is the cause**; it harbors organisms that are benign to you but drive her vagina crazy. Here's how to help:

~ Keep it to yourself for thirty days. Cuddle, massage, kiss, but no genital contact, not even rubbing or oral sex.

~ Do masturbate. Ejaculate as frequently as you can to clear organisms that may be hiding out in the prostate.

~ Drink cranberry juice and lots of water so you have to pee a lot and so your pee is acidic. This will kill infectious organisms lurking in your urethra.

• **Herpes** type two is a viral infection. It is passed by vaginal, anal, and oral sex, but *you can get it or spread it even with protection and even in the absence of sex.* It requires only bare skin contact to transmit. There is no definitive treatment for herpes, and more than three-quarters of infected men have no symptoms. Remedies to ease and eliminate herpes begin on page 160.

• **Gonorrhea** became far less threatening to health with the introduction of antibiotics in the mid-twentieth centuy. But now, new antibiotic-resistant strains are common in Asia, Indonesia, and Hawaii. **Herbal antibiotics** (page 342) **used in conjunction with prescription antibiotics** can give you the edge against gonorrhea's sophisticated stealth.

• **HPV** causes genital warts. Warts you can see are contagious but not problematic. The ones you can't see (unless you soak your penis in a mix of one ounce vinegar and one cup water for six minutes, which causes them to turn white) are contagious and can cause cancer, including cancer of the penis! (Remedies: page 176.)

• **Syphilis** is a high-risk infection *Antibiotics are the best medicine.* Read more about it, starting on page 166.

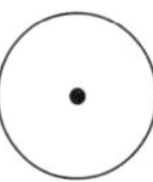

Circumcision

"It was my second scar," Grandfather Growth comments as we sit on the high ledge and watch the moon rising.

"The first, still not healed, throbbed on my belly where my connection to Mother had been cut. The second, just below, shocked me to my core. I was acutely conscious of my body: its weight, its hunger, its pain.

" 'Where is safety? Where is peace? Where is love?' If infants can have thoughts, I pondered these questions. I am an old, old man now, but I have not yet found the answers to those questions. Have you?"

Step 0. *Do Nothing*

• Circumcision – the cutting away of the foreskin – is usually done on newborn boys. Some men feel deprived by this "senseless and risky mutilation;"[15] others prefer it.

Step 1. *Collect Information*

• Circumcision reduces the risk of infection by HPV and STDs by 35–60 percent, and the risk of getting HIV by half.[11, 12, 13]

• Uncircumscised men say their sexual response is heightened. Not so great when most men, according to surveys, can't keep an erection long enough to satisfy most women. Well, says herbalist

James Green: "Kegels [page 14] improve control! Sure beats circumcision as a way to prevent premature ejaculation."[14]

• In 2010, 33 percent of boy babies were circumcised in the United States and 20 percent of men worldwide.[16] African men are adopting it avidly as a way to cut their risk of AIDS.[17]

• Let a boy decide for himself when he is older? Infants rarely suffer infection, scarring, or penile damage; older boys can.

• Is circumcision like cutting off the labia or a breast or pulling a good tooth, as some male writers would have it?[18] Circumsized men say it is more like a tonsilectomy or appendectomy.

> ". . .this traumatic procedure is undeniably physically painful and psychologically stressful. . . ."[19]

Step 2. *Engage the Energy*

• Homeopathic *Arnica* counters pain and swelling from trauma.

Step 3. *Nourish and Tonify*

• Heal the wound with soothing oils like **calendula**, or wash the penis with **comfrey**, **plantain**, or **mallow** leaf infusion.

Step 4. *Stimulate/Sedate*

• If you leave your boy intact, *leave the foreskin alone.* It naturally adheres to the glans for four or more years. If there is irritation or infection (unlikely) swish the penis in warm water with a little salt, vinegar, or echinacea tincture added to it.

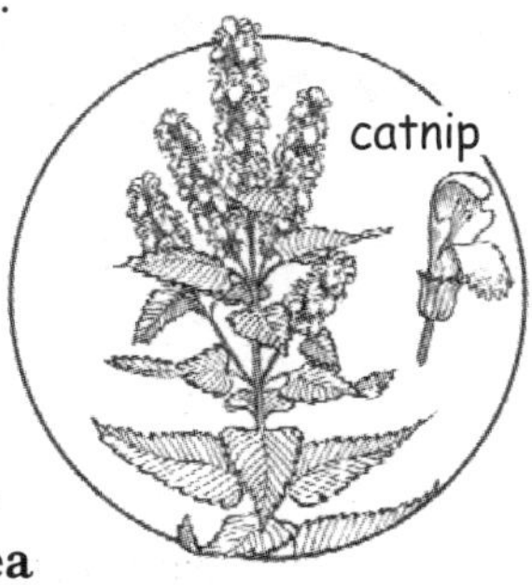

• If you do choose circumcision, it is best to wait until 10–14 days after the birth, if you can. These herbs can help:

~ Ease pain/crying by letting your newborn suck on a finger or pacifier dipped in dilute tincture or tea of **skullcap** or **catnip**.

~ To prevent infection and hasten healing, I apply tincture or ointment of **echinacea** root, **calendula** flowers, or **yarrow** herb.

catnip

Erectile Dysfunction

Step 0. *Do Nothing*

• Psst. It's a secret. Many women would rather cuddle, kiss, stroke, lick, be licked, and laugh than do the old "in-and-out." She is probably more interested in you than in your penis. Really!

Step 1. *Collect Information*

• Of the four primary causes of erectile disfunction (ED) – atherosclerosis, prescription drugs, diabetes, and hormones – atherosclerosis of the penile artery accounts for half of all cases.[20] Most blood-pressure, anti-anxiety, and antidepressant drugs lower libido and interfere with erections. Diabetes damages potency by narrowing the penile blood vessels. Estrogen-mimicking chemicals (organochlorines) in the environment may play a role as well.

Step 2. *Engage the Energy*

• **Homeopathic remedies** for ED or "lack of competence":
~ *Agnus castus*: genitals cold, testes swollen; no desire, no ability.
~ *Argentum nitricum*: genitals weak, shriveled.
~ *Baryta carbonica*: the older loner; lacks desire and ability.
~ *Caladium seguinum*: older; craves sex, but is unable.
~ *Conium maculatum*: avoids sex; ejaculation is painful.
~ *Kalium bromatum*: nervous, depressed; has no ability.
~ *Medorrhinum*: in too much of a hurry to be intimate.
~ *Phosphorus*: involuntary emissions; desire but no power.
~ *Sulphur*: penis cold; urethra burns after coition.

Step 3. *Nourish and Tonify*

★ **Oatstraw** infusion is my favorite sexual tonic, for both men and women. It improves blood flow, increases stiffness, amps up interest, and counters environmental estrogens. A cup or two a day helps lower cholesterol, too. For best results, alternate with **red clover** infusion to adjust hormones gently and build potency.

★ **Schizandra berry** tincture (1–2 dropperfuls) or infusion (2–4 cups), used as a regular tonic, strengthens the adrenals, counters inflammation, and increases sexual desire and vigor.

• Great-tasting **fenugreek tea** is a classic way to improve potency. Make it: Put 6 tablespoons of seeds in a quart jar, fill with boiling water, steep 15–20 minutes, strain, and drink freely.

★ Daily practice of **pelvic floor clenches** (Kegel exercises, page 14) helps you remain erect and stay continent.

• Foods like shellfish, fatty fish, eggs, **bee pollen**, and pumpkin seeds are known to improve potency. "Potency Potion Soup" (page 378) contains seven foods that aid erection: onions, savory, celery, lovage, lettuce, **burdock root**, and saffron.

• Two ounces of sunflower seeds supply 4 grams of erection-enhancing **arginine** (page 299). Other foods sources include: pine pollen, peanuts, sesame seeds (tahini and gomasio), almonds, Brazil nuts, lentils, chives, watercress, carob, and kidney beans.

Step 4. *Stimulate/Sedate*

• **Ginseng** improves sexual potency, especially when you are overworked or overstressed. Russian studies find it effective about 50 percent of the time.[21] It may counter hormonal disturbances, too.

★ **Ginger** aids sexual functioning. Regular use removes atherosclerotic plaque from penile blood vessels and increases circulation there. Snack on crystallized ginger, add ginger to food, make ginger tea. Yummy.

Help!
Erectile Dysfunction

Expect results in 2–3 months.

• Drink 1 quart each per week of **oatstraw**, **red clover**, **schisandra**.

• Do **pelvic floor clenches** daily.

• Eat more **ginger** or take **ginseng**.

• Tonify with an herb that counters ED (pages 298, 299).

★ It's an old joke that there isn't enough blood for both the penis and the brain, so a man can't think when he has an erection. That may explain why an herb that improves blood flow to the brain counters erectile difficulties, too. **Ginkgo** is especially effective when fat deposits or diabetes restrict blood flow, and in men whose blood flow is not improved by papaverine injections, or where potency is diminished by antidepressants.[22] Between 50–78 percent of men in trials using 60–240mg of standardized ginkgo daily for at least six weeks regained the ability to have regular erections.[23,24] Continue for 12–18 months. *Caution*: Avoid ginkgo before surgery and if taking blood-thinning drugs.

• **Potency wood**, muira puama, is a South American herb that stimulates arousal and erection in men who are tired, run down, and weak. From 50–70 percent of those taking tea or tincture (½ teaspoon twice a day) report intensification of libido and improvement in hardness.[25] *Caution*: May lower blood pressure.

★ **Yohimbe** bark, from tropical west Africa, improves blood flow to the penis and increases smooth muscle relaxation.[26] It has no effect on testosterone levels; instead, it acts to increase norepinephrine, which is essential for erections and which decreases with age. Yohimbe is especially helpful for those with diabetes or heart disease. Yohimbe hydrochloride is the only FDA-approved anti-impotence herbal drug. Its effects on men – and women – include: increased stamina, heightened sensation, and greater desire. Consistent use of yohimbe tincture helps 81 percent of impotent men.[27]

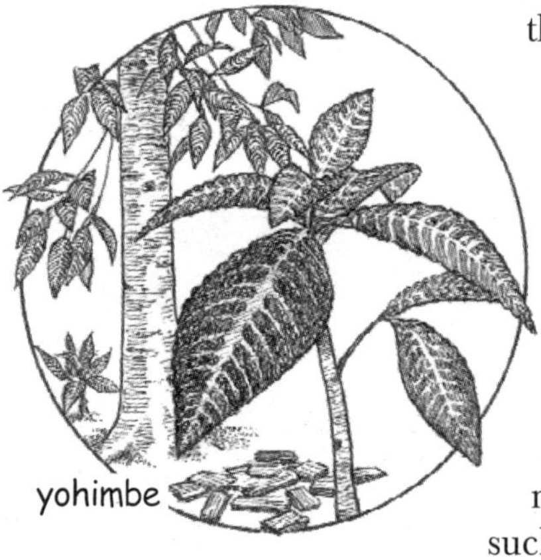

yohimbe

Cautions: Yohimbe can lower blood pressure or cause kidney problems. It is a short-term MAO inhibitor; do not combine with high-tyramine foods such as cheese, chocolate, nuts, beer, red wine, red grape juice, or aged meat; nor with tyrosine or phenylalanine supplements.[28] Nor should yohimbe be used concurrently with antidepressants, sedatives, antihistamines,

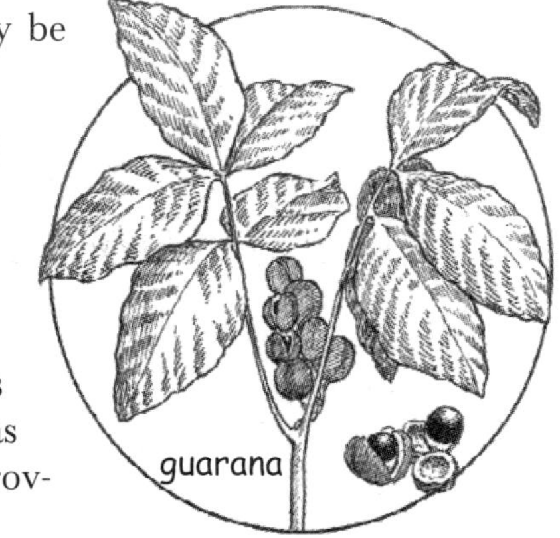

caffeine, or amphetamines. It may be agitating to the nervous system.

★ The favorite aphrodisiac and potency enhancer in Brazil is **guarana**. The peeled, dried, roasted, pulverized seeds of *Paullinia cupana* (or *sobilis*) are used. Guarana strengthens the nervous system, and helps prevent illness as well as increasing desire and improving performance.

• A cup of **damiana** leaf infusion – or a teaspoon of the tincture – improves her interest and his staying power.

★ When type-2 diabetes causes erectile difficulties, reach for the powdered **cinnamon**. Four tablespoonfuls a day has been shown to be effective in normalizing blood sugar.

• Men with diabetes who take 750–1500mg of **tribulus** daily report improvement in libido and erection.[29]

• Tobacco and beer contribute to erection problems. Smokers are twice as likely to have difficulty with erection. Beer raises prolactin and decreases testosterone levels.[30] Avoid herbs with strong estrogens like black cohosh, licorice, and hops (beer), too.

• Try erection-friendly **hawthorn berry** tincture, two dropperfuls twice a day instead of/in addition to blood pressure drugs.

Step 5a. *Use Supplements*

★ Supplements of **L-arginine** increase the effectiveness of ginkgo and other herbs.[31] L-arginine is a precursor to nitric oxide, which is essential to vasodilation and erection.[32] Daily use of 1–3 500mg pills twice a day slowly corrects erection problems. For an extra boost, as many as 36 pills (18g) can be taken 45 minutes before sex. Arginine cream is used directly on the penis, too.

Cautions: Diabetics should avoid L-arginine. Use worsens shingles and herpes outbreaks (but does not trigger them).

Drugs Can Ruin Your (Sex) Life

Problem	OTC Drug	Presc. Drug	Side Effect	Herbal Alternative
Allergies	Benadryl, Zyrtec, Claritin	Clarinex, Allegra	Inhibits arousal Dries vagina	Osha tinct. Eyebright tinct.
Depression	*	SSRIs: Paxil, Prozac, Zoloft Tricyclics: Elavil	Decreases desire Inhibits orgasm	St. Joan's wort tinct.
Anxiety	–	Xanax, Valium	Decreases desire Delays orgasm	Motherwort tinct. Passionflower tinct.
Hypertension	–	Thiazide diuretics Beta blockers: Lopressor	Decreases desire Dries vagina Blocks orgasm	Hawthorn berry tinct. Motherwort tinct.
Hormonal Birth control	–	The Pill DepoProvera	Inhibits arousal Blunts desire	Wild carrot seed tinct. Wild yam capsules
Pain	Advil, Aleve, Motrin, aspirin	Numerous	Inhibits desire, arousal, & orgasm Dries vagina	Skullcap tinct. Willow bark tinct.

* *Although over 118 million prescriptions are written for antidepressants in the US each year, they "produce significant mood improvements only in the most severely depressed patients."*[31] *The majority of patients improve as much on a placebo as on a drug.*

★ L-dopa stimulates erections and desire.[33] **Fava beans** and their sprouts are the best food sources. Supplements of L-tyrosine and L-phenylalanine are precursors; a dose is 100–500mg of each daily. *Caution*: Increases blood pressure. Do not use with yohimbe.

• L-choline is another amino acid critical to erection. Supplementation with 1–3 g a day is effective.[34] *Caution*: Causes stiffness of the upper back and neck, headache, diarrhea.

• Taking vitamin B_5, pantothenic acid, with L-choline leads to "longer and more pleasurable orgasms."[35]

• Carolyn Dean M D, advises anyone taking therapeutic medications for relief of depression or anxiety to protect their libido by also taking a **magnesium** supplement.

Step 5b. *(Don't) Use Drugs*

• Drugs can ruin a wo/man's sex life. (See facing page.)

~ Orgasms need muscle tension; antihistamines, antispasmodics, and pain killers relax muscles.

~ High levels of serotonin (caused by SSRI antidepressants) squelch sexual interest, performance, and orgasmic ability.

~ Engorgement is central to arousal and performance; blood pressure- and cholesterol-lowering drugs block engorgement.

~ The central nervous system is critical to arousal and orgasm; any medication that warns you not to drive depresses the central nervous system and therefore your sexual response.

Step 6. *Break and Enter*

• Injections of papaverine work, but ginkgo works better.

☯ Men can carry organisms in their urethra, vas, prostate, bladder, and testes that can infect others without causing symptoms in the man. The perfect lover has his ejaculate cultured for possible infectious hitch-hikers – including chlamydia and ureaplasma – and gets rid of them with herbs or drugs. Get yourself healthy; don't pass infections. If your lover has PID (page 245), you may be the cause of it. A course of herbal antibiotics and abstinence from intercourse for two weeks will help both of you get well.

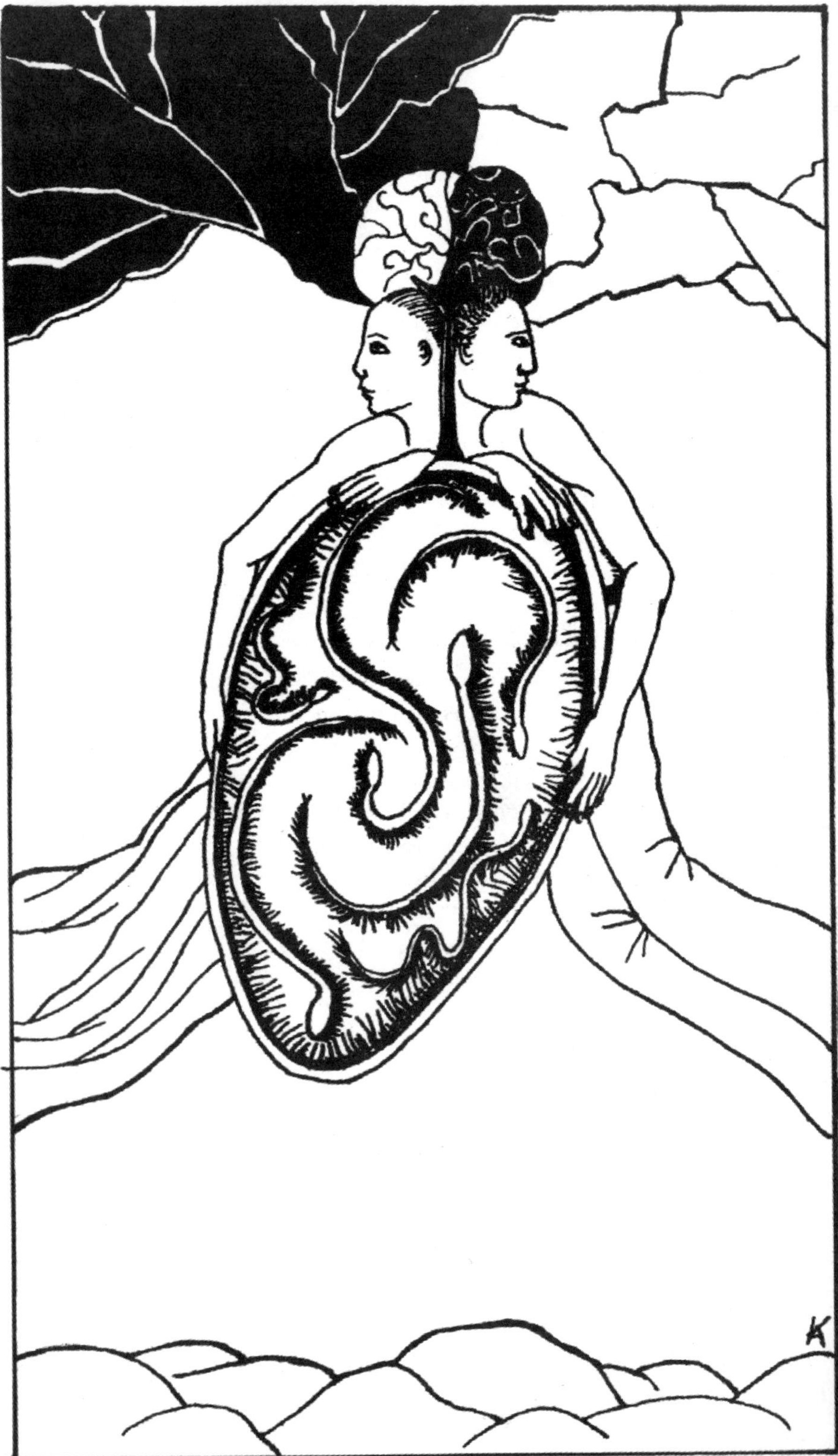

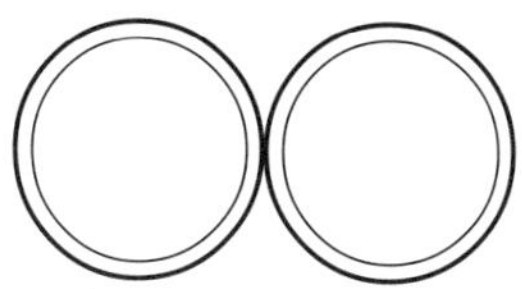

The Testes

We are the factory that never closes; our work never ceases. We are a garden of perpetual production. We are your dream of endless motion. Our clock ticks on, without winding, without batteries.

We don't take vacations, especially not to hot places; they make us weak and lethargic. We prefer to be cool, to swing in the breeze, to hang out and chill. We like to play ball. We are the essence of machismo.

We are not sluggards. Patience is not our virtue. We get the move on. We run the race. We are always ready to go. Our assembly line works day and night. We never rest.

We create the latest, the greatest, and the best of what can be. Our products are new and up-to-date. We are betting on the future.

Most of what we make is wasted. Like all natural things, we are profligate. We do not recycle or conserve resources. We use it all up like there is no tomorrow. And there is no tomorrow without our ceaseless effort. We fling ourselves into our work with total abandon.

With care, with attention, we initiate and watch over the process. Tick, raw materials are created. Tock, they mature in ninety days. Tick, a million a minute. Tock, day in and day out. We cherish redundancy. We cover all the bases.

We are the hive; we are the crêche; we are the heart of humanity. You owe your life to us. We are your father, and your father's father, and his father, too. We are your immortality. We are your testicles.

Healthy Testicles

The testicles, or testes, consist of two oval-shaped glands about 1½ inches long and 1 inch wide. They are the primary male sexual organs, akin to a woman's ovaries. They produce germ cells (sperm) and hormones (especially testosterone).

Fetal testicles, aided by the maternal placenta, begin producing testosterone at about ten weeks of gestation. Testosterone levels fall at birth and remain low until puberty, when they resurge, causing the penis, scrotum, and testes to grow about ten times larger. The testosterone they produce changes the prostate gland and seminal vesicles, increases facial and body hair, and has a stimulating effect on protein anabolism, bulking up muscles.

Each testicle contains several sections or *lobules*; inside each lobule are about five hundred long, narrow, convoluted *tubules.* If stretched out, the tubules would cover 750 feet. *Sertoli cells*, which make sperm and androgen-binding protein, live in the tubules. Every sixteen days, the Sertoli cells begin the production of sperm, which require a little over two months to mature fully. A man makes sperm almost continuously from puberty to death.

Sperm production is complicated: The hypothalamus secretes gonadotropin-releasing hormone (GRH), which triggers the pituitary to secrete luteinizing hormone (LH) and follicle-stimulating hormone (FSH). LH stimulates the testes to produce testosterone, and, in concert with FSH, induces immature sperm cells, called *spermatogonia*, to divide and grow. As they mature they are called, in sequence: *spermatocytes*, *spermatids*, and, finally, *sperm* or *spermatozoa.* Most men produce a thousand sperm a minute.

Sperm are easily injured by heat. In order to be viable, sperm must be cooler than the body by at least 2°F/1°C. To achieve this, the testes are suspended in a sac called the scrotum.

The epididymides lie in the scrotum, each *epididymis* adjoining its testicle. These narrow, elongated storage vessels hold the newly generated spermatozoa until ejaculation, when they usher them into the vas deferens and on their journey in the world.

A healthy man makes 31,536,000,000,000 sperm in the sixty years between the ages of 15–75.

Testicular Distresses

The testes are rarely bothered by infections, but they may become inflamed, swollen, and painful (**orchitis** or **epididymitis**, page 307). Benign cysts – **spermatocele** (below), hydrocele, and varicocele – may grow on the testicles. Testes may fail to descend (**cryptorchidism**, page 306), fail to produce viable sperm (**infertility**, page 309), or fail to create enough testosterone (page 316).

Testicular cancer (page 314) may begin in infancy; moms especially, please read **preventing testicular cancer** (page 312).

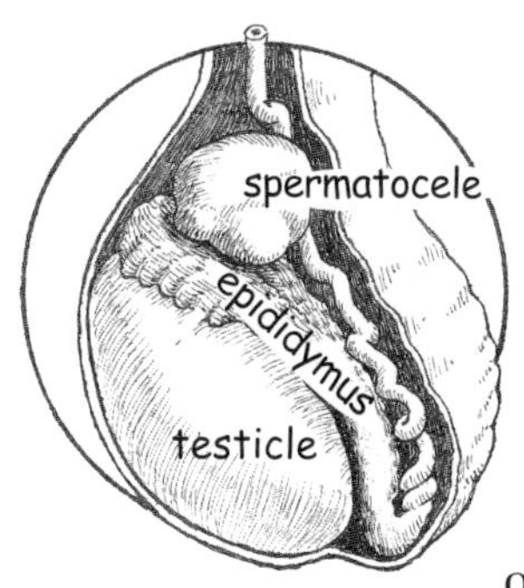

 Spermatocele 

A spermatocele is a cyst on the testicle, usually on or near the epididymis. It is usually about the size of a pea, smooth and firm, painless, and quite benign. Occasionally, a spermatocele may grow as large as a lemon; large ones will cause discomfort when the legs are crossed, or on walking or running. About 30 percent of men, increasing with age, have one.[1]

Treatment is rarely necessary, but if you want to remove a spermatocele without surgery, try dropperful doses of chickweed tincture, taken four times a day for as long as a year.

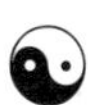 My Balls Hurt! 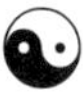

- **Fennel** seed tea is the specific for relieving testicular pain.
- So is **ejaculation**.
- **Homeopathic** remedies for men with swollen testes:
  - ~ *Pulsatilla*: testes dark red, congested, swollen, sensitive.
  - ~ *Hamammelis*: testes heavy, weighty, dragging.
- Sudden onset of pain, with heaviness: prostatitis (page 338).
- Pain with a hard, hot palpable lump: orchitis (page 307); also testicular cancer (page 314).
- Pain with swelling, heaviness: epididymitis (page 307).
- **Sciatica** can trigger testicular pain.

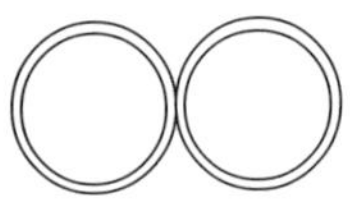

Cryptorchidism · Undescended Testes

"Warm and wet, we're hanging loose. Cold and dry, we're pulled up tight. The safer we feel, the more we relax. Coax us; don't threaten. Entice us; don't demand. Create space and we will fill it . . . in our own time."

"Yep," says Grandfather Growth, "That's what they say."

Step 0. *Do Nothing*

• The testes drop within a few weeks after birth. If not, read on.

Step 1. *Collect Information*

• About 10 percent of boys are born with undescended testes.[2]

• Men with uncorrected cryptorchidism are rarely fertile.

Step 2. *Engage the Energy*

• Fear contracts the testicles. Create safe space for your baby boy with plenty of skin-to-skin contact, nursing, sleeping with mom, swaddling, and soothing music.

Step 3. *Nourish and Tonify*

• Daily **moxibustion** near the pubic bone and across the lower pelvis is painless, safe, simple, and the top folk-medicine remedy for bringing down the testes. Ask for moxa sticks in Chinese pharmacies or health food stores. Hold the burning stick an inch from the skin. Move it in spirals until the patient reacts.

Help!
Undescended Testes

Let go of expectations.

• Birth–3 months: **Make safe space**. What does your baby boy need?

• 3–6 months: Add **moxibustion**.

• 6–12 months: Add **fennel** seed tea or steroidal herbs.

• 24 months: Consider surgery.

Step 4. *Stimulate/Sedate*

★ Herbalist Brigitte Mars uses delicious **fennel** seed tea to remedy cryptorchidism. It's great for babies and eases colic too.

• Herbs rich in sterols – such as saw palmetto, vitex, wild yam, or red clover – may encourage testicles to descend. Tinctures are easiest to use; the dose is one drop per five pounds of weight.

• Testosterone-nourishing **oatstraw infusion** safely aids the development, and descent, of healthy testicles in boys of all ages.

Step 5. *Use Drugs*

• Hormone therapies cause problematic side effects. Herbs rich in sterols (above) are safer.

• Sons and grandsons of women who took DES (page 202) are more likely to have undescended, undeveloped testicles, and benign cysts on the epididymides.[3] Maternal ingestion of hormones from plastics may increase the occurrence of cryptorchidism.

Step 6. *Break and Enter*

• If the testicles have not descended by age two, surgery is recommended. Left in the abdomen, the testicles get too hot, impairing future fertility and setting the stage for cancer.

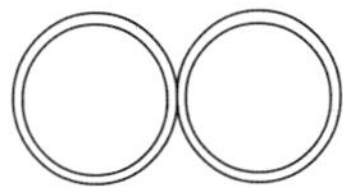

Orchitis & Epididymitis

"Strip!" orders Grandfather Growth.

"Follow!" he yells as he sprints down the beach, runs into the chilly water, and dives though the surf. Later, the two of you flop down on the sand, breathing deeply.

"And that's what I have to tell you about keeping your family jewels in good working order," he says with a grin.

Step 1. *Collect Information*

• Epididymitis and orchitis are caused by infections that require antibiotic treatment. Herbal treatment may be used concurrently.

• **Epididymitis** is usually caused by chlamydia. Untreated, it can lead to sterility. Symptoms include a tender, hard, hot lump in the back of the testicles, with a discharge or difficulty urinating.

• **Orchitis**, inflammation of the testicles, is often caused by gonorrhea, syphilis, or mumps. Symptoms include pain and swelling.

Step 2. *Engage the Energy*

• **Homeopaths** suggest *Serenoa* as an integrative remedy for men dealing with epididymitis or orchitis. Those with simple orchitis may also use homeopathic *Stramonium* or *Veratrum veridis.*

Step 3. *Nourish and Tonify*

★ Immune strengtheners like astragalus, eleuthero, and ginseng, as teas or tinctures, are allies for men with painful testicles.

Step 4. *Stimulate/Sedate*

★ A **hot sitz bath** will quell pain and increase circulation.

• Counter inflammation with **elevation**. Relax for no more than thirty minutes with a pillow under your hips (and testes).

• Single drop doses of poisonous **poke root** clear infection fast and counter inflammation. Poke combines well with echinacea, the herbal antibiotic. (Dosage on page 342.)

• Herbalist Michael Moore favors poisonous **Western peony** (*Paeonia brownii*) to counter orchitis. A dose is a cup of tea made with ½ teaspoon of the dried root, drunk nightly for a week.[4]

Step 5. *Use Drugs*

• Complement antibiotics with herbs, homeopathic remedies, and yogurt. Use daily for the full course of the antibiotics.

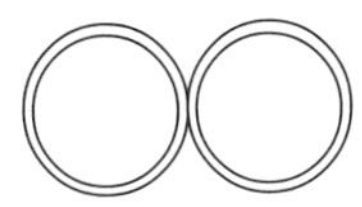

Fertility/Infertility

"To be fertile is to be potent. To be potent is to be a man. Man the lifeboats; survival is a man's skill.

"Some say," chuckles Grandfather Growth, "that the penis is an extension of a man's ego. But that honor really belongs to his children, the extension of his line, his life, his success. Find the part of you that desires immortality and feed it. Find the part of you that wants to be king and crown it. Find the part of you that you love the most and make it real."

Step 1. *Collect Information*

- It is estimated that 6 percent of men are infertile.[5]

- A couple is infertile if they are not able to achieve pregnancy after two years of unprotected intercourse.

- Causes of men's infertility include genetic and physical abnormalities, infections, androgen insensitivity, malnutrition, and exposure to heat, stress, environmental estrogens, or tobacco smoke. These cause low sperm count, low sperm motility (or comatose sperm), abnormal sperm, and clumping sperm.
  ~ Low sperm count (*oligospermia)* is less than 20 million/mL.
  ~ Low motility is less than 50 percent of the sperm moving.
  ~ Abnormal sperm is less than 30 percent normal.

Help! Infertility

Expect results in 7–9 months

- Ally with **pumpkin seeds**.
- Drink **oatstraw infusion**.
- Eat more **shellfish**.
- Experiment with **astragalus**.

★ It takes two months for sperm to mature. For best results, use infertility remedies for at least three months, nine is best.

Step 2. *Engage the Energy*

- The **homeopathic remedy** for fertility problems is *Serenoa.*

Step 3. *Nourish and Tonify*

> "Mice showed a significant increase in sperm production merely from adding garlic juice to their food."[6]

★ **Astragalus** increases sperm motility.[7] Add the powdered root to food or use up to four dropperfuls of the tincture daily.

• Several cups of **oatstraw infusion** a day will free up bound testosterone, increase desire, and improve sperm motility.

★ **Red clover infusion** is the single best remedy I know of for increasing fertility. It is not estrogenic, but sterolic, allowing the body to create the specific hormones it needs.

★ **Zinc-rich foods** like oysters, free-range eggs, and pumpkin seeds are what herbalist and men's health specialist, Ryan Drum, suggests for men intent on reproducing.

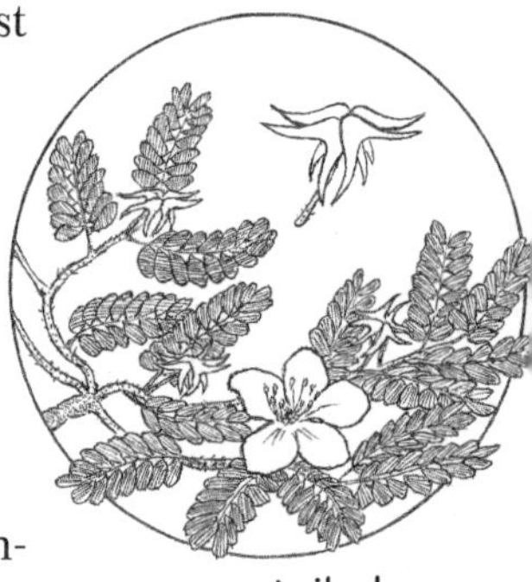

★ The invasive weed *Tribulus* – puncture vine, caltrop, goathead, toritos, bai ji li, bindii, or gokshura – has a world-wide reputation as an aphrodisiac and fertility aid. It promotes libido, increases erectile strength and duration, and "significantly improves sperm production and mobility."[8] Best as a strong tea or capsules of the powdered fruits/leaves.[9]

tribulus

★ Drinking 1–3 cups of Chinese dogwood fruits – one ounce steeped in 2 cups boiling water for twenty minutes – can increase sperm motility 68–120 percent.[10] You may also notice a heightening of libido, improved erections, and easing of incontinence and frequent urination.[11] Honey improves the sour taste.

• The ancient Aztecs called the avocado *ahuacatl* ("testicles"). Like figs, they are considered ideal for nourishing sperm.

Step 4. *Stimulate/Sedate*

• **Ginseng** increases the pituitary gland's secretion of luteinizing hormone, which increases testosterone and improves fertility.[12] Large doses, about three grams a day, are required for effect.

• A series of **acupuncture** treatments to deal with "damp heat" and "kidney insufficiency" can often improve fertility by increasing the number and the motility of sperm.[13] Acupuncture appears to be especially helpful for men with infections and inflammation in the reproductive organs.[14]

• English herbalist Penelope Ody favors He-shou-wu (fo-ti) as a stimulant to sperm production.[15] She steeps the roots in red wine for two weeks. The dose is a small glass of wine a day. (page 312)

• Herbalist Ryan Drum increases dietary zinc, decreases pesticide/herbicide exposure, and cools the testes to improve fertility.

★ **Heat** interferes with fertility: tight-fitting pants, underwear, or swimsuits, hot tubs, saunas, laptops. Sperm start to degrade after being next to an active cell phone for an hour (in your pocket).[16] Native Americans refrained from sexual relations – sometimes for months – after sweat lodge ceremonies.

• A health worker from India says men can limit family size by sitting in extremely hot water for fifteen minutes each night. She claims the ejaculate is non-fertile after the first ten treatments.

• **Cottonseed oil** is a source of the "powerful male antifertility compound gossypol, which inhibits sperm production."[17] Check the labels of processed foods you eat; lose the cottonseed oil.

Step 5a. *Use Supplements*

• Supplements of **vitamin E** (at least 10 percent gamma tocopherol), **zinc**, **vitamin B$_{12}$** and **selenium** can increase sperm motility and improve their symmetry and beauty (morphology).[18]

★ Supplemental **ascorbic acid**, even as little as 200mg per day, doubles sperm count. In one study, none of the placebo takers, but all of those supplementing, achieved conception.[19]

★ Four grams of **L-arginine** daily can double sperm count in two weeks and increase motility, too.[20] (Cautions: page 299.)

• Supplements of one gram of L-carnitine taken three times a day for three months with **alpha-lipoic acid** increase sperm count and motility in 78 percent of the men taking it.[21]

Step 5b. *Use Drugs*

• Sons and grandsons of women who took DES (see page 202) are more likely to have abnormal sperm and fertility problems.

• Fluoride, certainly in high doses and possibly in low ones, can damage sperm, lower sperm count, and reduce fertility. It reduces circulating testosterone, and it harms the Sertoli cells.[22]

Step 6. *Break and Enter*

• Intracytoplasmic sperm extraction coupled with in vitro fertilization (IVF) can help a couple conceive a child with their own sperm and eggs. These procedures can impair your health.

The Legend of He-shou-wu

He-shou-wu lived in China during the Tang dynasty.

"I was 58 and felt like half a man, for I was father to no children. Deep into my sense of failure, one day I drank myself into a stupor. I awoke on a mountainside, surrounded by twining vines. My curiosity urged me to dig one up.

"So I did. I took it to an old herb doctor. 'A fabulous restorative!' he exclaimed. Following his instructions, I cooked the root and began to drink the broth. Within days my virility was restored. Over the next ten years, with the root broth as my constant drink, I fathered a fine family. Look at me now. I still drink my root brew, my He-shou-wu. My hair has never grayed and I am 130 years old."

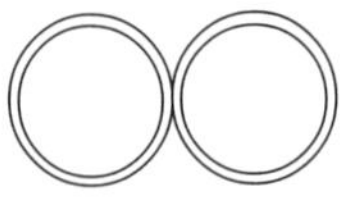

Preventing Testicular Cancer

"There is much in your life that you can control; but some things just happen," Grandfather Growth mutters as he strides purposefully along. "Do what you can, grandson. Live in truth and beauty. Treat all of life, including yourself, with respect. Work hard. Rest easy. Believe in my love. This is my plan for preventing cancer. What's yours?"

Step 1. *Collect Information*

"No one knows what causes testicular cancer."[23]

• The risk of testicular cancer varies widely. Danish men are five times more likely to have it than men in neighboring Finland. In America, white men are seven times more likely than black men to be diagnosed with testicular cancer.[24]

• You are at risk for testicular cancer if your father or brother has been diagnosed with it or if you are a white man under the age of 35 with one or more undescended testes.

• Unlike prostate cancer, which is more common as men age, testicular cancer is more likely in young men. Among American men aged 15–35, testicular cancer is the most common cancer.

★ Like breast cancer, testicular cancer can be felt even when small. Stay in touch with your testicles. During a relaxing hot shower or bath, lather up your scrotum and gently roll each testicle between fingers and thumb, feeling for lumps, thickening, enlargement, or fluid buildup. Pay special attention to the epididymis and vas deferens, both of which ought to feel firm and smooth with no lumps. Any pain in your testicles is an indication of inflammation, not cancer.

• Testicular cancer arises from *carcinoma in situ* (CIS) cells that are present in fetal testicles. Lifestyle choices and life experiences determine whether CIS goes on to become cancer.

Step 3. *Nourish and Tonify*

★ Because testicular cancer starts before you are born, you will have to **ask your mother to**:

~ Avoid estrogenic hormones while pregnant.
~ Eat organic foods while pregnant.
~ Use cloth diapers. Disposable diapers increase the temperature of the testes enough to impair later fertility and to "facilitate the development of testicular cancer."[25]
~ Eliminate plastic baby bottles, cups, and toys.
~ Breast feed.
~ Avoid soy-based formulas.

Step 4. *Stimulate/Sedate*

• Exercise lowers the risk of developing testicular cancer. The more a man exercises, the lower his risk.[26]

Step 5. *Use Drugs*

★ Men whose mothers took estrogen, DES, or any other female hormone during pregnancy are eight times more likely to be diagnosed with testicular cancer than those whose mothers were not exposed to hormones.[27] Estrogenic chemicals in the environment are probably responsible for the "dramatic increases" in testicular cancer over the past fifty years.

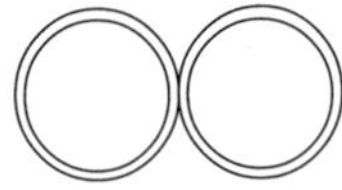

Testicular Cancer

"There is a moth in the granary, a rat in the corn, a pretender to the throne. Act quickly! Strike deeply! Commit yourself wholly to the task and stay focused, my grandson," admonishes Grandfather Growth.

"Take no prisoners; fight to win. Cede what you must; keep what is most precious. Count each breath a blessing. Your strength is sourced in the will of thousands. We stand by you, brother."

Step 0. *Do Nothing*

• Cancer in one testicle could be in the other. Is it best to wait and see if cancer does develop, or to biopsy th other one right away? Only 2–5 percent of men have cancer in the other testis.[28] Waiting preserves fertility and potency. Biopsies often find a precancerous condition – cancer in situ (CIS), which may, or may not, develop into cancer. We don't know how long CIS takes to become cancerous, or even in which men more it is likely to go on to become cancer. CIS can be treated with radiation, which destroys fertility, but leaves the testicles able to make testosterone. Once cancer develops, the affected testicle, and its spermatic cord, must be removed.

Step 1. *Collect Information*

★ The incidence of testicular cancer is rising in the USA. The number of men diagnosed increased 400 percent between 1975 and 2000 (when there were about 8000 cases).[29,30]

• Testicular cancer, like most cancers, is considered "curable" if found very early. However, it often spreads rapidly and lethally.

• Ninety percent of the 8,000–10,000 American men diagnosed each year with testicular cancer survive at least five years.

• Men diagnosed with testicular cancer have a five-fold greater risk of developing melanomas, lymphomas, and leukemias.[31]

Step 3. *Nourish and Tonify*

• Eat like your life depended on it: make friends with miso and seaweed, shitake and astragalus, burdock and garlic. Exercise like there's no tomorrow: yoga, tai chi, long walks with loved ones.

Step 5. *Use Supplements*

• There is a growing body of evidence that taking supplements neither prevents cancer nor retards its growth. Worse, some studies show vitamin supplements shelter the cancer from harm.

Step 6. *Break and Enter*

• When a woman has a suspicious lump in her breast, a biopsy removes a piece of tissue to be examined for cancer cells. When a man has a suspicious lump in his testicle, the entire organ is removed.

Help!
Testicular Cancer

Expect results quickly.

• After surgery: homeopathic *Arnica*.

• Before chemo: **milk thistle seed**.

• Against radiation damage: carrot juice, sweet potatoes, 5–10 grams of sargassum seaweed powder daily.

Why not do a biopsy? Because ". . . biopsying a tumor-bearing testicle runs the risk of dislodging any cancer cells that may have turned metastatic. . . ."[32] Hmmm.

• The experts say men retain the ability to have an erection even if they have both testicles surgically removed. Whew! Most men regain potency and desire within six months of surgery.

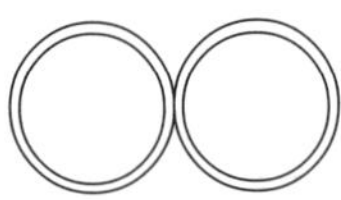

Testosterone Supplementation?

"Have you ever imagined youself to be an old man like me?" Grandfather Growth queries with a wink. "Can you see yourself being on the sidelines, coaching? Can you feel the hardening and stiffening in the places that ought to bend, and the lack of it where you want it the most? Do you have gray hair? Or no hair? Do you have a grandson? Or do you believe you will be forever young? Pan? Peter Pan?

"You are perfect, dearest grandchild, now and every day, young and old. Eat from the Earth Mother's riches; use her herbs as elixirs; allow yourself to change; welcome age. New vistas are opening. Look!"

> ". . . the attempt to reverse the gradual decline in testosterone levels in aging men can't be considered the treatment of a disorder: it amounts to a vast, uncontrolled experiment, whose consequences remain uncertain."[33]

Step 0. *Do Nothing*

★ The National Institutes of Health 2001 panel concluded that the andropause hypothesis is unproven, and testosterone supplementation is uncalled for and unnecessary for most men.

Step 1. *Collect Information*

• Supplemental testosterone is today's elixir of youth. It is supposed to delay or prevent erectile dysfunction, loss of muscle mass, and other ills of elderly men. Some men may benefit from testosterone supplements, but who and how much is unknown.

• Up to 15 percent of healthy men over 21 have testosterone levels that are more than 50 percent below the lower limit of "normal" as set by those who promote supplementation.[34]

• The tests doctors use to measure testosterone levels are "notoriously" unreliable. Furthermore, a man's testosterone levels can be markedly different at different times of the day or the year.[35]

★ The largest and longest-term study showed no improvements in energy level, sexual performance, or strength in men given transdermal testosterone supplements.[36]

• Testosterone supplementation does elevate the risk of prostate cancer. In men older than 45, those with the highest testosterone levels were twice as likely to be diagnosed.[37] In those younger than 45, the risk was three times as great.

• As men age, their blood contains more testosterone-binding proteins.[38] The amount of active, bioavailable testosterone is increasingly lower than the total amount of testosterone as the years add up. Perhaps to protect against prostate cancer?

Step 2. *Engage the Energy*

• We take on the shape of what we imagine. Imagine yourself as a vital, vigorous, curious, sharp-looking old man. Collect images of thriving older men. Find a role model for healthy aging.

Step 3. *Nourish and Tonify*

★ The safest and most effective way I know to maintain healthy levels of bioavailable testosterone is to drink **oatstraw infusion**. Drinking 1–2 quarts/liters a week can keep your libido purring, your heart smiling, your bones strong, and your energy going. (Herbalist Ryan Drum says **oysters** and raw meat are even better!)

Step 4. *Stimulate/Sedate*

★ The herbs most often recommended for increasing testosterone are those rich in steroidal saponins: **eleuthero**, **guarana**,

maca, **saw palmetto**, **tribulus**, and **yohimbe**. Fermentation in our guts transforms plant sterols into special non-cancer-inducing forms of hormones, including testosterone.

★ **Pine pollen** is a natural form of testosterone.

Step 5a. *Use Supplements*

• Supplements of L-taurine are reported to boost testosterone levels.

Step 5b. *Use Drugs*

• Testosterone supplements aren't new, but the delivery system is. Testosterone injections have been available for decades, but not widely used. Testosterone pills are "toxic to the liver."[39] Patches often irritate the skin. When rub-in testosterone gel was introduced in 2000, there was an immediate 30 percent increase in testosterone use.[40] Since then, use has soared.

• Supplementation may be useful for severely depressed men 30–65 years of age.[41] After eight weeks, those receiving an antidepressant plus testosterone gel felt significantly better than those who got the antidepressant plus a placebo gel.

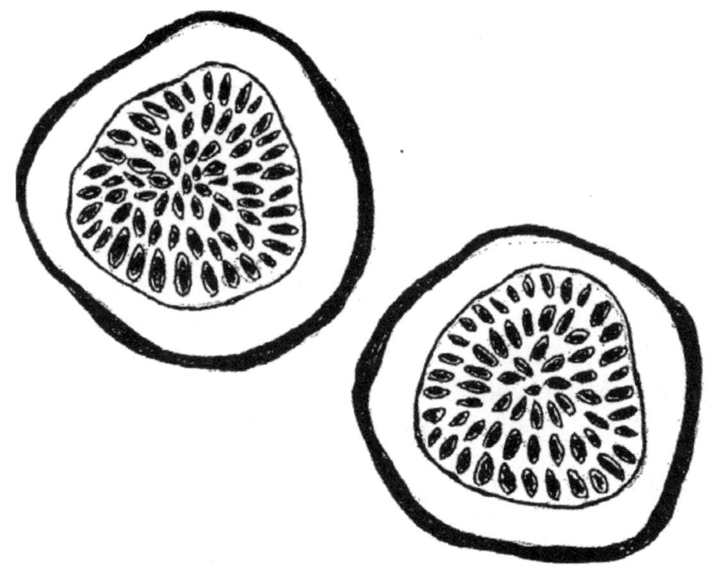

☆ Testosterone Star: Pine Pollen 

Pine pollen is a rich source of male hormones including androstenedione, testosterone, dehydroepiandrosterone, and androsterone.[42] It also contains the amino acids arginine (the precursor of nitric oxide, an erection stimulant), phenylalanine and tyrosine (precursors to L-dopa).[43] The neurotransmitter L-dopa facilitates erections, increases sexual interest, and promotes activity; it is specific for treating anorgasmia in women.[44]

Pine pollen has been in use in China for over two thousand years as a health restorative, longevity tonic, antiaging nutrient, strengthener, memory aid, immune system nourisher, and tonic to the lungs, the skin, the digestive and sexual organs.[45] Scientific research confirms that pine pollen counters fatigue, increases stamina, moderates stress, protects the liver and increases its ability to deal with alcohol and chemicals, reduces cholesterol, increases HDL, lowers LDL, protects blood vessels, and increases libido.[46]

Tincture the male catkins at the peak of their pollen production (early spring) in 198 proof alcohol, or buy ready-made tincture.

"When taken as a tincture, the pollen constituents enter the bloodstream almost immediately . . . [producing an] upsurge in energy, and, over time, an increase in strength, vitality, libido, and optimisn. Sexual stamina and erectile function both increase."[47]

The dose is a dropperful of tincture up to three times a day. No overdose level has been found, and there are no known interactions with any drug.[48]

If you are allergic to other pollens, you may wish to start slowly, with small doses, to be sure that you are not among the very few who cannot tolerate pine pollen.

Pine pollen has been used as a permanent adjunct to the diet for thousands of years by generations of Koreans and Chinese with no recorded toxicity.

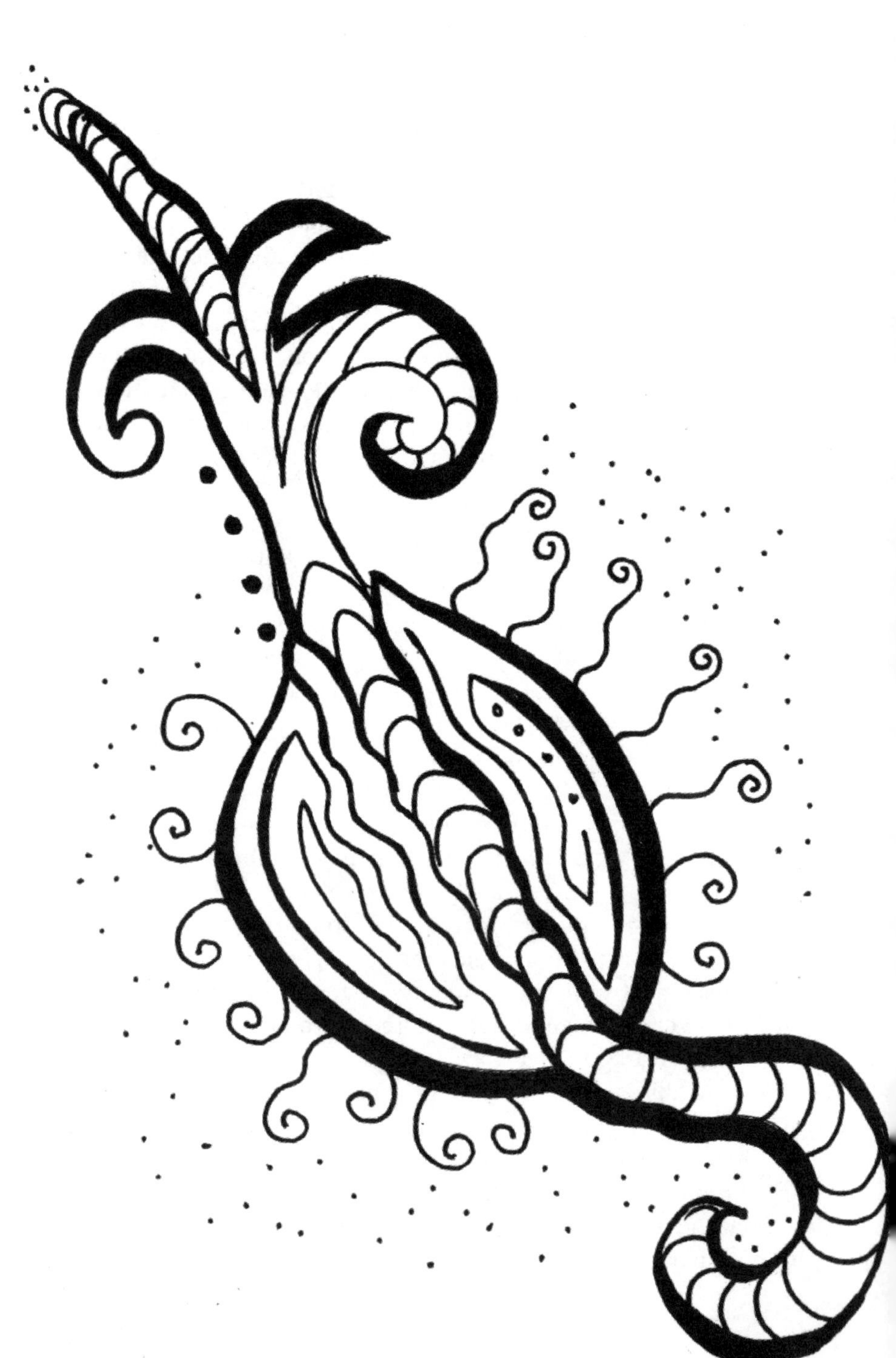

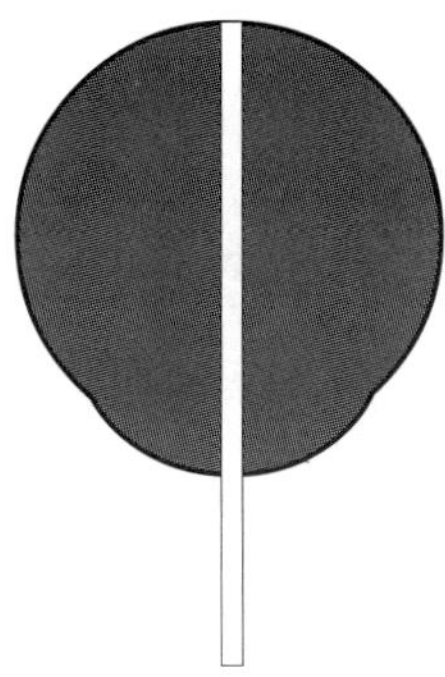

Prostate

I am the center of the future. I am the glory of the past. I am the wormhole that joins the generations and spans the universes.

I am eternal. I am designed by competition. Your ancestors' ancestors' ancestors bequeathed my subtlety and strength to you. I help you win the race. I help you continue the race.

I protect you. I join with your immune system to keep you safe. I speak through gut feeling, intuitions, emotions.

When threatened, I swell. When angered, I inflame. When sad, I choke up and ache. When pleased, I warm you like an inner fire. When delighted, I guide you like an angel of mercy.

Move me, move me, move me. Rock me back and forth. Rock me, rock me, rock me. Sway me side to side. Walk me, run me, stroll me, dance me. Just don't sit on me all day. I crave motion.

I crave activity. I am your craving. I thrive on lust; I am your lust for life. I am filled with desire; I am your desire to cheat death.

I am ready for the challenge. I am prepared for the task. I am steady. I am up for the journey. Trust me to hurl us into what is to come, what must be brought forth. I am your center. I am your prostate.

Healthy Prostate

The prostate gland lies immediately under the urinary bladder and above the testes in the abdominal cavity, very near the rectum. The fetal tissues that become the prostate in a man are the same as those that become the uterus in a woman. The prostate, like the uterus, is sensitive to hormones, environment, diet, and emotions.

The prostate doubles in size during puberty. The healthy prostate of a twenty-year-old weighs about one ounce. It is the size of a "golf ball" or "walnut," but with a hole in the middle, like a bagel or a donut. The tube that carries urine and semen out of the body (the urethra) passes through this hole.

From puberty until middle age (40–60), the cells of the prostate become quiescent and stop repairing and replacing themselves. Then, during the period I call "second puberty," the prostate wakes up and starts to grow. This can lead to problems.

The prostate is encased in a fibrous capsule. Within are three zones: the outer or *peripheral zone* (70–80 percent of the prostate), the *central zone* (20–25 percent), which lies between the front of the urethra and the peripheral zone), and the *transitional zone* (5 percent) which surrounds the urethra. It is the central and transitional zones which enlarge as a man ages.

The prostate gland produces prostatic/seminal fluid (the primary component of semen), functions as a valve to keep urine and sperm moving in the proper direction, and pumps semen into the urethra during orgasm. **Seminal fluid** is slightly alkaline and milky. It is rich in minerals, especially calcium, phosphates, and citrates. Seminal fluid nourishes the sperm and moistens the lining of the urethra, keeping infective bacteria out.

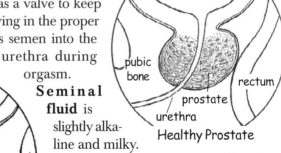

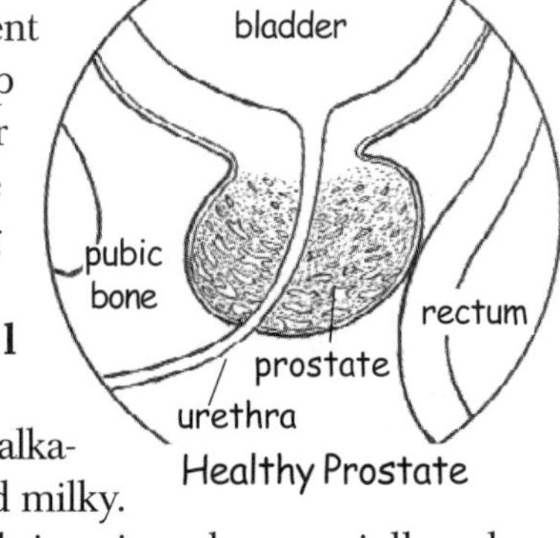

Healthy Prostate

BPH

Prostate Distresses

For the first half of a man's life, the prostate is invisible, unnoticed, unimportant. At midlife, however, normal hormonal changes cause the number of cells in the prostate to increase, enlarging it. Testosterone, the primary male hormone, interacts with an enzyme called 5-alpha-reductase, to form dihydrotestosterone (DHT), which prompts cellular proliferation in the prostate.

Normal, age-related prostate enlargement often occurs without symptoms. But symptomless prostate enlargement may also be caused by early stage prostate cancer. Modern medicine, through tests such as **PSA** (page 324), attempts to distinguish benign swelling from malignant changes. If your PSA is elevated, you may be urged to have further tests. Wait! Injecting dye into your bladder, inserting a tiny telescope through your penis, even being catheterized, can be irritating, painful, counterproductive, and damaging. Before agreeing to invasive **diagnostic tests**, try the effective herbal and food remedies collected here (page 327).

Men who don't have cancer, but do have symptoms, have **BPH**, benign prostate hypertrophy (page 329), or overgrowth of prostate cells. The prostate's tough outer covering forces it to expand inward, constricting the urethra and causing **lower urinary tract symptoms** or **LUTS**. Herbal remedies are at least as effective as drugs in relieving BPH (page 331) and LUTS (pages 55 and 330).

Not all prostate swelling is BPH. It may be chronic nonbacterial prostatitis, also called **prostatodynia** (prostate pain) or chronic pelvic pain (page 15). When prostate growth slows circulation or prevents complete emptying of the bladder, bacterial **prostatitis** (page 338) becomes more likely.

Most older men have prostate cancer. Between puberty and midlife, prostate cells lose their ability to repair DNA damage. But the prostate is "continuously – and increasingly – bombarded by free radicals." As a man ages, these damaged cells constitute a cancer "time bomb."[1] A few small changes in your diet, lifestyle, and beliefs (see *The Biology of Belief*, Bruce Lipton) can help you **prevent prostate cancer** (page 343).

When the diagnosis is **prostate cancer** (page 351), consider all your choices: watchful waiting, herbal allies, surgery, and radiation.

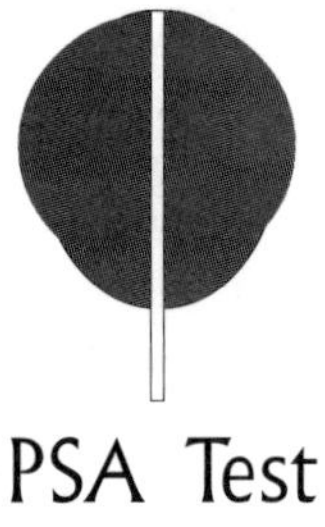

PSA Test

"Who can be trusted?" asks Grandmother Growth. "You can trust your inner wisdom. Call upon Grandfather Growth. Listen to him."

> "PSA starts the wheels turning on a treadmill that can drag patients into further diagnostic testing, . . . and, finally, into invasive surgery — all of it often unwarranted."[2]

Step 1. *Collect Information*

• Like the mammogram, the PSA test, entrenched as the best way to find early cancer, isn't. PSA tests increase needless surgery that can cause functional problems that may persist for the rest of your life, and don't decrease mortality. Recent studies of PSA screening and mortality involving a quarter of a million European and American men found "no reduction in deaths from prostate cancer after . . . 10 years of screening. By 7 years, the death rate was 13 percent lower for the unscreened group."[3]

> ". . .for breast or prostate cancer, screening simply might identify low-risk, non-life-threatening cancers that then are treated inappropriately with aggressive therapy."[4]

• Prostate-specific antigen (PSA) is an enzyme (a protein) produced by the prostate. It liquefies the ejaculate so sperm can move freely. It generally spills into the blood only when there is irritation, inflammation, infection, injury, disease, or cancer in the prostate.

★ The ability of a PSA test to predict cancer is about 2 percent. This makes it, according to its developer, Dr. Thomas Stamey, Doctor of Urology at Stanford, "worthless" as a screening tool.[5]

> "[With a PSA test]. . . you are 47 times more likely to be harmed . . . than to have your life saved."[6]

• PSA is a "smoke alarm," not a cancer diagnostic. If your PSA level is high, or rising, you will be urged to have a surgical procedure, a biopsy, to look for cancer cells. About 90 percent of prostate biopsies find no cancer, but can be "debilitating."[7,8]

> "The benefits of prostate cancer screening are modest at best, with a greater downside than any other cancer we screen for."[9]

• PSA tests, like Pap smears and mammograms, can seem to indicate a problem when there is none, that is, be falsely positive. False positives trigger hundreds of thousands of unnecessary, painful, and expensive biopsies every year. Will a PSA test increase your health and set your mind at ease, or will it increase your anxiety and scare you into agreeing to further tests and treatments? Just because everybody else is doing something, it doesn't mean you have to do it too. (Your mother told you that, didn't she?)

> ". . . the economic and psychological costs of false-positives are huge."[10]

• Act on a false positive PSA and you may have lifelong urinary and/or erectile problems. (*See* My Story, page 328.)

> "[Some men] may not want to expose themselves to a test that may force them to undergo possibly needless treatments with known risks. [This] decision is reasonable."[11]

• If you choose to have a PSA test:

Do not ejaculate within 48 hours before the test. Ejaculation may cause a false positive result, especially in men over 50.[12]

Ask for copies of the results so *you* can track changes.

• Results of the PSA test in relation to cancer risk, according to conventional standards in nanograms per milliliter:

Normal: 0–4ng/mL	*Cancer risk 0%*
Slightly elevated: 4–10ng/mL	*Cancer risk 20%*
Moderately elevated: 10–20ng/mL	*Cancer risk 50%*
Highly elevated: Above 20ng/mL	*Cancer risk 90%*

> "PSA levels fluctuate naturally throughout the day and rise in response to ejaculation, prostatitis, or injury. . . ."[13]

• Among 8,595 Japanese men older than 50, only 8 (0.18 percent) of those with PSA under one ng/mL were diagnosed with prostate cancer during an eleven-year follow up.[14]

• PSA normally increases with age. Age-adapted normal levels are up to 4.5ng/mL for men 60–69; up to 6.5ng/mL for men 70–79.

> "Some men naturally produce so little PSA that their levels are below 4 with a tumor, while others excrete so much that their levels are high even when the gland is cancer-free."[15]

• Twenty-five percent of men with prostate cancer have PSA levels that are below 4ng/mL.[16,17]

> ". . . with 4 as a cut-off point, a surprising 82 percent of prostate cancers are missed in men under the age of 60."[18]

★ It is not the absolute number of the PSA that indicates cancer, it is its movement. *The rate of PSA increase is more predictive of cancer than the numeric score.*[19]

• Any consistent rise in PSA levels is cause for action.[20] Men with rapidly rising PSA levels – more than 0.75ng per year – are about 20 times more likely to die of prostate cancer.[21] Slower rises usually indicate slow-growing, small cancers, giving you more time to implement preventative strategies (page 343).

• PSA level changes are one of the best ways to measure the effectiveness of prostate cancer treatments.

• **PCA3Plus** tests for early prostate cancer with a look at PSA (in the blood), plus a look at PCA3 (in a urine sample, taken after a doctor massages the prostate to dislodge cells). PCA3 is genetic material that increases sixty-fold in men with prostate cancer.

★ Three new tests: (1) **EPCA-2** ("early prostate cancer antigen"); highly predictive, with very few false positives.[22] (2) **AMACR** (alpha-methylacyl coenzyme A racemase) over-expression; correct 100 percent of the time in ruling out cancer, and 97 percent of the time in identifying it.[23] (3) Comparisons of **free-floating PSA** to total PSA (lower ratios indicate higher risk for cancer); less cost and less risk than a biopsy.[24]

★ A digital rectal exam (DRE) allows a medical professional to touch the prostate through the thin tissue of the rectum. It is easy to feel swelling and surface tumors, but not easy to categorize them without unnecessary biopsies and damaging treatments.

For early detection of prostate cancer, DRE – beginning at age 40, or earlier if you are at high risk – is strongly recommended.

Step 2. *Engage the Energy*

• Blue light calms the prostate and lowers PSA. Imagine vivid blue light bathing the prostate first thing in the morning and just before going to sleep to help normalize PSA in six weeks.

• Having a biopsy will "piss off your prostate," says herbalist James Green. "This anger may feed any latent cancer."

Step 3. *Nourish and Tonify*

★ Consuming one ounce/30g of ground, cooked **flax seeds** daily can reduce PSA levels by one-third.[25]

★ Flax, plus a low-fat diet, can "significantly decrease" or normalize PSA readings.[26] Results may be evident within 30 days.[27]

★ **Lycopene** in cooked tomatoes, frozen watermelon, and pasteurized pink grapefruit juice, but not from pills or raw food, reduces PSA levels, and reduces DNA damage in the prostate.[28,29]

★ **Pomegranate** juice, rich in anticancer polyphenols, lowers PSA levels – sometimes by up to 85 percent – in 30 percent of men who drink 8 ounces a day.[30]

• After three months, men eating two servings of **soy** foods daily lowered their PSA by 14 percent.[31]

Step 4. *Stimulate/Sedate*

★ Try echinacea (page 342) instead of antibiotics to lower PSA.

Step 5b. *Use Drugs*

• Four weeks of antibiotics returns PSA to normal in half of those with inflamed prostates.[32]

Help!
High PSA

Expect results in 1–2 months

Before you get a biopsy; before you take drugs:

1. Eat 1 ounce/30g of cooked, ground **flaxseeds** daily.
2. Eat **tomato sauce** daily.
3. Reduce dietary fat to 20%.
4. Consider **antibiotics**.

Retest after six months.

• Proscar (finasteride) prevents prostate cancer 25 percent of the time. But the cancers Proscar prevents are those men die with, not from. If a man does develop prostate cancer while taking Proscar, his cancer is likely to be very aggressive.[33]

• Men who take Proscar, the hair-growth drug Propecia, or the herb saw palmetto, as well as those who are obese, may get a false-negative PSA reading – a low result even though cancer is present. Greater body weight causes lower scores.[34,35]

Step 6. *Break and Enter*

"A biopsy of the prostate won't kill a man, but he won't forget it."[36]

• During a prostate biopsy, an ultrasound probe is inserted into the rectum to illuminate lumps and guide the biopsy tool. Snips of prostate tissue are taken from six or more sites, examined microscopically, and rated on a ten-point Gleason scale. "This gives us an educated guess," comments Joseph Oesterling MD, a Mayo Clinic urologist.[37]

His Story

Ray is a retired professor of English.

"At 62 I was told my PSA was 7.5. The doctor gave me a choice between waiting for six months and retesting, or doing an immediate biopsy. I was planning to be in a third world country for the next year, and he characterized the biopsy as 'a minor procedure' with few side effects, so I opted for peace of mind. Which I got: the biopsy was negative. Saw palmetto tincture keeps my PSA around 2.5. All is well, except . . . since the biopsy, it is very difficult for me to maintain an erection. I can ejaculate with enough stimulation, but my penis remains quite flaccid. Viagra helps somewhat, but the side effects deter regular use."

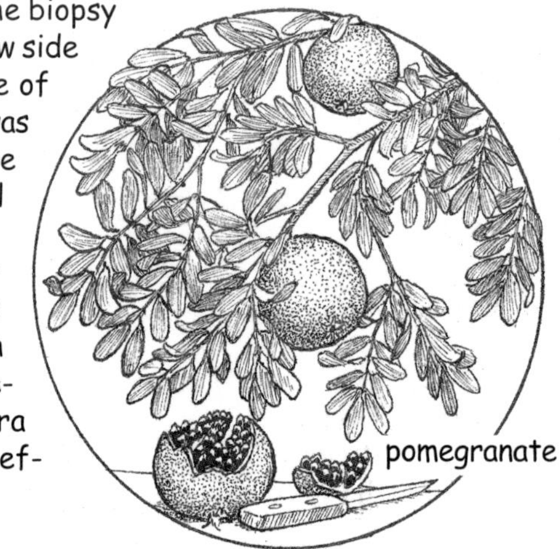

pomegranate

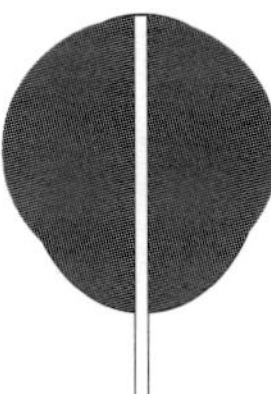

Benign Prostate Hyperplasia (BPH)

"Let us walk and talk together, grandson," suggests Grandfather Growth. "I sense a burning fury in you. I feel your tension. I know you are disappointed, sad, confused. You are good and hard working. But it has not brought you happiness. The work men do today is not the work our bodies crave, so we retreat to our minds and battle the wild animals of our own thoughts.

"I remember my own drive to succeed, to win, to overcome, to be the top dog, to lead the pack. I remember how much I worked. The long hours I sat at my desk, in my car, at meetings, on the phone. I pulled all my energy into my head and ignored the rest of my body. Except for sex, I paid no attention to all that stuff down there. It wasn't important, it didn't matter to me.

"When things didn't go well, I stuffed my distress. I kept a tight lid on my temper and all of my feelings. I had no idea I was jamming that energy into my prostate. I thought my feelings would just go away without bothering me.

"But little by little, it all caught up with me."

Step 0. *Do Nothing*

• The symptoms of BPH and the symptoms of prostate cancer are the same. Some men opt for diagnostic surgery. Others choose **watchful waiting** and alternative remedies.

• Possible complications of untreated BPH: acute urinary retention, kidney failure, bladder stones, urinary tract infections.

Step 1. *Collect Information*

• BPH, the most common prostate problem for American men, is virtually unknown outside North America and Europe.[38] In the USA, treatment of BPH costs over $2 billion annually and results in more than 300,000 surgical procedures.[39]

• Fifty percent of 50 year-old, 60 percent of 60 year-old, 70 percent of 70 year-old, 80 percent of 80 year-old, and 90 percent of 90 year-old American (and European) men have enlarged prostates.[40,41] Half will be symptomatic; one-third will require treatment.[42]

• Yes, black men are more likely to have BPH than white men, but it's not a given. BPH tends to run in families, too.

• Symptoms of BPH usually vary over time. They may gradually get worse, or mysteriously disappear, only to return months later. Symptoms don't relate to the size of the prostate. Some men who have very enlarged prostates have no symptoms; others, even with only a little swelling, have many aggravating symptoms.

• BPH symptoms are mostly LUTS/lower urinary tract symptoms (remedies, page 55) and often include an increased need to urinate at night (remedies, page 51).

• The causes of BPH are unclear. Perhaps it's too little testosterone . . . or too much prolactin . . . or too much 5-alpha-reductase . . . or perhaps all of these . . . or something else altogether.

Step 2. *Engage the Energy*

> "There is a strong placebo effect at work on symptoms associated with prostate enlargement. In drug trials, 40 percent of men getting dummy pills showed measurable improvement in symptoms."[43]

Help!
LUTS

Expect results in two weeks

• Take **saw palmetto** tincture twice a day.

• Use a **slant board**.

• Eat more foods high in **zinc**, or take a supplement.

• See pages 55 for more specific remedies.

★ **Affirmations**, **visualization**, and **prayer** are worth trying as a way to relieve prostate symptoms before resorting to more costly herbal remedies and more injurious drugs or surgery. Try this simple visualization at any time, even waiting for a red light to change. Take a slow, deep, belly breath. As you breathe out, vividly imagine a soft blue light glowing inside your prostate gland. Smile. Repeat frequently.

- **Homeopathic remedies** to relieve BPH include:
  - ~ *Sulphur*: prostate swollen, hard, painful after sex.
  - ~ *Thuja*: prostate chronically enlarged and inflamed.
  - ~ *Gaultheria procumbens*: prostate pain; constant sexual desire.
  - ~ *Selenium*: prostate pain worse with urine, stool, walking.

★ Lying on a **slant board** with the legs up and the head down may be the simplest and most successful treatment for men with BPH.[44] No slant board? Just lie on your back, bend your knees, bring the feet up close to the buttocks, and, keeping the feet close together, let the knees fall out to the sides. Use pillows to prop the knees if you wish. Relax into this pose for 5–10 minutes at a time to improve circulation and reduce inflammation in the prostate. Any **inclined position** (more examples on page 9) allows gravity to relieve pelvic and prostate pressure.

Step 3. *Nourish and Tonify*

• Men who eat the most fruits and vegetables have the lowest risk of BPH. Those with the highest vitamin C, beta-carotene, and lutein intakes (from food, not pills) are 7–16 percent less likely to have enlarged prostates. Particularly effective foods include orange juice, peas, peaches, and winter squash.[45]

★ For freedom from BPH, eat green and yellow produce. Men who eat ½ cup of **green** foods daily – spinach, kale, broccoli, Brussels sprouts, peas, or nourishing herbal infusion – have a 17 percent lower risk than men who eat a serving a week. Likewise, men who eat ½ cup of **yellow foods** daily – carrots, peaches, sweet potatoes, winter squash, papaya, cantaloupe, and apricots – have a 13 percent lower risk than men who eat a serving a week.[46]

Help!
BPH

Expect results in 4–6 weeks

- Take **saw palmetto** tincture or **rye pollen** several times a day.
- Drink 2–4 cups of **red clover infusion** every other day.
- Eliminate seed oils from your diet. Use **olive oil**.
- **Walk** or **dance** for 15 minutes a day.

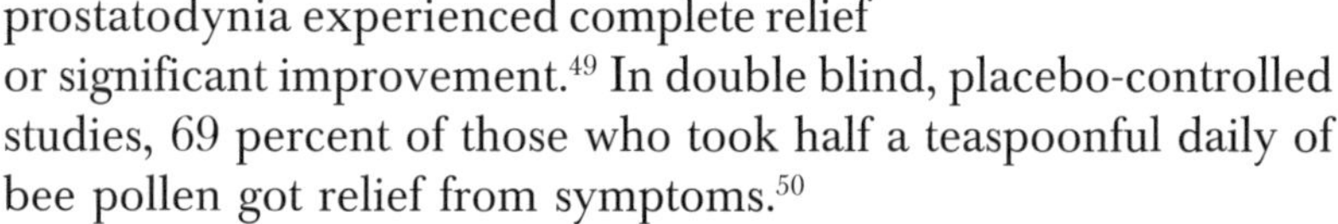

★ **Pollen** from the flowers of rye grass is a traditional European remedy for men with urinary and prostate problems. Some pollens are powerful anti-inflammatory and anti-androgenic agents.[47] On a daily dose of two 252mg tablets of bee pollen extract (sold as Cernitin),[48] more than three-quarters of men with uncomplicated prostatitis/prostatodynia experienced complete relief or significant improvement.[49] In double blind, placebo-controlled studies, 69 percent of those who took half a teaspoonful daily of bee pollen got relief from symptoms.[50]

• **Zinc** reduces prolactin secretion and calms swelling. Best food sources include **raw oysters** (30mg per ounce), **beef** and **lambshank** (2.5mg per ounce), **pumpkin seeds** (8mg per half-cup), lentils, peas, beans, garlic, whole grains, and organic dairy.

• **Isoflavones** block the action of 5-alpha-reductase and reduce prostate swelling. Minimally processed soy products, such as tamari, miso, tofu, edamame, and soy nuts, are one way to get isoflavones. So are most **beans** (legumes), especially lima beans, black beans, green beans, and lentils. Aim for 2–4 servings of beans a week. Or, drink a quart of isoflavone-rich **red clover infusion** several times a week.

• **Omega-3 fatty acids** are anti-inflammatory. Best sources are **flax seeds** (but not oil, *see* page 346), **purslane**, and oily fish, like **sardines**. Men who eat the most omega-3 fatty acids have smaller prostates, a stronger urine flow, and less retention of urine.[51]

• Omega-6 fatty acids are inflammatory. To get less omega-6, avoid seed/vegetable oils (corn oil, sesame oil, soy oil, flaxseed oil, cottonseed oil, sunflower seed oil, safflower seed oil, hemp oil, and canola oil). Instead use olive oil, avocado oil, and organic butter.

• The essential fatty acids gamma-linolenic acid (GLA) and eicosapentaenoic acid (EPA) block 5-alpha-reductase and reduce prostate swelling. Evening primrose oil, borage oil, and black currant oil are high in GLA and EPA. In one small study, two-thirds of those taking essential fatty acids had complete elimination of residual urine in the bladder and a reduction in nocturia.[52]

• **Belly fat** pushes on the prostate, reducing circulation. Obese men are much more likely to have prostate cancer and BPH.[53]

★ **Movement** – dancing, making love, yoga, tai chi, bowling, swimming, walking the dog – benefits the prostate. Moving the lower half of the body increases the circulation of nourishing blood to, and waste-removing lymph away from, the prostate, and minimizes the effects of stress hormones. Men who walk at least two hours a week have a 25 percent lower risk of BPH.[54]

• Pelvic rocking during intercourse benefits the prostate, easing BPH. Conversely, masturbation often pushes energy into the prostate. Counter this by keeping your hand still and moving the lower body rhythmically when you masturbate. It may take a while to make this work for you, and it is extra work, but it is work that will keep you potent and pain free for many decades.

★ Men in Bulgaria, Turkey, and the Ukraine use a handful of **roasted pumpkin seeds** daily to prevent and treat BPH. Pumpkin seeds contain essential fatty acids which reduce swelling, and cucurbitacins which prevent testosterone from changing to dihydrotestosterone (DHT). High DHT levels are associated with LUTS – and hair loss.[55] Perhaps their diuretic effect helps, too. And the abundant presence of three amino acids – alanine, glycine, and glutamic acid – nourishes the prostate.

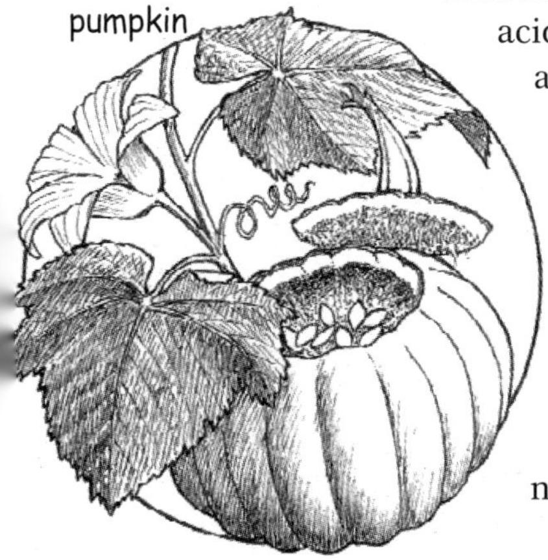

pumpkin

German herbalist Rudolf Fritz Weiss says "only a specially bred variety from the Near East is effective in medicinal use."[56] Most herbalists use ordinary – non-rancid! – pumpkin seeds. The effective dose is "never less than two heaping tablespoons morning and night, taken for months, even years."

Pumpkin seed increases the tone of the bladder muscles, relaxes the sphincter mechanism, decongests the prostate, and hastens recovery after surgery. (Try Amazonian Prostnut Butter: page 375.)

> ". . . there is no evidence that [herbal remedies for the prostate] . . . interact with prescription medications . . . ."[57]

Step 4. *Stimulate/Sedate*

★ **Saw palmetto** is widely regarded as the most effective treatment for men with BPH. It is featured in David Winston's male tonic combo (page 364). Saw palmetto works better than any drug to inhibit prostate cancer growth, reduce inflammation, and help the immune system. More on page 362. Reduce dose over time.

★ Stand up. Sitting on your butt cuts off the blood supply to your enlarged prostate. Avoid hard bicycle seats, too.

• Men with BPH who don't respond to saw palmetto may wish to ally with **pygeum** (page 337) or capules of **turmeric** root.

★ The **root** of the **annual nettle** (*Urtica urens*) has a "significant antiproliferative effect" on damaged prostate cells.[58] Some authors specify *U. urens*, but most regard the roots of the usual perennial nettle (*U. dioica*) as equal in effect. You can buy a standardized extract of nettle root. Or dig your own, dry it, and make an infusion (30g in a quart of boiling water). The dose is 1–2 cups a day.

★ When herbalists want to relax a muscle, they reach for **St. Joan's wort** tincture. It improves nerve functioning and relieves spasms. A dropperful dose 2–6 times a day can relieve symptoms as quickly as an alpha-blocker.

• **Alcohol** prevents the liver from removing prostate-irritating substances from the blood. And it depletes the prostate's friend, zinc. So, the standard advice for men with BPH is to avoid alcohol. Nevertheless, that advice is best ignored. When 30,000 men aged 40–74 were questioned about their drinking habits, researchers found those who consumed 1–3 drinks per day had a more than threefold decrease in the incidence of BPH.[59] "I agree," my 76-year-old tai chi teacher says with a bow. "One beer with dinner and I sleep through the night."

• Chinese herbalists recommend **American ginseng** to help men with BPH. The dose is up to four grams of dried root three times a day, alone or with other herbs.

Step 5a. *Use Supplements*

• Supplements of **beta-sitosterol**, 30–120mg per day, are used in Germany and other parts of Europe to treat men with BPH.

• There is more **zinc** in the prostate than in any other part of the body. In one study, 14 of 19 men who took 45mg of zinc daily reduced the size of their prostate and improved their ability to urinate.[60] If you decide to supplement – you're better off getting zinc from food – be aware that taking over 100mg daily for extended periods depresses the immune system, interferes with copper absorption, and actually increases the risk of prostate cancer.[61] Taking vitamin B_6 at the same time increases the absorption of zinc.[62] (*See* page 332 for zinc-rich foods.)

• No pill provides prostate health. *Supplements can't compete with real food, nor make up for a poor diet.*

> "Overproduction and accumulation of DHT seems to be a crucial element responsible for different pathologies, such as BPH, acne vulgaris, . . . male pattern baldness, and hirsutism."[63]

Step 5b. *Use Drugs*

★ Drugs work, sometimes slowly, or in as little as three days, to relieve BPH and LUTS, but must be taken indefinitely, often in combination. Please try herbal allies first. If you do choose drugs, using herbs at the same time can cut down on side effects.

• To shrink the prostate, a combination of an **alpha-blocker** (to relax bladder muscles) and a **5-alpha reductase inhibitor** like Proscar (finasteride) or Avodart (dutasteride) is commonly used. Inhibiting 5-alpha reductase – an enzyme which catalyzes the conversion of testosterone into dihydrotestosterone (DHT) reduces symptoms – but accelerates the incidence and growth of high-grade, aggressive prostate cancers.[64,65,66] It takes 6–12 months for 5-alpha reductase inhibitors to reduce symptoms. Suspicions that long-term use could increase the risk of hip fracture have not been shown, even after a decade of regular use.[67] There are side effects: 10–12 percent of men report decreased libido, poor quality of erection, and ejaculation difficulties.

Proscar gives "no greater relief than the placebo."[68]

Pregnant women should not touch Proscar or have unprotected sex with a man who is taking it. (His semen could damage the fetus.)

• Drugs such as gonadotrophin-releasing hormone analogs/agonists, progestogens, and nonsteroidal anti-androgens block the testicular hormones necessary for BPH. While they reduce the size of the prostate very well, their acceptance is limited due to their side-effects ("I'd call them front-effects," quipped one reader): impotence and loss of libido.[69]

★ Avoid over-the-counter cold and cough medications. They can cause prostate swelling and worsen LUTS.[70] Instead, treat your cold to a hot cup of soothing **sage** or **linden** tea with a spoonful of honey. Umm. For the flu I rely on dropperfuls of the tincture of fresh or dried **elder berries**.

Step 6. *Break and Enter*

• TUNA, TURP, TUMT, and TUIP are not sandwiches but surgeries; see page 57.

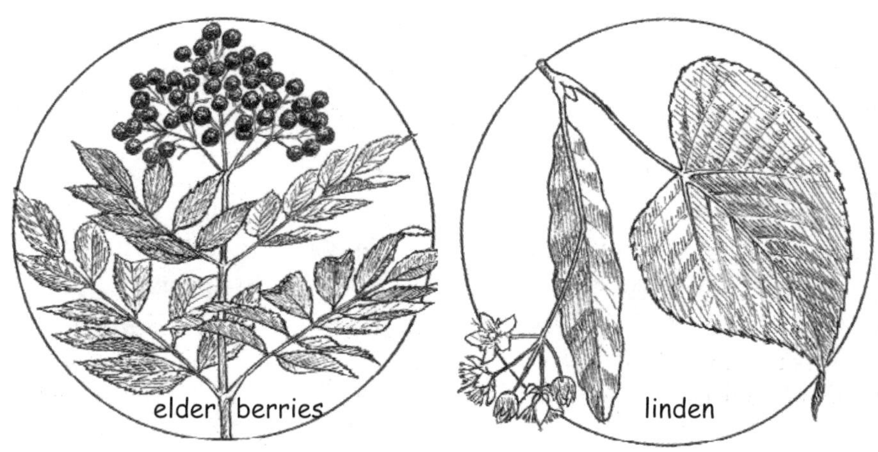

 Prostate Star: Pygeum (*Prunus africanum*) 

"[Pygeum]. . . involves impoverished farmers, deteriorating rainforests, international regulation, and big business . . . ."[71]

Pygeum, also known as Malagasy Medicine Tree or African prune, is an evergreen of elevations over 3000 feet. It is found in isolated populations in Africa and Madagascar, where it is regarded as the best herb for "old man's disease" (BPH) and bladder pain. Pygeum has become too popular for its own good. One kilogram of bark produces only 100 doses of extract, obtained through chloroform extraction and standardized to 12–13 percent beta-sitosterol.[72] Overharvesting has nearly doomed pygeum, so *let us use it sparingly, and only when other herbs won't do.* **Turmeric** is a substitute for pygeum.

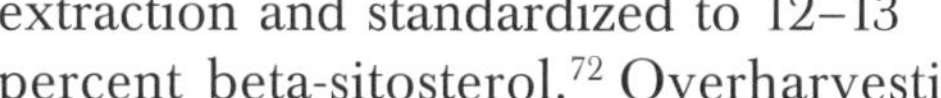

Pygeum contains anti-inflammatory phytosterols, decongestant pentacyclic triterpenes, and prolactin-reducing ferulic esters. It reduces prostate problems by interfering with, inhibiting, or blocking proliferation of fibroblasts and the accumulation of prostaglandins, prolactin, and cholesterol in the prostate. (Fibroblast proliferation drives BPH.[73] Prostagladins inflame; prolactin increases uptake of testosterone; cholesterol provides binding sites for DHT.) Pygeum's phytosterols also increase bladder elasticity.

A two-month, three-center study done in Poland reported a 32 percent reduction in nocturia and a 40 percent reduction of most symptoms. The improvements exceeded those observed with placebo, and were maintained for 30 days after treatment ceased.[74]

The usual **dose** is 50mg once or twice a day for 6–8 weeks, with a break of 1–4 weeks before continuing.[75] **Side effects** such as nausea, vomiting, diarrhea, and indigestion deter 13 percent of men from using pygeum.[76]

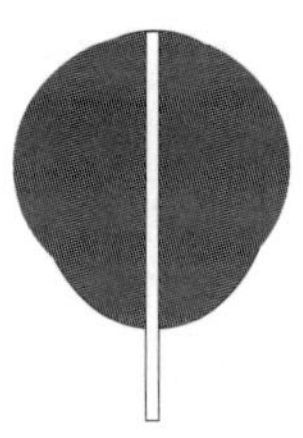

Prostatitis

"Finally," continues Grandfather Growth, "I had to choose between medical intervention and a long, hard look at myself.

"Drugs seemed like an easy fix, but I was more distressed by their side effects than by my symptoms. Herbs relieved my symptoms. And they helped me begin to realize that my prostate was sending me a message. It was telling me that I wasn't really happy, that I wasn't really fulfilled.

"It was difficult to accept that my body needed more than food, sex, and sleep. I had to learn to be human. I studied tai chi. I ate less steak, fries, coffee, soda pop, and alcohol. I even learned to dance.

"Those changes were hard for me, but even more demanding was the work I did to open my heart to my own distress. Gradually, with effort, I began to acknowledge my own fears, to honor my fear and pain, to ask for, and receive, gentle nurturing. Slowly, I began to release the tight grip I had on myself, to relax the unrelenting internal pressures.

"I began to honor the irritation I felt instead of stuffing it inside. I began to consciously move energy from between my legs up into my heart and then into my wisdom mind. I began to circulate the energy of creation throughout my body instead of always using it for sex.

"I hear your heart, brave one. And I know you hear me. I am here, behind you, supporting you. Shall we explore together?"

Step 1. *Collect Information*

> "BPH . . . rarely causes pain. Any man who has BPH but also has pain may want to get checked by a urologist for prostatitis."[77]

• "Itis" is an inflammation. Prostatitis is inflammation of the prostate. It will affect half of all men at least once in their lives.[78] Most common between the ages of 30 and 50,[79] prostatitis is a growing problem among older men as well.

• Prostatitis may be a bacterial infection, acute or chronic, with symptoms. Or it may be non-bacterial, usually chronic, sometimes asymptomatic.[80] About 80 percent of prostatitis cases are chronic nonbacterial.[81] Previously called "prostatosis," "prostatodynia," or "urinary sphincter hypertonicity," chronic nonbacterial prostatitis is now "chronic pelvic pain" (page 15).

• Symptoms of prostatitis include urinary difficulties, pain in the lower abdomen, groin, scrotum, testes, penis, or lower back, ranging from a constant ache to intense, erratic stabs. Sitting usually makes it worse. Some men with prostatitis have severe pelvic pain after ejaculation; others find ejaculation relieves their pain.

• Prostatitis, even if bacterial, is not contagious. Nor is it an STD, although in some cases, chlamydia may be present.

Step 2. *Engage the Energy*

"[If t]he man is uptight, . . . so is his urinary sphincter."[82]

• **Homeopathic remedies** for men with prostatitis:

~ *Chimaphila*: acute; feels like a ball in the perineum.
~ *Nux vomica*: acute; pain relieved by passing urine.
~ *Pulsatilla*: severely painful, spurting stream of urine.
~ *Sulphur*: inflamed, hard prostate; urinary burning.

★ **Visualize** (imagine) your prostate being held by loving hands. **Say**, to yourself or aloud: "I am safe. I offer myself ease."

★ **Reiki** energy healers say it is "extremely effective" in removing prostate pain. Do it yourself or ask someone to do it for you.

Step 3. *Nourish and Tonify*

★ **Corn silk tea** or infusion heals and soothes irritated prostates.

★ Tincture of flowering **cleavers** tincture is a specific against prostatitis. Try a dropperful dose 2–4 times a day. (Make it: page 367.)

**Help!
Prostatitis**

Expect results in 3–6 weeks

• Learn (and do) prostate massage.

• Take **cleavers tincture**.

• Use **reiki** to counter pain.

• Drink 2–4 cups of **nettle leaf infusion** every other day.

• Eliminate seed oils from your diet; use **olive oil** instead.

• Vegetable oils promote inflammation. To calm an inflamed prostate, use only **olive oil**, avocado oil, and butter.

• Herbalist Rudolf Fritz Weiss favors tincture or infusion of **couch grass** root to treat men with prostatitis and prostate edema.[83] Also called "witch grass," it is a common garden weed. (Make it: page 373.) The dose is a dropperful of tincture, or a cup of infusion, several times a day.

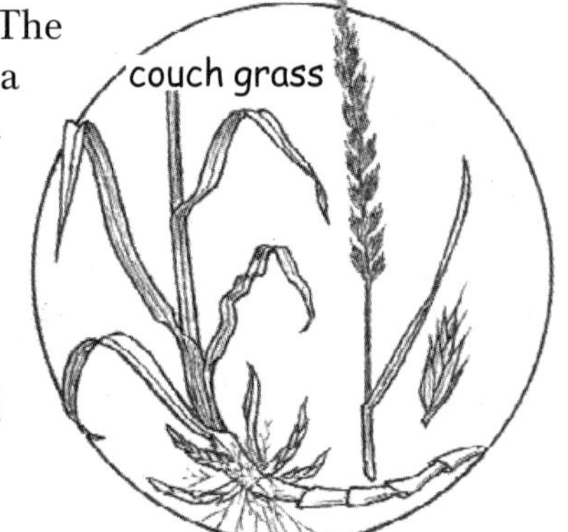

• If couch grass isn't effective in two weeks, Weiss adds a twice daily dose of two large tablespoonfuls of ground pumpkin seeds plus a dropperful each of tinctures of goldenrod flowers and aspen leaves.

Step 4. *Stimulate/Sedate*

★ Eliminating coffee, cayenne, black pepper, and alcohol from your diet may eliminate prostate pain from your life.

• David Hoffmann, herbalist and author of many herbals, gathers six of the most effective herbs for men dealing with prostatitis into one **Big Guns** formula. (Make it: page 377.)

★ **Prostatic massage**, or prostatic drainage, can relieve the symptoms of prostatitis. Many men find it uncomfortable and unpleasant, but not painful or difficult. Some find it erotic when done in conjunction with fellatio. **How to:** Three times a week, insert a clean, lubricated finger into the anus and gently press on the prostate for 1–2 minutes.

★ **Quercetin,** a bioflavonoid, significantly reduces prostate pain and improves quality of life for two-thirds of the those who take it, compared to one-fifth of those taking a placebo.[84] Urinary symptoms do not improve. Side effects, including rashes, headaches, and tingling in the extremities, were mild and disappeared quickly.[85] Combine quercetin with the enzymes bromelain and papain, and 82 percent of men report improvement.[86] Quinolone-class antibiotics block the effectiveness of quercetin.[87]

Get quercetin from **oak bark** tea, **green tea**, apples, grapes, citrus fruits, berries, cherries, beans, tomatoes, broccoli, garlic, and leafy greens, including nettle leaf infusion. The highest amounts are in the peels of onions;[88] boil them, add broth to soups.

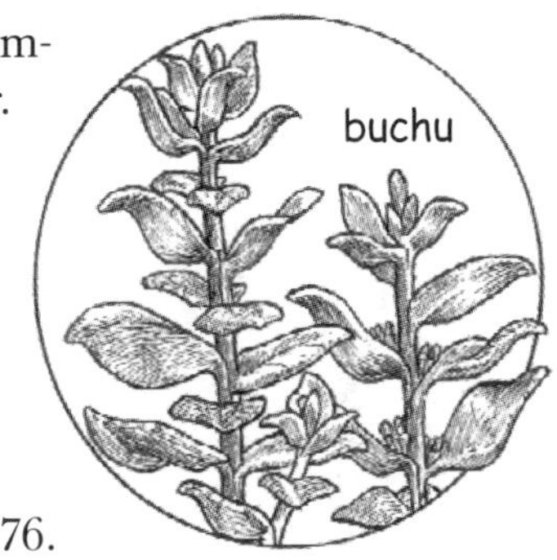

★ **Buchu** infusion "heals all chronic complaints of the genitourinary tract," says Dr. Christopher.[89] (Make it: page 370.) Taken cold, it increases the flow of urine, soothes the pelvic nerves, and relieves urgency. Drunk warm, it shrinks the prostate and ends inflammation. Large doses of the tincture can be used, but with less success.

• Try **Prostate Power Combo**, page 376.

★ **Sitz baths** relieve pain down there from non-bacterial prostatitis. Try warm water, or warm water with salt or Epsom salt in it, or an infusion of an astringent herb such as **oak bark**, **witch hazel**, **tormentil**, or **wild geranium**. (Make it: page 368.) For fastest results, switch back and forth: a hot water sitz bath for 10–15 seconds. then a cold astringent herb sitz bath for 5–10 seconds.

★ **St. Joan's wort** tincture is my favorite for easing muscle spasms and nervous tension. Dropperful doses may be taken every 2–4 hours. Relief is usually prompt.

• To ejaculate or not is the question for men with prostatitis. Doing it helps move energy, redistributes fluids, and relieves pressure. Not doing it helps avoid the pain of doing it. Your choice.

"[Chronic] prostatitis is notoriously difficult to treat."[90]

Step 5. *Use Drugs*

• High-dose antibiotics – taken for 4–6 weeks – counter acute bacterial prostatitis; or – taken for 3–4 months – counter chronic bacterial prostatitis. So do antibiotic herbs, page 342.

• Finasteride, tamulosin, nonsteroidal anti-inflammatory drugs (NSAIDs), antidepressants, and even epilepsy drugs have been tried in efforts to counter non-bacterial prostatitis.

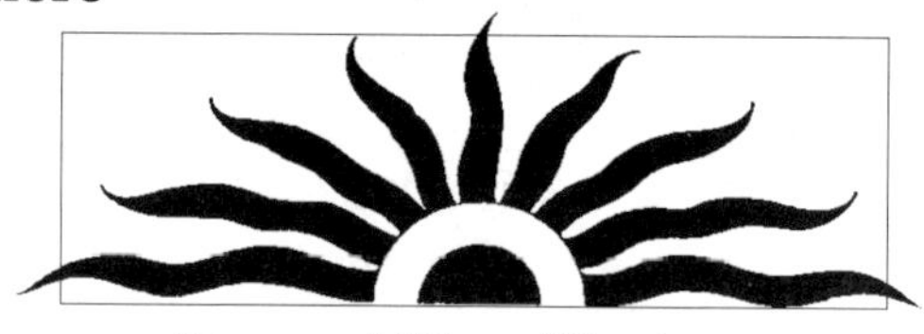

Expand Your Horizons

Instead of Antibiotics

There are good reasons to use antibiotic drugs. That said, it is agreed that they are often overused. If the infection is not life-threatening, you may wish to try herbs instead of, or in addition to, regular antibiotics.

Of the most-often used herbal anti-infectives – calendula, chaparral, echinacea, goldenseal, myrrh, poke, usnea, and yarrow – it is the lovely purple coneflower that I most often turn to.

I find **echinacea** as effective as antibiotics (dare I say sometime better than!) if *E. angustifolia/augustifolia*), not *E. purpurea*, is used; **tincture**, not capsules or teas, is used; the **root**, and only the root, is used; and very large doses are taken very frequently.

To figure your dose of echinacea, divide your body weight (in pounds) by 2; take that many drops per dose. There are about 25 drops in a drop-perful; round up to full droppers. If you weigh 180 pounds, take 90 drops/4 dropperfuls. There is no known overdose of echinacea tincture.

With *acute* infection, I take a full dose every 2–3 hours. When *chronic*, a full dose every 4–6 hours.

Most infections can be countered by echinacea alone. But, when there is a deeply entrenched infection in the pelvic area, I add one dropperful of **poke root** tincture to my one- ounce bottle of echinacea. Poke is an especially effective ally for men with prostatitis, women with chronic bacterial vaginal infections or PID, and anyone dealing with an STD/STI or UTI.

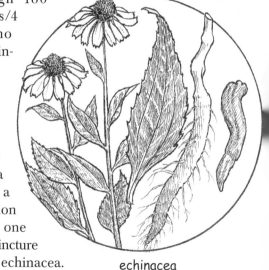

echinacea

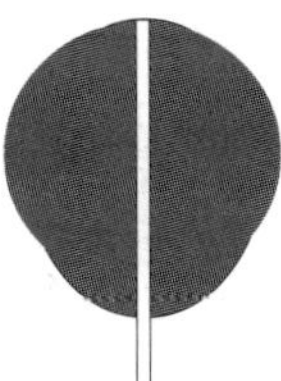

Preventing Prostate Cancer

Step 0. *Do Nothing*

• Sit quietly and listen to the Wise Healer Within. Practice.

Step 1. *Collect Information*

• Prostate cancer is the most common cancer among American men.[91] The US rate of prostate cancer is six times greater than it is in Japan.[92] African-American men are more than twice as likely as white men to be diagnosed with prostate cancer.[93]

• Between 1980 and 2009 the lifetime risk of prostate cancer for a white man doubled: from 1 in 11 to 1 in 6.[94]

Step 2. *Engage the Energy*

• Activating the energy at the base of the spine is fundamental for a healthy prostate. Get into your root any way you can: meditate or go fishing, do yoga or dance, practice pelvic floor clenches (page 14), visualize healing energies vibrating in your prostate.

Step 3. *Nourish and Tonify*

> "The best diet for preventing prostate cancer is one that is low in fat and high in vegetables and fruits, and avoids high-calorie intake and excessive meat, dairy products, and calcium."[95]

• Many **foods** protect against prostate cancer.[96] The most important ones are those that contain **sulforaphane** (cabbage, garlic), **lycopene** (cooked tomatoes, apricots), **quercetin** (apples, tea), **selenium** (nuts, seeds), or **phytoestrogens** (lentils, red clover). Flax seeds, kelp, avocados, pecans, and fatty fish also reduce risk.

• Three or more servings a week of vegetables in the **cabbage family** reduce your risk of prostate cancer by 50 percent.[97,98]

Cook 'em! Raw broccoli, cauliflower – everything in this family contains enzyme inhibitors which prevent the conversion of indole-3-carbinol into cancer-preventing DIM (diindolylmethane).[99] Other compounds in cooked cabbage family plants help the body get rid of cancer-promoting substances created by grilling meat.[100]

• **Cooked tomatoes** are a tasty way to prevent prostate cancer, according to more than fifty studies.[101] Two servings a week reduces risk by 23–36 percent.[102,103] Four servings a week reduces risk by 35 percent.[104] Ten servings a week reduces risk by 45 percent.[105] In animal studies, tomato consumption lowers testosterone levels.[106] " . . . lycopene and other biochemical constituents have greater bioavailability [when] bound in an oil base."[107] Dried tomatoes, olive oil, and garlic team up for prostate health in **Dried Tomato Paté** (page 377).

• Pour tomato sauce on broccoli for a one-two punch against any possible prostate cancer; they work better together.[108]

• **Lycopene**, found in cooked tomatoes, dried apricots, guavas, watermelon, and pink grapefruit, prevents prostate cancer, repairs damaged cells, shrinks tumors, and slows the spread of active prostate cancer.[109] Lycopene supplements don't.[110] A large European study found a 60 percent lower risk of advanced prostate cancer in men with the highest lycopene levels in their blood.[111]

Prevent Prostate Cancer

Results last a lifetime.

• Drink a quart of **red clover infusion** at least once a week.

• Eat a quart of **tomato sauce** a week.

• Limit meat at breakfast and lunch. Eat more **fish**.

• Snack on **pumpkin seeds**, **avocados**, Brazil nuts, peanuts.

• **Apples** contain *quercetin*, a compound that discourages cancer.[112] Quercetin may even be able to slow down established prostate cancer.[113] Applesauce is an especially good source. Other good sources on pages 52 and 341.

★ **Pomegranate's** anti-cancer, antioxidant polyphenols are stronger than those in blueberries, green tea, or supplements of A, C, or E.[114] Regular use lowers PSA levels, slows cancer growth, induces cancer cells to kill themselves, and delays progression.[115] Pomegranate seeds have the highest concentration of estrone (a real estrogen, not a phytoestrogen) of any plant.[116]

• **Green tea** contains the potent antioxidant polyphenol epigallocatechin-3-gallate, which inhibits the growth of prostate cancer cells, kills them if they are present, and slows the spread of established cancers. Men who drink the most green tea (up to four cups a day) reduce prostate cancer risk by 85 percent compared to those who drink the least.[117] One cup a day reduces risk by 15 percent; three cups reduces risk by over 70 percent.[118] Black tea may be as effective; bottled teas are not.

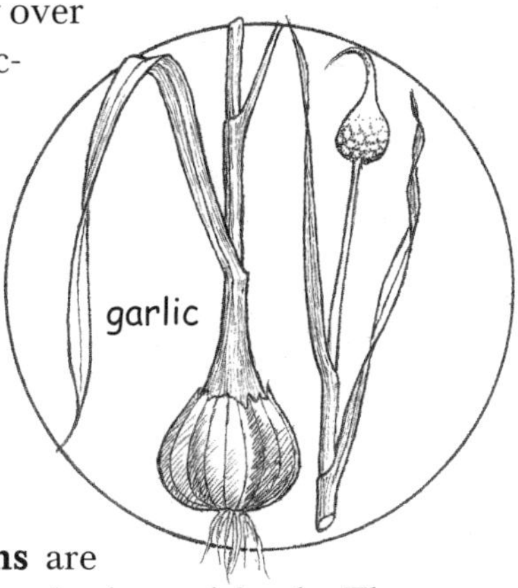

garlic

★ High concentrations of sulphur compounds, flavonols, and phytosterols in garlic, onions, and leeks counter cancer. Even two servings a week, cooked or raw, reduces risk. Three cloves of **garlic** or several onions a day cuts risk by 50 percent.[119]

• **Phytosterols** and **phytoestrogens** are hormone-like compounds found in many herbs and foods. They decrease oxidant activity at the tissue level, decease cell turnover, and decrease new blood vessel formation. In men, they counter prostate cancer.[120] Good sources of phytoestrogens include **red clover infusion** (Make it: page 367), lentils, beans, flax seeds, and whole grains.

★ A study of 12,000 Californians found those who had two servings of **soy beverage** a day were 70 percent less likely to be diagnosed with prostate cancer than those who never drank it.[121]

★ **Selenium** is *the* anticancer mineral.[122] It is critical for proper functioning of the immune system and may kill cancer cells directly. Men with the highest blood levels of selenium are 65 percent less likely than those with the lowest levels to develop advanced prostate cancers.[123] Those with high blood levels who also consume at least 28 IU of vitamin E a day have a 40 percent lower risk of any type of prostate cancer.[124] A daily serving of **Brazil**

nuts, fatty fish, whole wheat bread, lentils, wild rice, or sunflower seeds provides enough vitamin E and enough selenium – 150mcg, or twice the Daily Value[125] – to reduce your risk.[126,127]

★ Eating **fatty fish,** such as salmon, sardines, herring, and mackerel, two or more times a week, halves the risk of prostate cancer.[128] Microscopic examination of prostates of Inuit men – whose diets are rich in fatty fish – found only 1 out of 65 with cancer.[129] Non-fish eaters have 200–300 percent more prostate cancer than those who eat even moderate amounts of fatty fish.[130] **Note:** No protection against prostate cancer has been found in men taking fish-oil supplements.

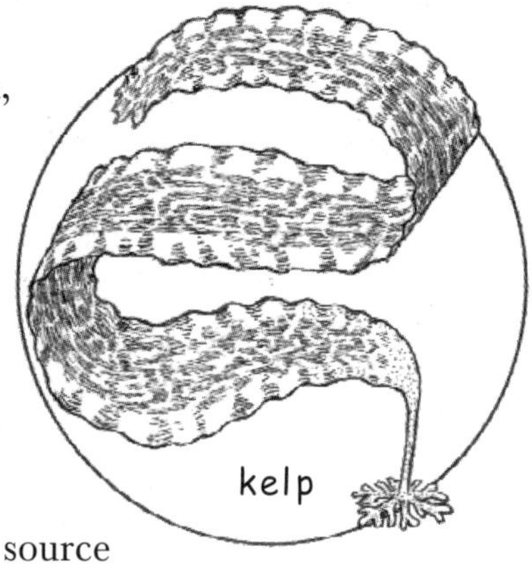

★ **Kelp** such as wakame, kombu, or nereocystis – not powdered, not pills, but real seaweed – cooked into beans, grains, soups, or stews, is especially effective in reducing prostate cancer risk. Men with prostate cancer often have elevated levels of mercury, cadmium, and lead; seaweed removes these heavy metals.

kelp

★ **Avocados** are an exceptional source of beta-sitosterol, a proven protector against prostate cancer. When eaten with other foods, avocado boosts the absorption of cancer-preventative carotenes. Three tablespoons of avocado added to a serving of salsa or salad puts thirteen times more beta carotene, eight times more alpha-carotene, four times more lutein, and four times more lycopene into the blood than eating either alone.[131] **Pumpkin seeds** are another good source of beta-sitosterol.[132]

• **Flax seeds**, ground and cooked, interrupt the chain of events that leads cells to become cancerous. Flax oil, however, appears to increase risk.[133] Alpha-linolenic acid (ALA), a fatty acid abundant in **flax** oil, **canola** oil, and **soy** oil, is the culprit. Men who consume the most ALA are twice as likely to be diagnosed with advanced prostate cancer as those who consume the least.[134]

• **Walnuts**, **pecans**, and **sesame seeds** contain a unique form of vitamin E, gamma tocopherol. Unlike the alpha-tocopherol found in supplements, this form of vitamin E is very active against cancer cells, especially those arising in the lungs and prostate.[135]

• **Nettle** has a "significant antiproliferative effect" on damaged prostatic epithelial cells; no cytotoxic effects were observed.[136] That means it stops hyperplasia without harming you. My favorite way to ingest it is as infusion. Make it: page 367.

• After nine years, among 175,000 men aged 50–71, the risk of advanced prostate cancer was 30 percent higher in those who ate: the most red meat (5 ounces vs. 1 ounce a day), the most processed meat (2 ounces vs. 1 ounce a day), the most iron, the most benzo[a]pyrene (found in grilled and barbecued meat), and the most nitrates or nitrites (found in processed meats).[137] Recent studies find no association with the amount of red meat eaten nor the method of cooking it, but find any meat eaten "well-done" to raise risk.[138]

• After "a comprehensive review of the research," the American Institute for Cancer Research found "insufficient" evidence to link milk and prostate cancer.[139] Concerns that calcium or dairy foods might promote prostate cancer have not been confirmed.[140,141]

• Meat and milk from grass-fed and wild animals are rich in conjugated linoleic acid (**CLA**), a substance which inhibits the growth of tumors.

★ **Vitamin D**, the sunshine vitamin, affects about 200 genes important in the prevention of cancer, including ones that control cell proliferation, cell differentiation, and cell death.[142] For cancer prevention, 2000 IU a day is a good goal. Ten minutes of bright sun on the arms and face can provide 10,000 IU. Since the body stores the surplus, exposure to sunlight during the late spring, summer, and early fall can provide vitamin D for the entire year.

Supplements of D_3 (rather than cod liver oil) are preferable; they have a protective effect against prostate cancer in animals. Caution: Men with the very highest blood levels of vitamin D have more prostate cancer.[143]

• 5-HETE – a breakdown product of arachidonic acid, found in large amounts in the meat (and in smaller amounts in the milk) of grain-fed animals – feeds prostate cancer and helps it spread.

• Green tea, olive oil, saw palmetto berries, turmeric, and **ginger** prevent arachidonic acid from being coverted to 5-HETE. Eicosapentaenoic acid (EPA), which is found in wild fish, also prevents the formation of 5-HETE.

• BPA (bisphenol-A) is used to line most food and beverage cans, or formed into baby bottles, sippy cups, and sturdy water bottles. Numerous animal studies have found exposure in early life, even at low doses, to cause cell and tissue changes, alter immune function, and increase risk of breast and prostate cancer.[144]

★ **Boron** is a trace mineral that helps prevent prostate cancer. Those who eat the most boron are one-third less likely to be diagnosed than those who eat the least.[145] This association is "very specific to prostate cancer" and does not apply to any other cancers. Fruits and nuts are the best sources. A glass of wine, a handful of peanuts, or a serving of non-citrus fruit provide generous amounts. Caution: Supplements of boron can damage health.

 Protect Your Prostate 

Best Bets: Cabbage family plants, cooked
Lycopene, from cooked tomatoes
Nettle infusion, two quarts a week
Omega-3 fatty acids, from walnuts, leafy greens, fish
Organic meat and milk
Physical activity, 30 minutes a day
Selenium, from foods; Vitamin D, from the sun
Sterols from lentils, split peas, and black-eyed peas

Limit: Alcohol to no more than two drinks a day
Caffeine to no more than two cups daily
Calcium to 1200mg daily; avoid supplements
Commercial, grain-fed, meat to once a week or less
Flax seed oil; it increases cancer risk[146]
Multivitamins, especially if eating enriched foods
Spicy, peppered foods; or avoid them completely
Stress; counter it with meditation or relaxation
Tobacco; better yet, eliminate it altogether
Zinc supplements

• Eat foods high in **zinc** to prevent prostate cancer.[147] Insufficient zinc in the prostate allows normal citrate-producing cells to turn into citrate-oxidizing cancer cells. Zinc sources, page 332.

Step 4. *Stimulate/Sedate*

• Exercising for three hours a week helps prevent prostate cancer. Regular, moderate activity gives "significantly lower risk,"[148] mostly for men over age 65, though: "In younger men, there was no effect on prostate cancer related to exercise at any level."[149]

• Men in their twenties who ejaculate at least five times a week are one-third less likely to develop aggressive prostate cancer later on.[150] So fire away boys! For the sake of your health, of course.

• **Farming** is the "most consistent occupational risk factor for prostate cancer."[151] Why? **Pesticides**, especially methyl bromide, a grain fumigant, and insecticides like permethrin. Those who apply them are 14 percent more likely to be diagnosed.[152,153]

• Alternating between daytime and nighttime shifts on the job can triple the risk of prostate cancer, according to a Japanese study of 14,000 men.[154] Working at night did not increase risk.

Step 5a. *Use Supplements*

> "It may be time to give up the idea that the protective influence of diet on prostate-cancer risk . . . can be emulated by isolated dietary molecules given alone or in combination. . . ."[155]

• ***Consider*** **antioxidant** supplements. Why? Men with normal PSA levels benefit from low doses of vitamin C (no more than 120mg a day), vitamin E (no more than 45 IU a day), selenium (no more than 100mcg a day), and zinc (no more than 20mg a day). Why not? Antioxidant supplements increase risk in men with elevated PSA.[156] You can easily get these amounts of antioxidants from food and nourishing herbal infusions.

• ***Avoid*** **multivitamins.** Why? Taking more than one multivitamin a day, or a multi plus enriched foods or extra selenium, zinc, or beta carotene, increases the risk of advanced prostate cancer by 32 percent and doubles the risk of it being fatal.[157,158]

• ***Avoid* zinc** supplements. Why? Men who take 100mg or more a day have twice the risk of being diagnosed with prostate cancer.[159] Why not? Low doses may help prevent prostate cancer.

• ***Avoid* lycopene** supplements. Why? They don't work.[160] Eat tomato sauce (pizza) and baked sweet potatoes instead.

• ***Consider* selenium** supplements. Why? Men with the lowest blood levels of selenium are four to five times more likely to have prostate cancer than those with the highest levels.[161] Supplemental selenium reduces risk more in those whose intake of vitamin C and carotenoids is low.[162] In one study, 200mcg daily of high-selenium yeast decreased prostate cancer incidence by an "unheard-of" two-thirds.[163] Why not? Too much selenium (800mcg a day) is as bad as too little.[164] High blood levels are associated with high risk of aggressive cancer.[165] *Men with adequate levels of selenium get no benefit from supplements.*[166] A study of 35,000 men given 200mcg of selenium or 400 IU of vitamin E, or both, daily, for seven years, found no decrease in prostate cancer in the selenium group, but more type-2 diabetes.[167,168]

• ***Avoid* vitamin E** supplements (alpha tocopherol). Why? They increase the risk of prostate cancer by suppressing the absorption of cancer-fighting gamma tocopherol.[169]

• ***Avoid* calcium** supplements. Why? They appear to increase prostate cancer.[170,171] Nourishing herbal infusions are safer sources of calcium. Schuessler homeopathic cell salts are another option.

• ***Avoid* DHEA.** Why? Even in doses as small as 25mg per day, it raises IGF-1 levels. And men with elevated levels of IGF-1 are 4.5 times more likely to be diagnosed with prostate cancer.[172]

Step 5b. *Use Drugs*

> ". . . one study that pooled the worldwide data from 18 studies and over 10,000 men, found NO association between the risk of prostate cancer and serum levels of sex hormones."[173]

• Finasteride use reduces overall risk of prostate cancer by 25 percent, but *increases* the incidence of the most fatal types of prostate cancer.[174,175] Side effects include loss of sex drive.[176]

• **Aspirin** has anti-inflammatory effects that inhibit the action of an enzyme that encourages the growth of prostate tumors.[177] **Warning:** Daily use of aspirin can cause internal bleeding.

• Men who take **statin drugs** are half as likely to have advanced prostate cancer as men who don't take statins.[178] An especially strong link has been established between high total cholesterol (200 or more) and advanced prostate cancer in men 65 and older.[179]

Step 6. *Break and Enter*

• A recent analysis of 200,000 men found no link between having a **vasectomy** and being diagnosed with prostate cancer.[180]

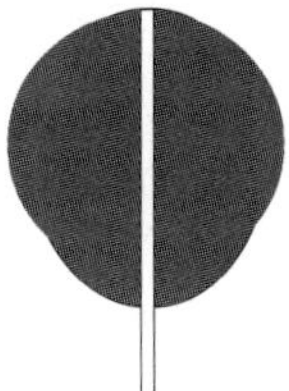

Prostate Cancer

"Can you hear me, grandson?" Grandfather Growth calls to you. "You are distressed at the thought of cancer in your body, between your legs. You feel betrayed. You are angry, hurt, even afraid. What lies ahead?

"I know you want to shut your eyes and block your ears and submit passively to whatever treatment the doctor recommends. But that is not the path to health. Nor is it the path to your wholeness.

"Open your heart to me. Allow me to walk this challenging path with you, dear child. I am here; I stand with you. Although this path may lead to your death, it might also lead to a reawakening of your life. Dare you explore the possibilities with me?"

Step 0. *Do Nothing*

"Men are at least ten-fold more likely to be harmed than helped by treatment of early-stage symptomless [prostate] cancer."[186]

★ It may seem irresponsible to do nothing when diagnosed with cancer, but it isn't. Wiser decisions come after the waves of emotion have washed through us. Modern medicine plays on our fears by urging us to act fast. But men who wait up to three months between diagnosis and treatment fare no worse than those who start treatment immediately.[187] Nor does use of hormone therapy during that interval improve the outcome.[188]

> "Not all men with prostate cancer should receive the same treatment – in some cases, no treatment may be the best option."[189]

• For early stage prostate cancer, drugs and surgery are no more effective in extending life than watchful waiting.[190]

• A 15-year study concluded that "two-thirds of prostate cancer patients do not require urgent treatment. . . ."[191] Men who do not display Hsp-027, a protein that indicates that the disease will progress rapidly, are best served with careful monitoring.

• A Swedish study found surgical removal of a cancerous prostate did reduce mortality, but worsened the quality of life. After five years, there was no significant difference between surgery or watchful waiting in terms of overall survival.[192]

• Of 223 men with early-stage prostate cancer who received no treatment at all, only11 percent of them died of it within 15 years, and only 25 percent of them died of it within 20 years.[193]

> "Choosing a treatment for prostate cancer is a tricky business."[194]

Step 1. *Collect Information*

> "Men diagnosed with prostate cancer . . . often neglect their own preferences because of biased, incomplete or confusing information. . . . Doctors give falsely optimistic information about effectiveness and tend to downplay side effects. . . ."[195]

• Worried about prostate cancer? Prevent it, starting on page 343. High or rising PSA level? Get it down, page 327. Told you need a biopsy? Before you agree, check out page 328. Diagnosed with prostate cancer? Read on.

• Three-quarters of men aged 80 have cancer cells in the prostate.[196] In the vast majority of cases (80 percent), prostate cancer grows so slowly that it is not the cause of death.

• One out of every six American men will be diagnosed with prostate cancer. It is fatal in only one out of 34 men diagnosed.[197]

• Each year, a quarter of a million American men are diagnosed with prostate cancer, and 27,000–32,000 die of it.[198,199] It is the second most common cancer (skin cancer being the first), and the second most likely to kill (lung cancer being the first).[200]

• Race affects your risk more than 50-fold. Asian men, particularly Chinese men, have the lowest rates.[201] African American men have the highest incidence in the world (236 per 100,000).

• If your brother *or* father had prostate cancer (*or* if your sister *or* mother had breast cancer), your risk doubles; if any two of them were diagnosed, your risk quadruples.[202]

• The symptoms of prostate cancer are the same as LUTS or BPH with the addition of blood in the urine and frequent pain or stiffness in the lower back, hips, or upper thighs.[203]

• Most **prostate cancer** (85 percent) starts in the peripheral zone.[204]

• The earliest evidence of prostate cancer? The mummy of a 3,000-year-old Scythian prince in southern Siberia? Or the prostate tumor found in remains from 40,000 years ago?

Step 2. *Engage the Energy*

• Homeopathic support for men with prostate cancer: Dilutions of *Thuja*, *Conium*, *Sabal serrulata*, or *Lycopodium* alternating with *Scirrhinum* using Ramakrishnan successions (page 244).

• Men treated for prostate cancer fare better mentally and physically when they have the support of a partner, "regardless of age, ethnicity, disease stage, or treatment type."[205]

Help!
Prostate Cancer

Expect results in 2–4 months

• **Reduce dietary fat.**

• Eat one ounce of ground, cooked **flax seed** daily.

• Include **tomato sauce** or **juice** in every meal.

• Increase phytoestrogens: eat more **beans** and **lentils;** drink **red clover infusion**.

• **Walk** for 30 minutes daily.

• Do yoga, **meditate**, or attend a support group.

Step 3. *Nourish and Tonify*

> "Overall intake of tomatoes, tomato sauce, tomato juice, and pizza was associated with fewer cases of advanced prostate cancer."[206]

★ An **ultra-low-fat diet** (10 percent of calories), combined with moderate exercise, meditation, and yoga, reverses or slows the growth of prostate cancer according to Dean Ornish MD.[207] Add generous helpings of tomato sauce, ground flax seed, and fatty fish and you may well survive your diagnosis by many years.

• A serving of **tomato sauce** every day for three weeks can reduce PSA by 20 percent and prevent DNA damage, too.[208]

★ Men who eat one ounce/30g/three tablespoons of ground, cooked **flax seed** daily, with or without a low-fat diet, reap lots of benefits. They have the slowest rate of tumor growth, the lowest proliferation rates, an increase in cancer cell death rates, and lower PSA scores, too.[209,210]

★ Men with prostate cancer who regularly eat **fatty fish** – such as salmon, mackerel, sardines, or herring – are 33 to 48 percent less likely to die of cancer.[211,212] Twice a week consumption can reduce the growth of prostate tumors by 17 percent.[213]

• A Canadian study found those who consumed the most saturated fat were three times more likely to die of prostate cancer within five years of diagnosis than those who consumed the least.[214]

• Less androgens, less lethal prostate cancer. **Red clover** infusion causes changes in prostate cancer cells "indicative of androgen deprivation and typical of a response to estrogen therapy."[215,216,217]

★ Even one serving of cabbage family plants per week cuts the risk of developing aggressive prostate cancer by half.[218]

> ". . . throughout the world . . . [i]n autopsies of men who die of other causes, a third of those over 30 have microscopic clusters of prostate cancer cells."[219]

• When mice who are genetically prone to prostate tumors were fed the equivalent of 8 cups of green or black **tea** a day plus 250mg of **soy**, their tumor growth rate was slowed, the spread to lymph nodes was inhibited, hormone concentrations linked to prostate cancer decreased, and angiogenesis was reduced.[220]

• Even high doses of green tea failed to reduce PSA levels in patients with metastatic, androgen-independent prostate cancer, and it caused severe adverse effects.[221] Foods that prevent prostate cancer aren't always capable of reversing it.

• **Obesity** is related to aggressive, fatal prostate cancer.[222] Obesity not only increases the chances of being diagnosed with aggressive cancer, it increases the risk of death once you are diagnosed.[223]

• Men who consume the most calcium have a "significantly" increased risk (2.12 times more likely) of being diagnosed with advanced prostate cancer.[224] The largest study to date found that men getting more than 2000mg of **calcium** a day from supplements and foods are 60 percent more likely to develop prostate cancer than those who average less than 700mg a day.[225] Interestingly, high consumption of fructose and high blood levels of vitamin D can "neutralize" the risks of ingesting excess calcium.[226]

Step 4. *Stimulate/Sedate*

★ **Licorice** infusion, 1–2 cups a day, or 1–2 deglycrrhizinated tablets a day, suppresses testosterone quite quickly.[227] Caution: Avoid licorice if you have kidney problems or are taking blood-pressure or blood-thinning drugs.

★ **Cayenne** pepper causes prostate cancer cells to self-destruct, slows tumor growth, and keeps tumors small in genetically susceptible populations.[228] A dose is 400mg three times a week, in capsules. Other peppers, including black pepper, irritate the prostate, and are best avoided.[229]

cayenne

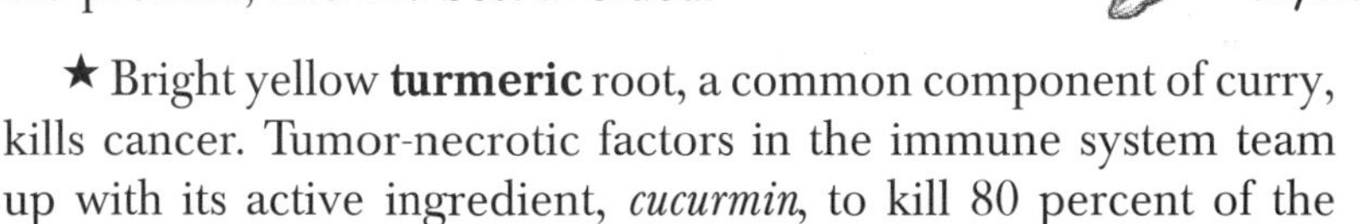

★ Bright yellow **turmeric** root, a common component of curry, kills cancer. Tumor-necrotic factors in the immune system team up with its active ingredient, *cucurmin*, to kill 80 percent of the prostate cancer cells they find.[230] A dose is a teaspoonful a day. Fortunately, turmeric is tasty enough to eat regularly, and capsules are an effective way to take it.

Step 5a. *Use Supplements*

★ Incidence of prostate cancer was reduced by one-third, and mortality from advanced prostate cancer was reduced by 41 percent, when men in their fifties and sixties took 50 IU of **Vitamin E** daily.[231,232,233] Smokers need 100 IU daily to decrease their risk of developing metastases.[234]

★ **Avoid zinc supplements**; they increase blood levels of testosterone.[235] Men who take more than 100mg a day are twice as likely to develop advanced prostate cancer.[236]

• In a study of 1000 men with a history of skin cancer, those who took 200mcg of **selenium** were 63 percent less likely to be diagnosed with prostate cancer than those taking the placebo.[237]

• **Modified citrus pectin** slowed the progression of recurrences in a small study of men who had undergone conventional treatments including radical prostatectomy.[238]

★ Ralph Blum, prostate cancer survivor, uses **colloidal silver** to stop blood flow to his tumor and prevent metastases.

> "Prostate cancer is one of the most over-treated diseases in American medicine, both because patients insist and many radiation oncologists and urologists are too willing to oblige."[239]

Step 5b. *Use Drugs*

> "Prostate cancer is very chemotherapy resistant."[240]

• Androgens feed prostate cancer. **Androgen deprivation therapy** (ADT) is "chemical castration." Drugs, rather than a surgery, "remove" the testes. Side effects include: low libido, impotence, osteoporosis, hot flashes, breast enlargement, periodontal disease, anemia, fatigue, and cognitive changes.[241]

Long-term use is associated with up to 50 percent increase in the risk of bone fracture, **diabetes**, coronary artery disease, **heart**

attack, and sudden cardiac death.[242] The drugs stop working after 2–3 years.[243] *The side effects of ADT outweigh the benefits,* except for men with cancer cells in the lymph nodes after prostatectomy.[244]

Nonetheless, ADT is routinely given to men whose cancer is localized (confined to the prostate), and its use has steadily increased, with no increase in men's longevity.[245] Men with prior health problems are twice as likely to die if they use ADT.[246]

> "Inevitably, [advanced prostate cancers] become hormone independent, and then there's no effective therapy. . . ."[247]

• The anti-breast-cancer drug **raloxifene** slowed the development of prostate cancer in 28 percent of a small group of men with advanced prostate cancer.[248]

• PSA levels fell by at least half for 100 percent of men with advanced hormone-sensitive prostate cancer who took **PC-SPES**.[249] It lowered PSA levels by half for three-quarters of other prostate cancer patients as well, providing significant decreases in pain.[250] Some remained cancer-free for a year afterward.

PC-SPES, developed by a Chinese-American chemist, Dr. Sophie Chen, contains eight herbs, including saw palmetto and *Panax* (Chinese) ginseng in addition to hormonal drugs. Side effects include enlarged breasts, nausea, and diarrhea.[251]

• A new "therapeutic cancer vaccine"– **Provenge** – increased the lifespan of men with late-stage prostate cancer by about four months with "modest" side effects. [252,253] Specialized cells are collected from a patient's blood and mixed with a protein found on most prostate cancer cells. The resulting "vaccine," given as three infusions two weeks apart, alerts the immune system, countering the cancer.

• **Fasting** may "not only minimize chemotherapy's toxicity but also make cancer cells more susceptible to chemotherapy."[254] Thomas Cravy, a retired ophthalmologist with metastasized prostate cancer, resisted chemotherapy "for a long time because I so feared its side effects." Now, he fasts for about 64 hours before his treatment and another 24 hours afterward. He admits to losing mental acutity while fasting, but claims the technique has left him feeling vigorous and "virtually free of chemo side effects."[255]

• Worried about **surgery-related impotence**? Men who take erectile dysfunction drugs nightly after prostatectomy fare no better than those who take them only as needed.[256] (Herbs, page 296.)

Step 6. *Break and Enter*

> "No one knows which treatment option is the best . . . radical prostatectomy, radiation therapy and watchful waiting are all acceptable . . . there is no clear-cut evidence for the superiority of any one of them."[257]

• Diagnosed with prostate cancer? Modern medicine suggests: watchful waiting (this page), ADT (page 356), radical prostatectomy (this page), external radiation therapy (page 360), and radioactive seed implants (page 361). New treatments are being developed as well (page 357). Examine all your options. Opt for what works best for *you*, not for your doctor.

• Is **watchful waiting** safe? In one group of 700 men under the age of 75, all diagnosed with prostate cancer, 90 percent of those who had surgery, and 85 percent of those who didn't, survived for ten years or died of other causes.[258] In another group, ten-year survival was 72 percent of those opting for watchful waiting, 75 percent of those who chose radiation therapy, and 83 percent for those who had a prostatectomy.[259]

> "Try to imagine your life after a radical prostatectomy, where you are impotent. Try to imagine your life after radiation therapy, where you suffer with urinary or bowel irritation. Then imagine that you've done nothing, just been closely monitored. . . . Which bullets are you willing to take?"[260]

• **Radical prostatectomy** removes the entire prostate under general anesthesia. Men younger than 70 and men with aggressive tumors who chose prostatectomy are half as likely to die.[261] One percent of men die as a result of prostatectomy.

• **Impotence**, the most common side effect of radical prostatectomy, is experienced by 50–70 percent of men.[262,263] The nerves that promote an erection lie under the prostate, in a neurovascular bundle. If the surgeon tugs on or stresses these nerves, they die. Regeneration, if it occurs, takes about three years. If the neurovascular bundle is not removed or damaged, half of men in their sixties with no erection problems prior to surgery can have erections 9–12 months after prostatectomy – with the help of erectile dysfunction drugs,[264] or with herbal allies (page 296).

> "Men who have their prostate gland removed become incontinent immediately after surgery. Regaining urinary control can take several weeks to a couple of years, and some men remain incontinent indefinitely."[265]

• **Incontinence** follows prostatectomy. Patients have a urinary catheter for 1–2 weeks after surgery. On removal, fifty percent of men will be incontinent on stress.[266] The upper, most active urinary sphincter goes with the prostate, and 5 percent of men have "serious" problems controlling urination afterwards. Over 25 percent have "bothersome" problems.[267] About 6 percent will be permanently incontinent.[268] The degree of continence is dependent on the surgeon's skill. A year after surgery, more than 90 percent of the patients of the most experienced surgeons – those who have done at least 250 prostatectomies – are continent.[269,270]

★ The lower urinary sphincter, usually untouched by the surgery, can be trained to provide continence most of the time. Of men who did 90 **pelvic floor contractions** daily (page 15), 88 percent regained urinary control within three months of a prostatectomy; only 56 percent of the placebo group did.[271]

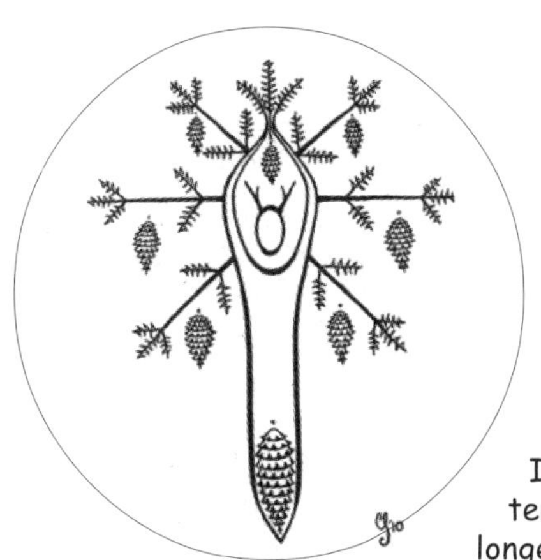

His (Posthumous) Story

Mitch was an electrical engineer. "I asked my doctor for a PSA test when I was 49. He said my insurance wouldn't cover it unless I was fifty, so I let it go until I was 53. My PSA was really high. The biopsy was positive for prostate cancer. The scan found metastases.

"I threw myself into the good fight. I did it *all*. I lived for seven years after my diagnosis. But I wonder how much longer I would have had if I'd followed my desire to be tested 4 years earlier."

• Radical prostatectomy leaves cancer cells behind 10 percent of the time. It also injures the rectal tissues of 3 percent of men and constricts the flow of urine in 10 percent.[272]

• Radical prostatectomy has been done successfully for men of every age, even octogenarians.[273]

• In 15 percent of men, PSA rises after prostatectomy. Only one-third of them have metastatic prostate cancer, and they generally live for another 13 years.[274] The faster your PSA rises and the quicker this happens after surgery, the more likely that follow-up hormone treatment will be more helpful than harmful.

• **HIFU**, high intensity focused ultrasound, heats and destroys prostate cancer without the incontinence and impotence common after surgery or radiation.[275] Countires including Canada, Mexico, and England permit HIFU, but not the USA.

★ Taking aspirin (or any NSAID) prior to radiation therapy improves survival. After ten years, 91 percent of those who did were alive, compared to 68 percent of those who didn't.[276]

★ Shrinking the prostate before radiation therapy with hormonal drugs (or foods such as soy, flax meal, or tomatoes), improves the effectiveness of radiation therapy.[277]

• **Radiation** may be done externally or internally. It is less likely (3 percent) to cause incontinence than surgery (6 percent).

~ *External* radiation uses x-ray beams, which tend to spread out and damage tissues even at low intensities. More than half of those who choose radiation against prostate cancer will gradually, over years, permanently lose their potency.[278] In 56 percent of men, the radiation causes rectal inflammation and bleeding.[279] (Rectal bleeding is reduced to 37 percent when targeted **conformal radiation** is used.[280]) Up to 30 percent of all radiated men suffer permanent damage to the blood vessels of the rectum, leading to bowel urgency and painful hemorrhoids.[281,282] Radiation causes constricted urine flow in 8 percent of men, urinary incontinence in 4 percent, and death in .5 percent.[283] External radiation leaves cancer cells 40–60 percent of the time.[284]

~ **Intensity modulated radiotherapy** (IMRT), a new technique, breaks radiation up into thousands of tiny beams that enter the body from many angles and intersect at the tumor, allowing a lethal dose to be delivered to the tumor while causing less (but not no) damage to surrounding bladder and rectal tissues. After eight years, 89 percent of those treated with IMRT were cancer-free.[285]

~ **Proton Beam Therapy** (PBT) uses a very narrow, high-intensity proton beam focused with the aid of MRI or CT scans. No trials have compared it to the less expensive and equally effective IMRT. Side effects include the usual: rectal and bowel problems (in 5–18 percent), bladder irritation (in 5 percent), and erectile dysfunction (up to five years after the treatment) in 30–50 percent.[286]

~ *Internal* radiation is **brachytherapy**. Sixty or so radioactive cesium-131 pellets are implanted in the prostate, usually under general anesthesia. The rate of sexual, urinary, and bowel problems is the same as after surgery.[287] Among 2000 men in their fifties who had brachytherapy, 85 percent were cancer-free ten years later.[288] ". . . men are radioactive for three months rather than almost two years [as with idoine seeds]."[289]

• **Cryosurgery** destroys tissue with freezing. Used initially to "salvage" prostate cancer patients who failed to respond to radiation, or whose cancer recurred, it is now an alternative for initial treatment. "Morbidity remains high"[290] and cancer cells persist in a fairly high proportion of men treated.[291]

His Story[292]

Jason is a surgeon.

"I have come to feel that there is great loneliness among men who carry the diagnosis of prostate cancer. The illness arises and is tackled in a male world, one in which feelings are not readily revealed and burdens are often shouldered in isolation. . . . Perhaps it takes a doctor-turned-patient to share the emotional experience of having prostate cancer, to reveal everyone's sense of vulnerability and fear through his story. . . . Every traveler forges his own path through a thicket of information, decisions, hopes, and consequences. Nothing, not family and friends, nor knowledge, nor level of education, nor money, nor power on earth totally insulates a man from the anguish caused by the threat contained in the word 'cancer.'"

 Prostate Star: Saw Palmetto (*Serenoa repens*) 

"Concentrated extracts of saw palmetto are the most widely prescribed prostate medications in Germany, France and other European countries. . . ."[293]

Saw palmetto berries are an old man's friend. Regular use, it is said, invigorates desire, rejuvenates ability, improves sexual performance, reduces prostate swelling, and improves urinary functioning. Really?

Yes. Saw palmetto berries are rich in phytosterols such as beta-sitosterol, stigmasterol, and campesterol. They are loaded with fatty acids, including lauric, linoleic, linolenic, capric, caproic, caprylic, palmitic, oleic, myristic, and stearic acids. And they contain lipase and tannins among other constituents. But saw palmetto, "like so many other herbal medicinals, is more than the sum of its chemical parts," Dr. James Duke reminds us.[294]

Studies show[295,296] saw palmetto:

★ Blockades androgen receptors, to interfere with DHT's ability to stimulate the growth and division of prostate cells.

★ Inhibits 5-alpha-reductase, to reduce the conversion of testosterone into DHT (just like the drug Proscar/finasteride does).

★ Disrupts the arachidonic cascade, to counter inflammation and relieve LUTS.

★ Competes for estrogen receptors, to prevent prostate cancer.

★ Decreases LUTS; reduces residual urine, urinary frequency, nocturia, and dysuria, and shrinks the whole prostate.[297,298]

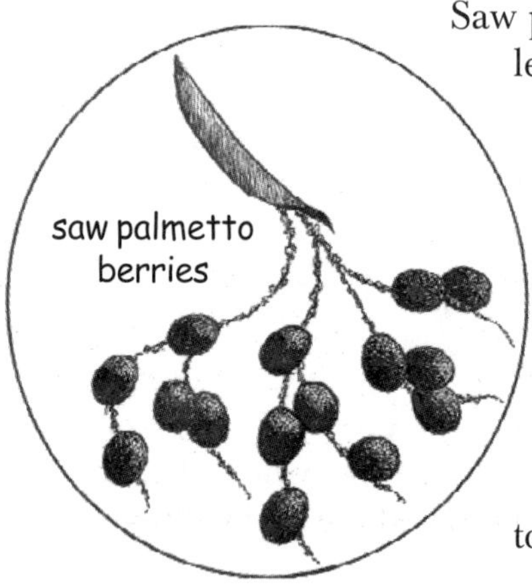

Saw palmetto "not only works on more levels than the synthetic [drugs], it works much quicker and for a greater number of people."[299]

Saw palmetto relieves symptoms in 90 percent of men after three months of use; Proscar has a 50 percent response rate after six months.[300]

In a strictly controlled German study, 88 percent of the men who took saw palmetto extract, and 88 percent of their physicians, said they saw results within 90 days of starting to take saw palmetto.[301]

In five out of seven placebo-controlled studies, saw palmetto relieved symptoms better than the placebo.[302] A meta-study including over 3000 men, found those who used saw palmetto for six months improved the force of their urination by 50 percent compared to those on a placebo.[303]

Generally more than one-third of those using saw palmetto for at least six months report complete elimination of urinary symptoms (LUTS). In a study of 1000 men, saw palmetto was as effective as Proscar in relieving urinary symptoms.[304] Only 1 percent of those taking saw palmetto experienced erection difficulties, compared to 5 percent of those taking Proscar/finasteride.[305]

Some studies find saw palmetto ineffective. Men with more enlarged prostates often have less reduction in size and symptoms from using saw palmetto than those whose prostates are not so swollen. Also, different preparations engender different results. Fat-soluble extracts out-perform water-based preparations. Tincture and extract work well for most men, while capsules, pills, tablets, infusion, and tea work less well.

A **dose of tincture** or standardized extract (85–95 percent fatty acids) is 2–4 dropperfuls twice a day. Dosing usually begins at high levels and is reduced as symptoms abate.

The **dose of infusion**, using one ounce/30g dried berries in 1 quart/liter of water, is 2–4 cups a day. Be warned: the berries smell weird and the infusion (but not the tincture) tastes weirder.

A 320mg dose of saw palmetto berry extract is *three times stronger than the standard dose of finasteride.*[306]

A commitment of 3–6 months is reasonable before deciding saw palmetto does, or doesn't, work for you. That's about 8 ounces/2 cups/500ml of tincture. (Make it: page 367. It takes less than five minutes and saves you a bundle of money.)

Millions of European men and more than two million American men currently take saw palmetto.[307]

Saw palmetto is a scrubby palm found throughout Florida. Harvesting the berries, even in immense quantity, neither harms the plant nor interferes with its profligate ability to reproduce. However, killing frosts in the areas of Florida where saw palmetto grows have reduced availablity. Who knows what will happen as baby boomer prostates start to put greater pressure on supplies.

Is saw palmetto an aphrodisiac? Men taking saw palmetto may not experience an increase in libido, but they certainly don't report, as do those taking drugs to address their prostate problems, reduction of sexual desire and erectile difficulties.

Other effects: Saw palmetto berries stimulate circulation to the genitals, improve thyroid functioning, reduce fluid retention, improve immune system functioning, and strengthen the kidneys. *King's American Dispensatory*, published in 1898, recommends the berries for men with low libido and impotence. Homeopaths rely on it to counter all types of testicular problems.

Women benefit from saw palmetto, too. A daily dropperful can increase desire, alleviate cystitis and interstitial cystitis, shrink enlarged ovaries, and ease irritations of the uterus and ovaries, including PCOS, fibroids, and CPP.

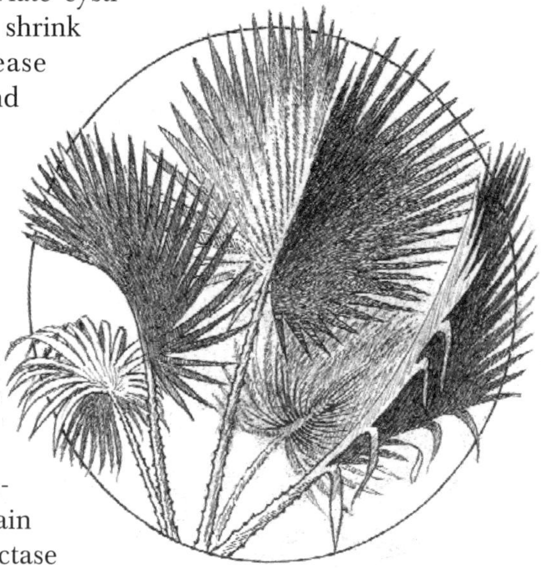

Cautions: Critics claim that taking saw palmetto "artificially" lowers PSA. Dr. James Duke isn't worried. "To one degree or another," he says, "all plants contain PSA-reducing sterols. For instance, most beans contain genistein, an alpha-reductase inhibitor. Where is the advisory against eating these foods?"[308]

saw palmetto

Side effects: Like Proscar, saw palmetto can trigger breast growth. Could it cause birth defects? Herbalists don't think so, but no one really knows for sure.

> "I am loathe to prescribe either pygeum or saw palmetto unless absolutely necessary. Saw palmetto in particular seems to have a distinctly erosive feminizing effect on the male body."
>
> herbalist Ryan Drum, 2010

The Herbal Pharmacy

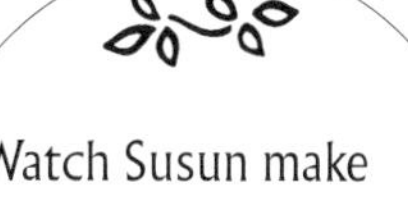

Watch Susun make herbal preparations on You Tube.

Sources for Herbs

- **Avena Botanicals** 1-866-AT-AVENA
  www.avenabotanicals.com
- **Blessed Herbs** 1-800-489-HERBS
  www.blessedherbs.com
- **Catskill Mtn. Herbals** 1-845-657-2943
  www.catskillmountainherbals.com
- **Frontier** 1-800-669-3275
  www.frontiercoop.com
- **HerbPharm** 1-800-348-4372
  www.herb-pharm.com
- **Herbalist and Alchemist** 1-908-689-0-9020
  www.herbalist-alchemist.com
- **Mountain Rose Herbs** 1-800-879-3337
  www.mountainroseherbs.com
- **Pacific Botanicals** 1-541-479-7777
  www.pacificbotanicals.com
- **Red Moon Herbs** 1-888-929-0777
  www.redmoonherbs.com

A Word About Simples

I am a simpler. That means I prefer to use one herb at a time. I rarely mix herbs together, though I may drink an infusion of one herb and take a tincture of one or two others in any given day.

Simples build relationship with individual plants. Simples help us pinpoint herbs that may not agree with us individually. Simples remind us that herbal medicine is people's medicine; it is as near as the back door and so easy a three-year old can do it. Simples put the power of health care back in our own hands.

I do not believe that herbs need to be combined to be effective, nor do I believe that they are more effective in combination. I get great results using one herb at a time.

So why do I include combinations? Because many people enjoy concocting them. Because it can be a quest to find all the herbs. And because combinations are an important part of our herbal history, a window into how previous generations used plants.

Make It: Nourishing Herbal Infusion

Comfrey leaf, Hawthorn herb, Linden, Nettle, Oatstraw, Red clover blossoms, Raspberry leaf, Rosehips

Place 1 ounce/30 grams dried herb in a quart/liter jar. Fill jar with boiling water. Cap tightly. Steep for four hours or overnight. Strain, squeezing well. Refrigerate liquid; compost herb.

To make linden flower infusion, use ½ ounce of herb to a quart.

Make It: Tincture, Dried Herbs

Chasteberry, Echinacea root, Saw palmetto berries

Put 4 ounces/115 grams of dried saw palmetto or chaste tree berries or echinacea cut root in a quart/liter jar. Fill the jar to the top with 100 proof vodka. Cap tightly, label. Wait at least six weeks before use; I think they are best after a year.

Make It: Tincture, Fresh Herbs

Cleavers, Poke root, St. Joan's wort flowers, Wild carrot seeds

Fill any size jar to the top with cut-up pieces of fresh, just harvested herb, then add 100-proof vodka, right to the top of the jar. Lid well, label. Ready to use in six weeks.

Make It: Infused Oil/Ointment, Fresh Herbs

Calendula, Chamomile, Chickweed, Clover, Comfrey, Hyssop, Lemon balm, Plantain, Red clover, St. Joan's wort

Fill a dry jar with fresh herb, then fill jar with any food oil; cap tightly. Label (on lid) with name and date. Put the jar in a small bowl to catch oozing oil. Steep, out of direct sunlight, for six weeks. Pour the oil out, squeezing well. For **ointment**: Thicken infused oil by melting a tablespoon of beeswax into each ounce of oil.

Make It: Comforting Compress

Castor oil, Calendula, Comfrey, Plantain, Witch hazel

Saturate a clean cotton diaper or an old, but well-washed, cotton terry dish towel with the liquid of your choice: castor oil, comfrey leaf/root infusion or oil, plantain leaf oil, calendula oil, witch hazel lotion/infusion, or any other healing herbal oil or infusion you wish to use. *For a cold compress*: Apply to body as is. *For a hot compress*: Fold the saturated towel into quarters, wrap in foil, bake for 15–20 minutes until very warm but not too hot to handle.

Unwrap and apply the compress. To keep the heat in, cover with a heavy towel and/or a hot water bottle or heating pad. Remove when cool or after fifteen minutes.

For repeat oil compresses, add more oil to the same towel. *An oil compress may be used over and over again.*

When using infusion or witch hazel, refrigerate towel after use and wash every third day. *Infusion compresses can rot and smell bad.*

You can also make (or buy) an herbal pillow that can be heated in the microwave or chilled in the freezer and applied to the area to be compressed. (Instructions, page 379.)

Hot compresses are used to relieve pain, counter stagnation, dissolve growths (fibroids, cysts, polyps), and warm and strengthen the organs of the pelvis. They are not used when there is infection or fever.

Make It: Soothing Sitz Bath, Healing Bath

Mallow, Comfrey, Flax seed, Oatstraw

Soothes inflamed and tender tissues, heals trauma, lubricates

Soak 2 ounces/60g dried or 8 ounces/250g fresh mallow or comfrey roots, leaves, and/or flowers in 2 quarts/liters of cold water in a pot overnight. Then bring to a boil. Cover, remove from heat, and steep for 4–6 hours. Strain. Warm the liquid, pour it into a small tub and sitz in it. Alternately, pour it into a hot bath. Or refrigerate and drink it. A dose is a cup or more a day – heated or iced, sweetened or not – daily for at least ten days.

Make It: Astringent Sitz Bath

Avens, Bistort, Chamomile, Cranesbill, Meadowsweet, Oak, Witch hazel, Wild geranium, White pond lily, Yarrow

Tightens tissues, counters infections

Add 2 ounces/60g dried herb to 2 quarts/liters of cold water and bring to a boil. Cover, remove from heat, steep for 4–6 hours. Strain. Warm the liquid, pour it into a small tub and sitz in it.

Bladder Blast

A dose is one-quarter cup every two hours to relieve urgency/pain.

Add to one glass of **cranberry** juice, a dropperful of each of these tinctures: **goldenrod** root, **marshmallow** root, **nettle** seed, **parsley** root, **rose** buds or hips, **uva ursi**, and **willow herb**.

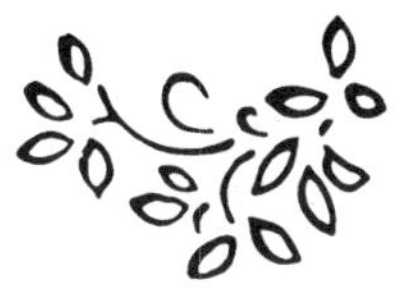

Sitting Pretty Salve

courtesy Mountain Rose Herbs

Especially effective against hemorrhoids

Witch hazel inner bark (*Hammamelis virginiana*)
St. Joan's wort flowering tops (*Hypericum perforatum*)
Horse chestnut bark, leaves, or seeds (*Aesculus hippocastanum*)

Infuse each fresh herb individually in olive oil at room temperature for six weeks using the directions on page 367. Or, add 1 ounce of each dried herb to a cup of olive oil and heat in a crock pot for several days. Strain. If desired, add beeswax to thicken.

Bladder Buddy Brew

I consider this safe for any woman of any age dealing with chronic cystitis – even women who are pregnant, lactating, or using chemotherapy or other heavy drugs that suppress the immune system (and make cystitis more likely), so long as the dose is not exceeded.

1/2 ounce/14g yarrow flowering herb (*Achillea millefolium*)
1/2 ounce/14g marshmallow root (*Althea officinalis*)
1/2 ounce/14g uva ursi leaves (*Arctostaphylos uva-ursi*)
1/2 ounce/14g echinacea root (*Ech. angustifolia* ONLY)

Soak the dried herbs in two quarts/liters of cold water overnight. Bring water and herbs to a boil, remove from heat, cover, and steep for four or more hours. Drink by the sip, about a cup an hour until symptoms abate. Continue drinking 2–4 cups a day for at least a week. For prevention, drink 1–2 quarts a week.

Bladder Helper Tea

by Rosemary Gladstar

1/4 ounce/7g nettle leaves (*Urtica dioica*)
1/4 ounce/7g dandelion leaves (*Taraxacum off.*)
1/2 ounce/14g corn silk (*Zea mays*)
1/2 ounce/14g uva ursi leaves (*Arctostaphylos uva-ursi*)
optional: 1/4 ounce/7g pipsissewa (*Chimaphila umbellata*) herb

Add dried herbs to 2–3 quarts/liters boiling water, cover and remove from heat. Allow to cool, strain, then sip as needed.

Traditional Chinese Medicine Formula To Counter Urinary Retention

Adapted to American herbs by S. Weed

Especially useful for men with BPH who frequently deal with retention

1/3 ounce/9g dried whole cinnamon (*Cinnamomum zeyl.*) bark
1/2 ounce/14g dried or fresh turkey tail (*Polyporus*) mushrooms
1 ounce/28g dried, cut peony (*Peonia lactiflora*) root
1 ounce/28g dried, cut dandelion (*Taraxacum off.*) root
1/3 ounce/9g dried fennel (*Foeniculi vulgaris*) seeds
1/3 ounce/9g dried plantain (*Plantago majus*) seed and husk
1/6 ounce/5g dried, cut licorice (*Glycyrrhiza glabra*) root
1/6 ounce/5g dried, cut astragalus (*A. membranaceous*) root

Add herbs to a gallon/4 liters of cold water. Bring to a boil; cover tightly; simmer one hour. (Or cook in a crock pot on high for 2–4 hours.) Strain, refrigerate. Dose is a cup a day for prevention, a cup an hour when blocked. Keeps well for a week or more.

Crotch Cream

by Gretchen Gould, the "Amazing Grease" Goddess

Relieves all crotch complaints, including herpes and yeast itch.

1 part dried black walnut hulls ((*Juglans nigra*) or oak bark
1 part fresh/dried calendula or chamomile flowers (*Matricaria*)
1 part fresh/dried dandelion roots (*Taraxacum officinale*)
1 part fresh/dried echinacea roots (*Echinacea angustifolia*)
1 part fresh jewelweed (*Impatiens pallida*) Omit if unavailable.
1 part fresh/dried yarrow flowering tops (*Achillea millefolium*)
½ part fresh/dried goldenseal root (*Hydrastis canadensis*), barberry root bark (*Berberis*), or Oregon grape root (*Mahonia*)

Mix and match these herbs. You don't need them all. Use what is available where you live. Fill your jar completely full with plants if you are using mostly fresh plants. If your plants are mostly dried, fill your jar only half full. Either way, pour olive oil into the jar, filling it to the very top. Label; let sit 6–8 weeks.

Strain, squeezing well. Measure one large spoonful of grated beeswax for each ounce of oil you have. Warm the oil over a low heat, then add the beeswax, stirring until melted. Pour into jars. Optional: Add 1–4 drops of **tea tree oil** to each jar.

Buchu Infusion

Counters incontinence, bladder/urethra irritation/inflammation, cystitis, prostate complaints, aching of the penis

Pour 1 quart/liter boiling water over 1 ounce/30g dried buchu in a quart/liter jar. Cap tightly, steep for 4–8 hours. Strain, refrigerate. *Dose is one ounce, three times a day, cold or hot, as desired.*

Fukepenkayen Pills Ingredients

Paeoniae rubra (red peony root)
Angelica sinensis (dong quai root)
Dioscorea batatus (wild yam root)
Curcuma zedoaria (zedoary root)
Salvia miltiorrhizae (red sage root)
Scirpus yagare (bullrush root)
Cyperus rotundus (sedge root)
Corydalis yahusuo (corydalis)
Euryale ferox (foxnut seeds)
Smilacis glabrae (smilax root)

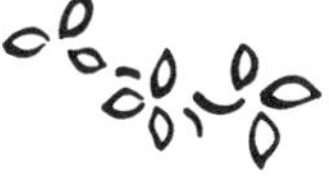

Anti-Adenomyosis Tincture

part of Tori Hudson ND's protocol

1 oz licorice (*Glycyrrhiza glabra*) root tincture
1 oz partridge berry (*Mitchella repens*) leaf tincture
1 oz blue cohosh (*Caulophylum thalictroides*) root tincture
1 oz geranium (*Geranium* spp.) root tincture
40 drops of cotton (*Gossypium*) root bark tincture

Combine tinctures. A dose is a dropperful twice a day.

Endo-Tea

by Rosemary Gladstar

3 ounces/85g dried dandelion (*Taraxacum off.*) root
3 ounces/85g dried wild yam (*Dioscorea* spp) root
2 ounces/55g dried pau d'arco (*Tabebuia avellanedae*) bark
1 ounce/30g dried Oregon grape (*Mahonia aquifolium*) root
1 ounce/30g dried vitex (*Vitex agnus-castus*) berries
½ ounce/15g dried dong quai (*Angelica sinensis*) root

Option 1: Add 4–6 tablespoons of mix, plus ½ ounce cinnamon, ginger, or orange peel to counter bitterness, to one quart of cold water. Cook for twenty minutes, strain. Dose is a cup a day.

Option 2: Put mixed herbs into two quart jars. Fill with 100 proof vodka. Label; let sit for six weeks. Use1–2 dropperfuls three times a day for six weeks; take the seventh week off.

Anti-Endo Formula

A heroic classic moderated to modern times and self-help. The response rate claimed is 75–85 percent when used daily for three months.

2 ounces motherwort (*Leonurus cardiaca*) flowering herb tincture
2 ounces dandelion (*Taraxacum officinale*) root/leaf tincture
2 ounces vitex (*Vitex agnes-castus*) berry tincture
2 ounces prickly ash (*Xanthoxylum clava-herculis*) root tincture
1/4 ounce poke (*Phytolacca americana*)* root tincture

Mix well. A dose is a dropperful, 2–3 times a day, plus, eat lots of fish high in omega-3 fatty acids.

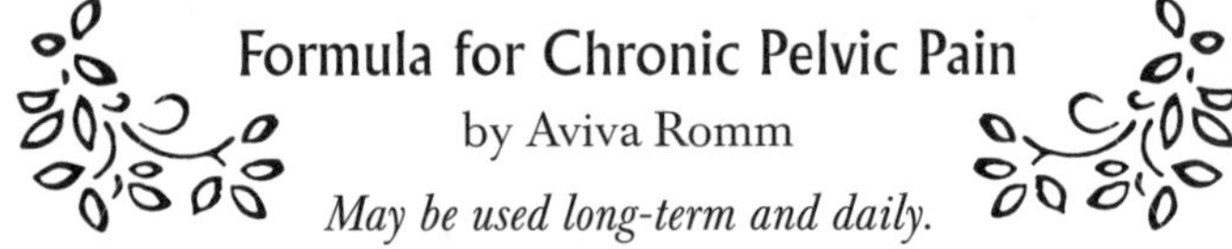

Formula for Chronic Pelvic Pain

by Aviva Romm

May be used long-term and daily.

2 parts blue cohosh (*Caulophyllum thalictroides*) root
2 parts cramp bark (*Viburnum opulus*)
2 parts peony (*Paeonia lactiflora*) root
1 1/2 parts motherwort (*Leonurus cardiaca*) herb in flower
1 1/2 parts horse chestnut (*Aisculus hoppocastanum*)*
1 part yarrow (*Achillea millefolium*) herb in flower

Mix tinctures together. Dose is a dropperful twice a day.

Lovers' Sitz Bath

by James Green

"Blessed relief" for lovers bothered by chronic non-specific vaginitis or yeast

1/2 ounce dried chaparral (*Larrea tridentata*)* herb
1/2 ounce dried oak (*Quercus* spp) bark
1/2 ounce dried spilanthes (*Spilanthes acmella* or *S. oleracea*)
1/4 ounce dried marshmallow (*Althea officinalis*) root
1/4 ounce dried yarrow (*Achillea millefolium*) herb in flower
Optional:1 ounce fresh periwinkle (*Vinca*) herb in flower

Boil one gallon of cold water. Add herbs, cover, turn off heat. Steep for 4–6 hours. Strain. Warm the liquid. Pour half (or a third) into each of two (or three) plastic dish pans. Bare those bottoms and sit – together – until the liquid cools. Make fresh for each use; do not reuse. Best if repeated daily for 7–10 days.

Heroic Anti-Syphilis/Gonorrhea Formula

2 teaspns Oregon grape (*Mahonia aquifolium*)root
2 teaspns red clover (*Trifolium pratense*) flowers
1 teaspn burdock (*Arctium lappa*) seed
1 teaspn burdock (*Arctium lappa*) root
1 teaspn yellow dock (*Rumex crispus*) root
1 teaspn cascara (*Cascara sagrada*)* bark
1 teaspn sarsaparilla (*Smilax officinalis*) root
½ teaspn blue flag (*Iris* species)* root
½ teaspn prickly ash *(Xanthoxylum clava-herculis*) berries
½ teaspn bloodroot (*Sanguinaria canadense*)*
1 teaspoon slippery elm (*Ulmus fulva*) bark
* considered poisonous.

Mix dried, finely cut herbs together. Soak in two quarts/liters of cold water for an hour, then bring to a boil and simmer for 15 minutes. Strain. The dose is 2 tablespoonfuls 3–4 times a day.

Classic "blood purifying formulae" are based on the (mistaken) belief that all infections, including sexual infections, arise from filth in the colon or toxins in the cells. If I had gonorrhea, syphilis, or any STD, I would not trust my health to these herbs. *Oregon grape is a source of antimicrobial berberine. Red clover and burdock aid the immune system, as does yellow dock, which is also a laxative. Cascara is a classic and powerful purgative; it literally gets the s__t out. No doubt the poisonous effects of the bloodroot and blue flag increase the purging. Slippery elm heals the intestines after all that. Whew. Sarsaparilla, blue flag, and prickly ash roots are native exotics, added for their aura rather than effect.*

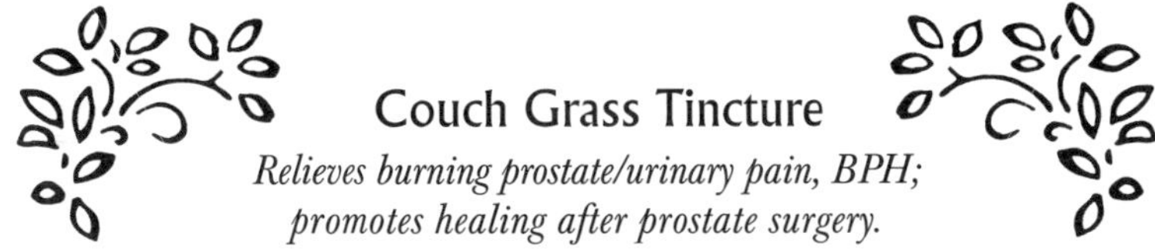

Couch Grass Tincture

Relieves burning prostate/urinary pain, BPH; promotes healing after prostate surgery.

Couch grass (*Agropyron repens*) is a weed in many temperate-zone gardens throughout the world, so it is fairly easy to find, but rarely for sale, so make your own. Fill a jar with fresh roots; pour100 proof vodka to the top of the jar. Cover tightly, label, ready in six weeks. The dose is 10–20 drops a day.

Penis Soaks

External Use Only

The idea of countering STDs by soaking the penis in a vase, a wide-mouthed quart jar, or a tall glass filled with herbal infusion, originated with Cascade Anderson-Geller.

Try this combination by James Green, from *The Male Herbal.*

1/4 ounce yarrow (*Achillea millefolium*) flowers
1/4 ounce sage (*Salvia officinalis*) leaves
1/4 ounce lavender (*Lavendula off.* or *Lavandin*) flowers
1/4 ounce chaparral (*Larrea tridentata*)* herb

Or Amanda McQuade Crawford's, from *Herbal Remedies for Women.*

1 ounce quassia (*Picrasma excelsa*)* bark
1 ounce chaparral (*Larrea tridentata*)* herb

Add 2 ounces of mixed herbs to 2 quarts of water, bring to a boil, lower heat and simmer for thirty minutes. Strain and return to stove. Gently simmer until there are only 3 cups of liquid left. (Alternate method: Add mixed herbs to a half-gallon canning jar, fill with boiling water, cap tightly – a two-piece canning lid is perfect as it can be removed more easily than a one-piece lid – and steep overnight or for at least four hours.) Strain, squeezing the herbs, and refrigerate the liquid. Warm what you need to fill your container of choice, retract foreskin, insert penis – and testicles if possible – and soak for 5 to 10 minutes, once or twice a day. Discard herbal infusion after use. (* Denotes an herb considered poisonous.)

> "No matter how absurd the image of this therapy [a penis soak] strikes you, in times when your female partner is stressed with reoccurring vaginal infection, discomfort, and pain, the most chivalrous act is a daily hygienic penis soak until the cycle of reinfection has been stopped." James Green

Men's Tonic

by David Winston, Herbalist and Alchemist

3 parts nettle (*Urticia urens* or *dioica*) root
3 parts saw palmetto (*Serenoa serrulata*) berries
2 parts collinsonia (*Collinsonia canadensis*) root
1 part white sage (*Salvia apiana*) herb

Combine tinctures. To reduce BPH, use a dropperful twice a day.

Reverse Cervical Dysplasia and *In Situ* Carcinoma

A naturopathic approach

Take daily for three months or as needed:

150,000 IU mixed natural carotenes
6000mg vitamin C
10mg folic acid
400mcg selenium
plus 1½ teaspoonfuls, twice a day, of a mixed tincture of:
- 2 parts red clover (*Trifolium pratense*) blossoms
- 3 parts dandelion (*Taraxacum officinale*) root
- 2 parts licorice (*Glycyrrhiza glabra*) root
- 1 part goldenseal (*Hydrastis canadensis*) root

Cautions: Goldenseal can stress the immune system and liver. **Antioxidant supplements** (unlike foods rich in antioxidants) **cannot reverse dysplasia**, and may even be cancer-promoting.

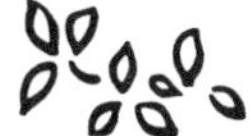

Female Restorative Roots Tincture

for women with PCOS

by Terry Willard

3 parts (12 drops or 1 oz) dong quai (*Angelica sinensis*)
2 parts (8 drops or 2/3 oz) Chinese peony (*Paeonia lacti-flora*)
1 part (4 drops or 1/3 oz) false unicorn (*Chamaelirium luteum*)
1 part (4 drops or 1/3 oz) black cohosh (*Cimcifuga racemosa*)
1 part (4 drops or 1/3 oz) wild yam (*Dioscorea villosa*)

Combine root tinctures and shake well. A dose is a dropperful, taken 2–4 times a day.

Amazonian Prostnut Butter

by Dr. James Duke

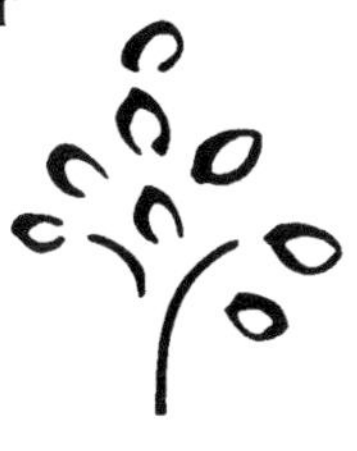

10 Brazil nuts
50–100 pumpkin seeds
½ cup cooked black beans or bean sprouts
1–2 teaspoonfuls tomato paste
2 capsules powdered saw palmetto berries

Blend ingredients together. The daily dose is a couple of tablespoons on crackers or bread. Do not be tempted to save time by doubling the recipe. "You want fresh phytomedicine," he cautions.

Australian Prostate Formula

Down Under heals Down There; reduces PSA levels, counters cancer

4 parts **saw palmetto** berries (*Serenoa serrulata*)
4 parts **willow herb** leaf (*Epilobium parviflorum*, not *Salix*); extremely active against abnormal prostate cells
2 parts grape seeds or skins (*Vitis vinifera*); anti-inflammatory, anticancer, inhibits cell proliferation
2 parts **hibiscus** flowers (*Hibiscus subdariffa*); anti-inflammatory, antioxidant, helps cell regeneration, good for gut flora
1 part licorice (*Glycyrrhiza glabra*)/counters testosterone
1 part passionflower (*Passiflora edulis*) seeds; hormonal effects
2400GDU bromelain powder; anti-inflammatory enzyme
200mcg selenium from yeast

Powder herbs and combine with supplements. Dose is one teaspoonful morning and night with a glass of water, one hour before or after food, other supplements, or medications. Not suggested for those taking antibiotics or anticoagulants, or those being treated for liver, heart, or kidney disorders. May cause upset stomach.

Except for the supplements, the exact amounts to use were not revealed by the authors of the original formula, so I estimated based on my knowledge of the herbs. This formula will be effective even if limited to the three most important herbs (in **bold**).

Prostate Power Combo

by Dr. Christopher

To reduce PSA, relieve LUTS, and counter prostatitis

1 ounce/30g buchu herb (*Barosma betulina*)
1/4 ounce/7g juniper berries (*Juniperus communis*)
1/4 ounce/7g cubeb berries (*Piper cubeba*)
1/4 ounce/7g uva ursi leaves (*Arctostaphylos uva-ursi*)

Place dried herbs in a half-gallon/2 liter jar. Pour six cups/1.5 liters of boiling water over them. Cap tightly; steep for 4-6 hours. Strain. The dose is 3-4 tablespoonfuls three times a day.

As is usual in the heroic tradition, these herbs are more stimulating than calming, more irritating than soothing, and more assertive than comforting. This formula would be well tolerated by men who have to be hit over the head with a two-by-four before noticing anything.

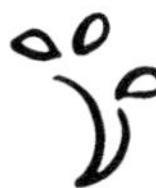

Big Guns Prostatitis Formula

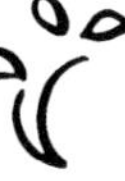

by David Hoffmann

To counter infection, inflammation, irritation in the prostate or bladder

1 oz antimicrobial uva ursi leaf (*Arctostaphylos uva-ursi*) tincture
1 oz soothing couch grass root (*Agropyron repens*) tincture
1 oz antiseptic buchu herb (*Barosma betulina*) tincture
1 oz anti-infective echinacea root (*Echinacea angustifolia*) tincture
1 oz wonderful saw palmetto berry (*Serenoa repens*) tincture
1 oz anti-inflammatory corn silk (*Zea mays*) tincture

Combine tinctures in an 8 oz/250ml bottle. Shake well. The dose is 1 teaspoonful/5ml three times a day. When the entire six ounces has been taken, if there is still a problem, remake the formula, adding an ounce of antibacterial, antiseptic yarrow (*Achillea millefolium*) tincture to increase the effect.

When the prostate swells, it pinches the urethra and interferes with the flow of urine. The bladder grows thicker and stronger to push against the resistance. But, eventually, it can't overcome the pressure. Then is can't empty completely and bacteria multiply in the stagnant urine. This leads to bladder infections, prostatitis, and, in extreme cases, kidney infection or failure.

This formula counters prostate swelling with saponins from couch grass and beta-sistosterol from saw palmetto. It soothes the bladder with corn silk. And it prevents and counters infection with buchu, echinacea, bearberry, and yarrow.

Dried Tomato Paté

Regular use can lower PSA readings and help prevent prostate cancer.

Pack **dried tomatoes** into a one-cup measure and add **boiling water** to cover. When they are soft, strain out the soaking liquid and save. Put half the soaked tomatoes in a blender or Cuisinart mini-prep. Add 1/4 cup **extra virgin olive oil**, 2 (or more) **cloves garlic,** chopped, plus a little **sea salt**. Blend well. Add the rest of the soaked tomatoes, more garlic, more salt, and more olive oil or soaking liquid. Blend very well. Kept in a tightly covered jar in the refrigerator, it is fine for up to a month.

Add some to an omlet, spread it on crackers or toast, spoon it into soups, use it as a dip, eat it by the spoonful.

Potency Potion Soup

Nourishing herbs that pack a punch down there

Sauté one large **onion** or the white part of one large **leek** in **olive oil** or **organic butter** over a low heat, stirring often, until soft and beginning to color; this will take about 20 minutes.

Meanwhile, slice: one fresh **burdock root** into thin rounds, four stalks of **celery** (and/or the same amount of **lovage**) into thin crescents, and one head of **romaine lettuce** into large pieces.

When the onion is cooked, add two quarts of cold water, all the vegetables, and two teaspoons of **sea salt** to the pan. Bring to a boil; lower heat and simmer for one hour.

When the soup is well cooked, add one teaspoonful of freshly ground dried **summer savory** or **wild thyme** or **basil**, and as much **saffron** as you can afford or desire, within reason. Simmer for another ten minutes. Serve hot. Makes four big bowls.

Belly Laugh Bowlful

Squash heals bellies; coconut soothes hormones; celery stirs interest

Choose a large **butternut squash**. Halve it; seed it; perhaps you will want to peel it, perhaps not. Cut into largish chunks and put into your soup pot. Add cold water to cover, bring to a boil, turn down heat, and simmer while you peel and chop 2 **onions**. Sauté them in some **olive oil**, at medium heat, stirring often.

When the onion is under way, wash a **celery root** (celeriac). Cut one half into tiny little pieces and saute it with the onion. Add the cooked onion and celery root mixture to the half-cooked squash in the soup kettle. Add more water if you wish. And do add a teaspoon or two of **sea salt** about now.

Cook the soup for another half-hour. Turn off heat and let it cool for a while. Using a stick blender (best) or a food mill, puree the soup. Return the puree to the soup kettle or store it in the refrigerator until ready to serve.

To serve, add one can of Thai Kitchen brand **coconut milk** to the pureed soup and heat until the coconut fat melts. Garnish with organic toasted coconut if desired. Serves 4–6.

Hot/Cold Herb Pillow

craft project that provides innumerable benefits

Your herb pillow will be filled mostly with flax seeds, buckwheat, or short-grain rice. Heat the seeds of your choice in the oven (300–350°) for one hour to dry them thoroughly and to kill the insect eggs present in all organic grains. Cool.

You will also want some dried aromatic herbs like lavender, cronewort, sage, or mint. Mix them in with the cooled grain.

Create a case for your pillow. You can stitch one up, or use the bottom six inches of an old pillowcase. Your finished pillow can be flat or round, but keep it fairly small; about 18 inches/45cm in length and 4–6 inches/10–15cm wide is a good size. If you wish to make a pillow specifically for your belly, make a round pillow 12 inches/30cm in diameter and about two inches/5cm in thickness. Heavy-weight cotton or silk are the best fabrics to use.

Use your grain/herb mix to fill the pillowslip – but not too full – and sew it shut with cotton or silk thread. (Avoid nylon or plastic.)

To use: Place the pillow in the freezer and apply to reduce inflammation. Or heat the pillow in the microwave, or wrap in foil and heat in the oven on the lowest setting, and apply to ease pain.

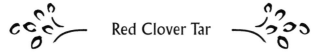

Red Clover Tar

A cancer-reducing salve created by Samuel Thomson (1769-1843)

Place fresh red clover blossoms in a double boiler, cover with spring water and cook for one hour. Remove blossoms, squeezing all the liquid from them back into the pan.

Add fresh red clover flowers to the liquid and cook for another hour. Remove those blossoms, squeezing all their liquid back into the pan, as before.

Now decoct the liquid, by slow simmering, until it becomes thick and tar-like. Patience! This part of the process takes hours.

To use: Spread the red clover tar on a gauze pad and apply to the cancer. Leave it on for 20–45 minutes, then remove and wash the area with dandelion root tincture. Repeat twice a day.

Skin irritation is normal, as is some pain, as the red clover tar slowly dissolves the tumor.

Ayurvedic Formulas for Women with Fibroids

Ayurvedic medicine groups individuals into three categories, with different herbs for each group. The original formulas used dried, powdered herbs. I prefer tinctures. A dose is a dropperful of mixed tincture, or 1 teaspoonful/3 grams of powdered herbs, taken between meals, twice a day with warm water and honey. Herbs marked are potentially poisonous.*

For **Vatas**

3 parts each of **black cohosh** root , **vitex**, and **St. Joan's wort** *plus*
2 parts each of **wild yam** root, **barberry** root bark, **turmeric** root, **myrrh*** resin, and **valerian** root
plus
1 part each of **calamus*** root, **cumin** seeds, **ginger** root, and **fenugreek** seeds.

For **Kaphas**

3 parts each of **vitex** and **myrrh*** resin *plus*
2 parts each of **black cohosh** root, **wild yam** root, **barberry** root bark, **dandelion** root, and **tumeric** root
plus
1 part each of **cumin** seeds, **ginger** root, and **black pepper**.

For **Pittas**

3 parts each of **vitex** and **St. Joan's wort**
plus
2 parts each of **barberry** root bark, **wild yam** root, **black cohosh** root, **gentian** root, **yellow dock** root, and **turmeric** root *plus*
1 part each of **cumin** seeds, **fennel** seeds, and **cinnamon** bark,
plus
a pinch of **saffron**.*

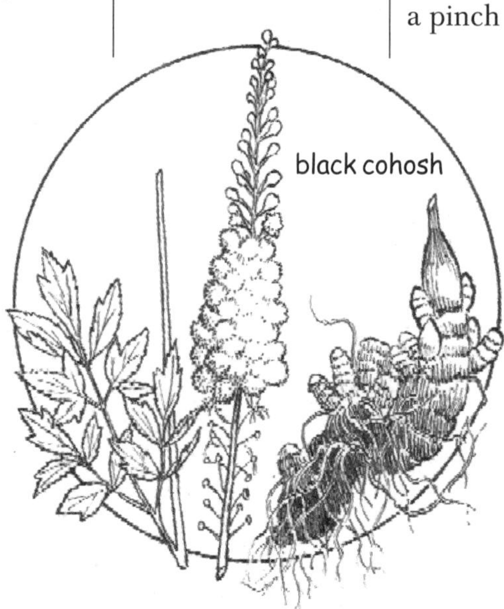

Glossary

To hear the spoken words, visit howjsayit.com

ablation (ab-LAY-zhun): the removal of tissue from the body.

adenomyosis (ADD-den-oh-my-OH-sis): a glandular derangement of the uterine muscle.

adhesions (add-HEE-zhuns): scar tissue that binds organs together. Common after pelvic surgery.

adnexal (add-NEX-ull): ovarian.

androgen (AN-droh-jen): hormone responsible for the development of male sex organs and secondary sexual characteristics.

angiogenesis (an-gee-oh-JEN-uh-sis): blood vessel (*angio*) growth (*genesis*) to a tumor, often leading to the spread of cancer to other areas of the body.

anterior colporrhaphy (ann-TEAR-ree-ur kol-POOR-uh-fee): surgery that attempts to pull the bladder back up into the pelvis by cutting, shortening, tightening, and repositioning muscles.

anti-androgenic (an-tee-an-dro-JEN-ick): against (*anti*) male hormones (*androgens*); counteracts the actions of testosterone.

antibiotic (an-tee-by-AH-tick): against (*anti*), life (*biotic*). A substance that kills bacteria.

anticholinergic (an-tee-kol-in-ER-jick): blocks the passage of specific nerve impulses.

antimuscarinic (an-tee-muss-cuh-RIN-ick): blocks normal nerve impulses.

anus (AY-nuss): the opening at the end of the large intestine where feces are released from the body.

aphrodisiac (aff-row-DEE-zee-ack): arouses or intensifies sexual sensations.

aspiration (ass-puh-RAY-shun): suctioning of fluids or gases from the body.

Bartholin's glands (BAR-toe-linz glanz): small glands that lie on either side of the entrance to the vagina.

benign (bee-NINE): non-cancerous, not harmful.

bilateral oophorectomy (by-LAT-uh-rul oh-oh-for-ECK-tuh-mee): removal of both ovaries; both (*bi*) sides (*lateral*).

bi-manual exam (BY-man-you-ul): examination done with two (*bi*) hands (*manual*): one on the abdomen and the fingers of the other in the vagina, so the uterus is between them.

biopsy (BY-op-see): surgical removal of tissues. A biopsy is examined under microscopic enlargement by a pathologist who looks for non-normal cells, especially cancer cells.

bolus (BOW-luss): a large pill, or a dose of a drug given quickly intravenously.

BPH: Benign Prostate Hyperplasia

brachytherapy (bray-kee-THAIR-uh-pee): a radioactive source is placed inside or next to the area being treated.

BRCA1, BRCA2: when mutated, these genes are associated with significant increase in breast cancer risk.

cancer (KAN-sir): abnormal cells growing without control. A general term that includes hundreds of different diseases.

candida (kan-DEE-duh): *Candida albicans.* A single-cell fungus that lives in healthy vaginas, intestines, and on our bodies. When vaginal pH is alkaline, it overgrows, causing a "yeast" infection.

carcinoma (kar-sin-OH-ma): malignant tumor; also any cancer that begins in the tissues covering or lining an organ, for example, the endometrium of the uterus or the lining of the bladder.

carcinoma in situ (in-SEE-too): a malignant tumor in its original place (*situ*).

catheter (KATH-it-ur): thin flexible tube inserted in the body to drain or inject fluid, or to keep a passage open.

catheterize (KATH-it-ur-eyes): to insert a catheter.

celibacy (SELL-i-buh-see): the state of abstaining from sex.

cervical (SIR-vuh-kull): of the cervix.

cervical erosion (ee-ROW-zhun): loss/degradation of tissues.

cervical eversion (ee-VER-zhun): inside out.

cervical os (oss): the opening of the cervix.

cervicitis (sir-vi-SIGH-tus): inflammation (*itis*) of the cervix.

cervix (SIR-viks): the lower, narrow neck of the uterus that connects to the upper end of the vagina.

chancre (KAN-kur): sore or ulcer from an infectious disease.

circumcise (SIR-kum-size), **circumcision**: removal of all or part of the foreskin from penis. Euphemism for clitorectomy.

clitorectomy (CLI-toe-REC-toe-me): removal of the clitoris.

clitoris (CLIT-or-iss): an organ devoted purely to pleasure. The visible portion (glans) lies above the urethral and vaginal openings, near the top of the vulvar lips. The rest, a network of erectile tissue, lies within the vulva.

colposcope (kol-puh-SKOPE): a lighted magnifying instrument used to examine the tissues of the vagina and cervix.

columnar cells (KOL-um-ner): cells that make up the inner surface of the cervix.

complete hysterectomy: surgical removal of uterus and ovaries.

cone biopsy: surgical removal of a large cone of tissue from the cervix, done under general anesthesia.

conformal radiation (kon-FOR-mull ray-dee-AY-shun): computers direct a high dose of radiation exactly at the cancer, minimizing damage to surrounding tissues.

contraceptive (kon-trah-SEP-tiv): anything used to prevent pregnancy, including barriers, IUDs, hormonal pills and patches.

contraindicated (kon-trah-IN-duh-kay-ted): against (*contra*) indications. A treatment or substance that should not be used.

corpus luteum (loo-TEE-um): the yellow (*luteum*) body (*corpus*), literally the egg yolk, which is left behind when the ovum ruptures out of its ovary. Source of progesterone and luteinizing hormone.

cryosurgery (kry-oh-SIRJ-uh-ree): surgery in which low temperatures are applied, usually to destroy tissue.

cyst (sist): thin-walled, closed sac filled with fluid or semisolid material.

cystectomy (sis-TECK-tuh-mee): surgical removal of the urinary bladder.

cystitis (sis-TIE-tus): bacterial infection of the urinary tract.

cystocele (SIST-oh-seal): protrusion of the bladder into the vagina due to a weakened vaginal wall.

cystoscopy (sigh-TOS-ka-pee): the insertion of a thin tube into the bladder. Used to diagnose and treat bladder woes.

D&C: dilatation and curettage. The cervix is opened (*dilated*) and a serrate-edged, spoon-shaped instrument (*curette*) is used to remove all or some of the endometrium.

DES or desPLEX is diethylstilbestrol (die-ethl-still-BESS-trull): an estrogen-like hormone prescribed for pregnant women, now known to cause rare reproductive cancers in their progeny.

DHT is dihydrotestosterone (die-high-droh-tess-TOS-tuh-rone): an androgenic hormone synthesized by the prostate, testes, hair follicles, and adrenals with the aid of 5-alpha-reductase. Cells absorb DHT more readily than testosterone. DHT increases facial and body hair but is the primary culprit in male pattern baldness.

diuretic (die-yur-ET-ick): agent that causes increased urine flow.

douche (doosh): A bath for the vagina. Not recommended, even for medicinal purposes. Finger baths or sitz baths are healthier.

dyspareunia (dis-puh-ROON-ee-uh): pain when attempting sexual intercourse.

dysplasia (dis-PLAY-zha): abnormal (*dys*) cells (*plasia*); pre-cancer.

dysuria (dis-YOUR-ee-uh): severe burning pain on urination.

egg tubes or Fallopian tubes: tubes stretching from the top of the uterus toward the ovaries, edged by the fimbria.

electrocautery (ee-lek-troh-KAW-tur-ee): process of destroying unwanted tissue with an electrically heated needle.

electromyography (ee-lek-troh-my-OG-ra-fee): a test that checks the health of the muscles and the nerves that control them.

embolization (em-bo-lie-ZAY-shun): the blockage of a blood vessel by an obstruction such as a blood clot.

endocervical curettage: (en-doe-SIR-vi-kull kure-uh-TAJ): scraping of cervical tissues (under local or no anesthesia) for examination by a pathologist.

endocervical glands/crypts (en-do-SIR-vi-kull glandz/kripts): a pit or recess (*crypt*) within (*endo*) the cervix (*cervical*).

endometrium (en-doe-MEE-tree-um): the inner lining of the uterus. It grows each menstrual month to allow a fertilized egg to implant; if none does, it is shed as menstrual blood.

episiotomy (eh-PEES-ee-otta-mee): incision made to enlarge the vaginal opening and prevent perineal tearing during birth.

epithelium (epi-THEEL-ee-um): a thin layer of cells covering the cervix; composed of columnar and squamous cells.

erysipelas (air-uh-SIP-uh-luhs): an acute infectious disease of the skin or mucous membranes caused by a streptococcus; characterized by local inflammation and fever.

erythematous (er-uh-THEEM-uh-tus): widening of small blood vessels near the skin's surface, reddening it. The drunkard's nose.

escharotic salve (ess-cuh-ROT-ick): a salve that burns tissue away; used to destroy cancer.

fascia (FASH-ee-uh): smooth, tough, stretchy connective tissue that envelops, separates, and binds together muscles, skin, organs, and other soft structures of the body. Faschia provides a way for all tissues in the body to communicate with each other.

fibroblast (FIE-broh-blast): a large flat cell that secretes proteins which form collagen and elastin and connective tissue fluids.

fimbria (FIM-bree-ah): waving fingers on the end of the egg tube that catch the egg as it leaves the ovary.

finger bath: standing in the tub, wet a finger in herbal tincture or infusion, and insert it into your vagina. Remove, rinse, repeat.

Five Element Theory: Oriental healing theory based on earth, air, fire, water, and wood elements.

flora (FLOOR-uh): literally the flowers. Gut flora are helpful micro-organisms that live in the intestines. Skin flora protect us.

follicle (FOLL-uh-kull): an immature ovum, including its covering sheet of cells, in the ovary. FSH helps mature it into an ovum.

frottage (fro-TAJ): a penis rubbing between thighs, buttocks, or breasts; or, between women, thighs rubbing against vaginas.

FSH: Follicle Stimulating Hormone.

functional ovarian cyst (FUNK-shun-ull oh-vary-in sist): sac that forms on the surface of an ovary. It holds the maturing follicle and, usually, melts away when the ovum is released.

fundus: the top of the the uterus.

Graafian follicles (GROF-ee-un): tiny potential eggs in the ovary.

glans: a small round mass or body; a tissue that can swell and harden; the tip of the clitoris or penis.

gynecological (guy-nick-uh-LOJ-uh-kull): relating to women's (*gyne*) reproductive health.

hemorrhage (HEM-uh-rij): large uncontrolled loss of blood.

hemorrhoid (HEM-uh-roid): a varicose vein of rectum or anus.

homeopathic (HOE-mee-oh-PATH-ick): treatment with minute doses of what would produce the disease if taken in a large dose.

hormone: from the Greek, "to arouse;" produced by endocrine glands like the testes, ovaries, adrenals, pineal, and pituitary.

hyperkeratosis (hi-per-KARE-uh-TOE-sis): benign thickening of the outer layer of skin.

hyperplasia (hy-per-PLAY-zha): too many (*hyper*) cells (*plasia*). Cells are still normal, but leaning ever so slightly toward cancer.

hysterectomy (hiss-ter-ECK-tuh-mee): surgical removal (*ectomy*) of the corpus and cervix of the uterus (*hyster*).

intravenous pyelogram (in-truh-VEEN-us pie-ELL-uh-gram): a contrast dye injected into a vein to make the bladder, ureters, and kidneys visible on an x-ray.

introitus (in-TROY-tus): entrance to the vagina.

labia (LAY-bee-uh): outer vaginal folds of a woman's vulva; from the Latin, meaning "lips." Singular is labium.

labial (LAY-bee-ull): of the labia.

laparoscope (lap-uh-RUH-skope): a small, flexible instrument equipped with a light and an optical lens that transmits a picture to a screen. Inserted through a small incision, laparoscopes are used to view internal organs and to guide surgeries such as biopsies.

laparoscopy (lap-uh-ROS-kuh-pee): use of a laparoscope to retrieve a tissue sample from the ovaries or pelvic organs for examination by a pathologist. Local or general anesthesia is used.

laparotomy (lap-uh-ROT-uh-mee): an incision down the middle of the abdomen. Requires general anesthesia.

LEEP: Loop Electrosurgical Excision Procedure. An electrified wire slices a button-sized disk off the cervix, under local (or no) anesthesia. Offered as a treatment for cervical warts, this is actually a biopsy. It takes 2–3 months for the cervix to heal.

lesion (LEE-zhun): a broken, infected, wounded, injured place.

leukorrhea (luke-uh-REE-yuh): white (*leuko*) flow (*rrhea*). Usually refers to an unwanted vaginal discharge.

lichen scleroses (LI-ken skler-OH-sees): a disturbance of the vaginal tissues that itches, burns, and sometimes fuses the labia.

lower urinary tract: the bladder and the urethra.

LUTS: Lower Urinary Tract Symptoms.

malignant (muh-LIG-nent): cancerous.

menorrhagia (men-or-AY-gee-uh): heavy or prolonged menstrual bleeding.

menstruation (men-strew-AY-shun): the monthly (*mens*) shedding (*struation*) of the endometrium from the uterus.

metastasis (muh-TAS-tuh-sis): spread of cancer.

metastudy: a study of many other studies.

mittelschmerz (MITL-shmertz): literally, middle (ovulation) pain.

monoclonal antibody (mon-oh-CLONE-uhl): antibody produced in large quantities by clones of an artificially created cell.

morphological (more-foe-LOJ-ih-kull): the form and structure of something.

myomectomy (my-oh-MECK-tuh-mee): surgical removal of fibroid tumors from the uterus, leaving the uterus in the pelvis.

myometrium (my-oh-MEE-tree-um): the muscular outer layer of the uterus.

necrotic (neh-KROT-ick): dead, as in dead tissue.

nocturia (nock-TOUR-ee-uh): urinary urges which disrupt sleep.

nosode (NO-sode): homeopathic dilution of a substance known to cause damage for generations, e.g., DES, syphilis. Taking the dilution is said to repair the damage.

omentum (oh-MEN-tum): a fatty layer of tissue that supports the abdominal organs.

onanism (OH-nuh-niz-um): masturbation.

oncologist (on-KOL-uh-jist): a specialist in treating cancer.

oophorectomy (oh-oh-for-ECK-tuh-mee): surgical removal of the ovaries, egg tubes, and all connective tissues.

ova, ovum (OH-vuh, OH-vum): eggs, egg; female reproductive cell/s that join with sperm to create a fetus.

ovary, ovaries (OH-vah-ree, OH-vah-reez): endocrine glands on either side of uterus.

Pap smear: a sample taken of cervical tissues.

papilloma (pap-ih-LOW-muh): benign tumor of the skin or mucous membranes; a wart.

paruresis (par-you-REE-sis): phobia in which a person is unable to urinate in the real or imagined presence of others.

pathologist (puh-THOLL-uh-jist): scientist specializing in disease.

pelvic exenteration (PELL-vick ex-EN-ter-ay-shun): radical hysterectomy plus removal of rectum and bladder; labia and clitoris are preserved.

perineum (peruh-NEE-um): area of skin between the vagina (or the scrotum) and anal openings.

peritoneal (peruh-toe-NEE-ull): around (*peri*), or inside, the abdominal cavity.

pessary (PESS-uh-ree): a device placed inside the vagina to counter prolapse and keep the uterus in place. Also a suppository of medication that is inserted into the vagina.

Peyronie's disease (pay-ROH-knees); also *induratio penis plastica* or CITA (chronic inflammation of tunica albuginea): a connective tissue disorder which causes penile curvature, indentation, lesions, and pain, especially on erection. The safest, most effective treatment is the Leriche technique surgery, available in Europe.

pH: (*potenz hydrogen*); acidity (1–6)/alkalinity (8 and above) scale.

phimosis (fie-MOH-sis): non-retractibility of the penile (or clitoral) foreskin; considered normal for intact pre-adolescent males.

priapism (PRY-uh-pizm): inability to lose an erection with in 4 hours of onset; complications include penile damage, impotence, and gangrene. *A medical emergency*. Ephedrine may relieve it.

phytosterol (fie-TOSS-tuh-rall): plant (*phyto*) steroid (*sterol*).

placebo (pluh-SEE-bow): an inert substance which has a curative effect.

polyphenol (pol-ee-FEE-nul): specialized chemicals found in plants characterized by many (*poly*) phenols (*aromatic rings*).

polyps (POL-ips): small stalk-shaped growths sticking out from skin or mucous membrane; most often benign.

prolapse (PRO-laps): something that has fallen out of its proper place in the body, such as uterine or bladder prolapse.

prophylactic (PRO-fuh-lack-tick): preventative.

PSA: Prostate Specific Antigen, a normal enzyme (protein) produced by the prostate to liquefy the gel surrounding semen. It increases when there are abnormal cells in the prostate.

pyelonephritis (PIE-uh-lo-nef-RYE-tus): bacterial infection of the upper urinary tract.

radical hysterectomy: surgical removal of the cervix, uterus, ovaries, fallopian tubes, lymph glands and surrounding tissues, and part of the vagina.

radical prostatectomy (pros-tuh-TECK-tuh-mee): surgical removal of the entire prostate gland and some of the tissue around it.

radical vulvectomy (vull-VECK-tuh-mee): surgical removal of the entire vaginal lips and clitoris, including the skin surrounding the vulva and associated lymph glands.

radio-immunoassay (im-mewn-oh-ASS-ay): a substance with a radioactive tracer attached to it is introducted into the bloodstream to measure levels of antibodies in the blood.

radiotherapy: treatment of disease using radiation X-rays or beta rays directed at the body externally, or internally from radioactive materials placed in the body. Also called radiation therapy.

rectal (RECK-tull): of the rectum.

rectum (RECK-tum): lower part of the large intestine between the colon and the anal canal.

salpingectomy (sal-pin-JEK-tuh-mee): salpingo-oophorectomy.

salpingo-oophorectomy (sal-PING-oh-oh-oh-for-ECK-toe-mee): surgical removal (*ectomy*) of the egg tubes (*salping*) and the ovaries (*oophor*); may be bilateral or unilateral.

sclerotherapy (SKLER-uh-THER-uh-pee): injection of a substance into blood vessels – hemorrhoids, varicose veins – to shrink them.

scrotum (SCROH-tum): skin and muscle surrounding the testes.

seminal fluid, semen (SEM-i-null), (SEE-men): watery mix of fructose and enzymes; promotes sperm survival and movement.

serum (SEER-um): clear watery body fluid. Plural: **sera**.

simple hysterectomy: a misleading term, as it is not simple, but total; see total hysterectomy.

simple vulvectomy: surgical removal of the skin of the major and minor lips of the vulva and, often, the shaft of the clitoris.

sitz bath: A bath for "down there."

speculum (SPEK-you-lum): an instrument used to widen the opening of the vagina so that the cervix is more accessible.

sperm, spermatozoa (sper-muh-tuh-ZO-uh): male reproductive cells.

sphincter (SFINK-ter): circular band of muscle surrounding a bodily opening; it narrows/closes the opening by contracting.

spontaneous remission (spon-TAY-nee-us ree-mish-un): the once-challenged, but now acknowledged, ability of the immune system to rid the body of cancer, even in advanced stages.

squamo-columnar junction (SKWAM-oh-KOL-um-ner): the place in the epithelium where the squamous and columnar cells meet; the transition zone. A common site for cervical cancer.

squamous cell (SKWAM-us): a cell that covers the outer surface of the cervix.

STDs/STIs: Sexually Transmitted Diseases/Infections, such as HPV, gonorrhea, syphilis, yeast, trich, chlamydia, and crabs.

stricture (STRICK-chur): abnormal constriction or narrowing of a body passage.

stroma (STROW-muh): hormone-producing ovarian tissue which replaces follicles as they mature; the older the woman, the more stroma she is likely to have.

substrate: a substance that is acted upon in a biochemical reaction, usually by an enzyme.

subtotal hysterectomy: supracervical hysterectomy; the uterus is surgically removed, but the cervix is not.

suppository (suh-POZ-uh-tory): a preparation designed to be inserted into the rectum, vagina, or urethra.

synthase (SIN-thays): various enzymes that catalyze the synthesis of a sustance without breaking high-energy phosphate bonds.

thrombosis (throm-BOW-sis): a blood clot which forms inside a blood vessel; it may block the flow of blood, causing a stroke.

topical (TOP-i-kull): used externally, on the skin.

total hysterectomy: surgical removal of the uterus and ovaries. Keep your ovaries!

transvaginal ultrasound: a non-surgical examination of the uterus, ovaries and surrounding areas with a small ultrasound wand placed into the vagina.

trich (trick): *Trichomonas vaginalis.* A benign parasite found in normal, healthy vaginas. Overgrowth is problematic. An STD.

trigger points: hyper-irritable spots in skeletal muscle that are associated with palpable nodules.

TUNA: TransUrethral Needle Ablation.

TURP: TransUrethral Resection of the Prostate.

ulcer (ULL-sir): an area of tissue erosion, a non-healing sore.

unilateral: on one (*uni*) side (*lateral*).

unilateral oophorectomy: surgical removal of one ovary.

upper urinary tract: the kidneys and the ureters.

ureters (you- REE-turz): long tubes connecting kidneys and bladder.

urethra (you-REE-thruh): the tube that connects the bladder with the outside.

urethritis (you-reeth-RYE-tus): inflammation of the urethra, usually caused by infection or drugs.

urethrocele (you-REETH-row-seal): protrusion of the urethra into the vagina.

urinalysis (you-rin-AL-uh-sis): analysis of the urine for levels of white blood cells, infective agents, sugar, protein, and acidity, as well as specific gravity,

vaginal hysterectomy: surgical removal of the uterus through the vagina.

vaginectomy (va-jin-ECK-tuh-mee): surgical removal of the vagina.

vermiform appendix (VERM-uh-form uh-PEN-dix): a tag of worm (*verm*)-like form, found on the large intestine in the lower right quadrant of the pelvis.

vestibular glands (ves-TIB-you-ler): Bartholin's glands.

vulvectomy (vull-VECK-tuh-mee): surgical removal of a woman's external genitalia.

Bibliography

Ayurvedic Healing for Women, Atreya; Weiser, 1999.

Before You Call the Doctor, Anne Simons MD, Bobbie Hasselbring, & Michael Castleman; Fawcett Columbine, 1992.

Botanica Erotica, Diana De Luca; Inner Traditions, 1998.

The Botanical Pharmacy, Heather Boon; Quarry Press, 1999.

Botanical Medicine for Women's Health, Aviva Romm; Elsevier, 2010.

The Clitoral Truth, The Secret World at Your Fingertips, Rebecca Chalker; Seven Stories Press, 2000.

The Complete Book of Essential Oils, Valerie Ann Worwood; New World Library, 1991.

Complete Guide to Herbal Medicines, CW Fetrow, JR Avila; Simon & Schuster, 2000.

C*omplete Woman's Herbal*, Anne McIntyre; Henry Holt, 1994.

Coping with Endometriosis, Robert H. Phillips PhD; Putnam, 2000.

Delmar's Integrative Herb Guide for Nurses, Martha Libster; Delmar, 2002.

Desk Reference to Nature's Medicine, Steven Foster & Rebecca Johnson; National Geographic, 2006.

Diet & Health, National Research Council; National Academy of Science Press, 1989.

Dr. Duke's Essential Herbs, James Duke; Rodale Press, 1999.

Encyclopedia of Natural Medicine, M. Murray ND & J. Pizzorno ND; Prima, 1991.

The Endometriosis Sourcebook, M. Ballweg; Contemporary, 1995.

The Family Herbal, Barbara and Peter Theiss; Healing Arts, 1989.

Fibroid Tumors & Endometriosis: Self Help Book, Dr. Susan Lark; Celestial Arts, 1993.

Fibroids: The Complete Guide, Johanna Skilling; Marlow & Co., 2000.

For Women of All Ages, Sheldon Cherry MD; Macmillan, 1979.

The Green Pharmacy, Dr. James Duke; Rodale, 1997.

Handbook of Obstetrics & Gynecology in Chinese Medicine, Yu Jin MD; Eastland Press, 1998.

Healing Foods, Amanda Ursell; Dorling Kinderley, 2000.

Heart of the Flower: Book of Yonis, A. Barnes & Y. Lumsden; Pangia, 2010.

Herbal Emissaries, Steven Foster, Yue Chongxi; Healing Arts, 1992.

Herbal Healing for Women, Rosemary Gladstar; Fireside, 1993

Herbal Medicine, Rudolf Fritz Weiss; Arcanum, 1988.

Herbal Medicine, Healing & Cancer, Donald Yance Jr.; Keats, 1999.

Herbal Remedies for Women, Amanda McQuade Crawford; Three Rivers Press, 1997.

Herbs for Health and Healing, Kathi Keville; Rodale Press, 1996.

Hold It Sister: The Confident Girl's Guide to a Leak-Free Life, Mary O'Dwyer; Redsok (Australia), 2009.

Healing Cancer Peacefully, Nancy Offenhauser; Round House, 2009.
Herbal Drugs and Phytopharmaceuticals, Max Witchl (Norman Grainger Bisset, ed.); CRC Press, 1994.
A Homepathic Approach to Cancer, Dr. A.U. Ramakrishnan, Narayana, Quality Medical Publishing, 2001.
Homeopathic Medicine for Women, Trevor Smith MD; Healing Arts, 1989.
How to Stay Out of the Gynecologist's Office, Federation of Feminist Women's Health Centers; Women to Women Pub, 1986.
Hysterectomy: Before & After, Winnifred B. Cutler, PhD; Harper Perennial, 1990.
The Male Herbal, James Green, Crossing Press, 2007.
Medical Self Care Book of Women's Health, Bobbi Hasselbring, Sadja Greenwood MD, Michael Castleman; Doubleday, 1987.
Mindfulness in Plain English, Bhante Gunaratana; Wisdom, 2010.
Mindful Therapy, Thomas Bien; Wisdom, 2010.
National Geographic Desk Reference to Nature's Medicines, Steven Foster and Rebecca Johnson; National Geographic, 2006.
Natural Healing in Gynecology, Rina Nissim; Pandora, 1986.
The Natural Testosterone Plan for Sexual Health and Energy, Stephen H. Buhner; HealingArts Press, 2007.
A New View of a Woman's Body, Fed. of Feminist Health Centers, 1981.
No More Hysterectomies, Vicki Hufnagel MD; NAL, 1988.
Nutrition Guide for the Prevention & Cure of Common Ailments & Diseases, Carlton Fredericks PhD; Fireside, 1982.
Overcoming Incontinence, Mary Dietrich RN & Felicia Froe MD; John Wiley & Sons, 2000.
Overcoming Bladder Disorders, Medical and Self-help Solutions, Rebecca Chalker & Kristene Whitmore MD; HarperCollins, 1990.
Our Bodies, Our Selves for the New Century, Boston Women's Health Book Collective; Touchstone, 1998.
The Patient's Guide to Medical Tests, Joseph C. Segen MD and Joseph Stauffer PhD; Facts on File Inc., 1998.
PDR Family Guide to Women's Health, Medical Economics, 1994.
PDR for Herbal Medicines: Second Edition, 2000
Pelvic Power, Eric Franklin; Elysian, 2002.
The Perfect Fit, Edward Eichel; Signet, 1992.
Positive Options for Polycystic Ovary Syndrome, Christine Craffs-Hinton and Adam Dalen MD; Hunter House, 2004
Resurrection After Rape, Matt Aktinson, R;R Publishing, 2008.
Saving the Whole Woman: Natural Alternatives for Pelvic Organ Prolapse and Incontinence, Christine Kent; Bridgeworks Press, 2003.
Sex for One, The Joy of Selfloving, Betty Dodson; Crown, 1974.
The Sexual Herbal, Brigette Mars; Healing Arts, 2010.

Sex Herbs, Beth Ann Roybal & Gayle Skowronki; Random House, 1999.
Take this Book to the Gynecologist with You, Gale Maeskey and Charles B. Inlander; Addison-Wesley Publishing, 1991.
Textbook of Modern Herbology, Terry Willard; Wild Rose, 2002.
Unwinding the Belly, A. Post & S. Cavaliere; North Atlantic Books, 2003.
The V Book, Elizabeth Stewart; MD, Bantam, 2002.
Vital Man, Stephen Harrod Buhner; Avery, 2003.
What Your Doctor May Not Tell You About Fibroids, Scott Goodwin MD & Michael Broder MD; Warner Bro, 2003. [abbreviated: *Fibroids*]
The Wellness Encyclopedia of Food & Nutrition, Sheldon Margen MD and the University of California; Health Letter Associates, 1992.
Wisdom of Menopause, Christiane Northrup MD; Bantam, 2001.
Woman, Natalie Angier; Houghton Miflin, 1999.
The Woman's Book of Orgasm, Tara Barker; Kensington Pub., 1997.
A Woman's Guide to Sexual Health, Mary Minkin MD and Carol Wright; Yale University Press, 2005.
Women's Anatomy of Arousal, Sheri Winston; Mango Garden, 2010.
Women's Bodies, Women's Wisdom, Christine Northrup MD; Bantam, 1994.
Women's Encyclopedia of Myths and Secrets, Barbara Walker; Harper, 1983.
Women's Encyclopedia of Natural Medicine, Tori Hudson ND; Keats, 1999.
Women Talk About Gynecological Surgery, A. Gross & D. Ito; Harper, 1991.
The Yoni: Sacred Symbol of Female Creative Power, Rufus Camphausen; Inner Traditions, 1996.

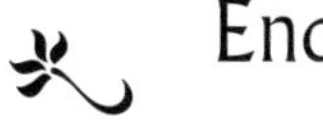

Endnotes

Key:
HWHW *Harvard Women's Health Watch*
JAMA *Journal of the American Medical Association*
JHML *Johns Hopkins Medical Letter*
NEJM *New England Journal of Medicine*
THNN *Tufts Health & Nutrition Newletter*
WHAd *Women's Health Advisor* (*Weil Medical College*)
UCBW *UC Berkeley Wellness Letter*
WHAct *Women's Health Activist*

Pelvic Floor

1. Lisa Sarasohn, *The Belly Book,* New World Library, 2006.
2. *Pelvic Power*, Eric Franklin, Elysian, 2002.

Pelvic Organ Prolapse

- **www.wholewoman.com** (help for women with prolapse)

3. "Prolapsed Bladder," *WHAd*, December, 2006.
4. *Saving the Whole Woman*, page 121.
5. *Ibid.* (whole book)

6. *Ibid.,* page 161.
7. "Pelvic organ prolapse & ending the epidemic of unnecessary hysterectomies," Pam Geyer, *WHAct,* Nov/Dec 2009.
8. *Ibid.*
9. *The Destroying Angel,* J. Money, Prometheus Books, 1985, page 116.
10. *Our Bodies, Our Selves for the New Century,* page 661.
11. *Pelvic Power,* Eric Franklin, Elysian, 2002.

Chronic Pelvic Pain

• www.pelvicpain.org (an interdisciplinary approach to CPP)
12. "Chronic Pelvic Pain," *WHAd,* Nov 2002.
13. *Ibid.*
14. *Ibid.*
15. "Endometriosis at midlife," *HWHW*, Feb 2006.
16. "Painful sex," *Women's Health and Fitness News,* Jan 1989.
17. *WHAd,* Nov 2002.
18. *Who Dies,* Stephen Levine, Anchor Books, 1989, page 134.
19. "Efficacy of static magnetic field therapy in chronic pelvic pain," Brown et al., *Amer J Obstet Gynecol,* 187(6):1561-7, 2002. (Active magnets [500G] applied to abdominal trigger points and left on the skin.)
20. "I broke my pelvis in 4 pieces when I was 16 (horseback riding). It wasn't a problem until menopause; then the pain drove me crazy. 'Biomedici' electro-magnetic therapy was the only thing that helped." (Correspondence, March 2010)
21. "Common Uterine Conditions," US Dept. of Health and Human Services, 2009. www.ahrq.gov/consumer/uterine1.htm
22. *WHAd,* Nov 2002.
23. *Ibid.*

Hemorrhoids

• www.hemorrhoidhelp.com
24. "Troubled by hemorrhoids?," *WHAd,* June 2005.
25. "Low down on hemorrhoids," *UCBW,* July 2004.
26. "Quick relief from hemorrhoid pain," Mark Stengler, *Very Personal Healthletter,* 2009.
27. *Natural Health First-Aid Guide,* Simon & Schuster, 1994, page 179.
28. "Low down on hemorrhoids," *UCBW,* July 2004.
29. *Ibid.*
30. "House call: hemorrhoids," *Health After 50,* Oct 2009.
31. "Troubled by hemorrhoids?," *WHAd,* June 2005.
32. *HWHW*, Nov 1996.
33. "Troubled by hemorrhoids?," *WHAd,* June 2005.
34. *Ibid.*
35. *Ibid.*
36. "Second opinion," *Mayo Clinic Health Letter,* Sept 2009

37. *Ibid.*
38. "Anal fissure," *HWHW*, Sept 2009.
39. *Ibid.*

Fenugreek

40. *Delmar's Integrative Herb Guide for Nurses*, pages 196-7.
41. *Ibid.*

Horse chestnut

42. *PDR for Herbal Medicines*, page 404. (Quote from *Commission E*)
43. *Ibid.*
44. *National Geographic Desk Reference to Nature's Medicines*, page 214.
45. *UCBW*, May 2007.
46. *PDR for Herbal Medicines*, page 404.
47. *Ibid.*
48. *The Complete Guide to Herbal Medicines*, page 276.
49. *PDR for Herbal Medicines*, page 404.

Bladder

- www.nafc.org (800-252-3337)
- 800-bladder
- www.simonfoundation.org (800-237-4666)
- www.aboutincontinence.org
- www.mypelvichealth.org
- *Overcoming Incontinence*, Mary Dietrich RN & Felicia Froe MD, John Wiley & Sons, 2000.
- *Hold It Sister: The Confident Girl's Guide to a Leak-Free Life*, Mary O'Dwyer, Redsok (Australia), 2009.

1. ". . . fibromyalgia and interstitial cystitis," Daniel Clauw, et al., *Journal of Psychiatric Research*, 31(1):125-131, Jan 1997
2. "Many effective treatments for urinary incontinence," *HealthNews*, Aug 2006.
3. "Urinary incontinence treatments that work," J. Vapnek MD, *Bottom Line Health*, 2007.
4. Overheard at a conference of health care professionals, 2006.
5. "Stem cells muscle in on bladder control," *New Scientist*, Dec 2004.
6. "Incontinence and women: usually curable, often ignored," Leah Thayer, *Women's Health Network News*, Sept/Oct 2002.
7. "Regain Control," Sarah Toland, *Delicious Living*, Jan 2005.
8. "Kegels hold up as urinary continence treatment," *HWHW*, May 2006.
9. *Ibid.*
10. "Pelvic organ prolapse runs in the family," *HWHW*, May 2007.
11. *International Urogynecology Journal*, Oct 2006.
12. *UCBW*, April 2009.
13. "Many effective treatments for incontinence," *HealthNews*, Aug 2006.

14. *Ibid.*
15. "Urinary incontinence may run in families," *WHAd*, Dec 2004. (*British Medical Journal*, 16 Oct 2004)
16. "Pelvic organ prolapse," Buchsbaum et al., *Obstetrics & Gynecology*, 108:1388-93, Dec 2006.
17. "Prevalence and associated risk factors of urinary incontinence: results from the Women's Health Initiative," WHI Investigator Group, *Abstracts: Twelfth Annual Meeting of NAMS.*
18. Nicolette Horbach MD, past president, American Urogynecologic Society, associate clinical professor of Ob/Gyn.
19. "Simpler solutions for incontinence," *HealthNews,* Sept 2002.
20. "Magnetic chair, spinal nerve stimulation help incontinence," *British Journal of Urology International*, March 2004.
21. *Hysterectomy: Before & After*, Cutler, page 269.
22. *HWHW*, May 2006.
23. "'Gotta go, gotta go?' Tips to help control overactive bladder," *Environmental Nutrition*, Aug 2003.
24. "The plastic panic," Jerome Groopman, *New Yorker*, 31 May 2010.
25. "When nature calls too often," *JHML,* Nov 2006.
26. "Hormones can worsen/cause incontinence," *HealthFacts*, March 2005.
27. "Urinary incontinence – one more purported benefit of hormone therapy disproved," *NEJM* 15 April 2005.
28. "Prevalence and associated risk factors of urinary incontinence," WHI Investigator Group, *Abstracts: Twelfth Annual Meeting of NAMS.*
29. "Hormone therapy increases the risk of urinary incontinence," *National Women's Health Network*, July/Aug 2005.
30. *JAMA*, 293:935-9048, 23 Feb 2005.
31. "Urinary incontinence risk increased with hormone therapy," *American College of Obstetricians and Gynecologists* conference, April 2003.
32. Jack Tsao MD, *Bottom Line Personal*, Jan 2009
33. "Dementia and incontinence treatments can lead to functional decline," *DukeMedicine*, Aug 2008.
34. "Stem cells muscle in on bladder control," *New Scientist*, Dec 2004.
35. "Oopsie daisy," Ranit Mishori MD, *AARP,* July/Aug 2006.
36. *Ibid.*
37. "Control of odor in urinary incontinence," *Nursing Homes*, 20(10):28, 1971.
38. Metastudy led by Jeanette S Brown MD, reported in *Bottom Line Health*, 1 Dec 2000.
39. *American Journal of Obstetrics & Gynecology*, Jan 2006.
40. "Handling the 'stress' and 'urge' of incontinence," *Johns Hopkins Health After 50*, Nov 2009.
41. "Exercising with incontinence," *Health*, 1999.
42. "Handling . . . incontinence," *JHML*, Nov 2009.
43. Leslie Talcott, MS, RN, dir.: Perineometer Research Inst., Stratford, PA.

44 "Stem cells may treat incontinence," *WHAd*, July 2006.
45. "Stem cells . . . bladder control," *New Scientist,* Dec 2004.
46. *Ibid.*
47. *Our Bodies ,Ourselves for the New Century*, page 574.
48. "Radio waves treat stress incontinence," *Journal of Urology*, March 2003. (*Health News,* June 2003)
49. "Renessa," *HWHW* , Oct 2009.
50. *Obstetrics & Gynecology*, Nov 2007, 110:1034.
51. *Obstetrics & Gynecology*, Dec 2006.
52. "Vaginal delivery not associated with urinary incontinence," *Women's Health Activist,* Dec 2005.
53. *Journal of Urology*, May 2002.
54. "Hysterectomy and urinary incontinence: a systematic review," *The Lancet,* 2000:356, 12 Aug 2000.
55. "Handling . . . incontinence," *John Hopkins Health After 50*, Nov 2009.
56. "Help for bladder problems," *More*, Jan 2008.
57. "Handling . . . incontinence," *John Hopkins Health After 50*, Nov 2009.
58. "Midurethral sling surgery for stress incontinence," *HWHW,* Sept 2010.
59. *Ibid.*
60. "Overcoming overactive bladder," *WHAd*, April 2007.
61. "Get it under control," *John Hopkins Medical Center*, 2007.
62. "Calming an overactive bladder," Mark Hyman MD, *Alternative Medicine*, April 2007.
62A. "Always sprinting for the loo?," *More*, April 2011.
63. "Best remedies for a healthy bladder," *Herbs for Health*, April 2006.
64. *Delmar's Integrative Herb Guide for Nurses*, page 551.
65. "Best remedies for a healthy bladder," *Herbs for Health*, April 2006.
66. *British Journal of Urology*, 61:490-493, 1988.
67. "Acupuncture aids overactive bladder," *Obst & Gyne*, July 2005.
68. *Delmar's Integrative Herb Guide for Nurses*, page 414.
69. *British Journal of Ob/Gyn*, 105:667-669, 1998
70. "Calming an overactive bladder," Hyman MD, *Alt Med*, April 2007.
71. *Ibid.*
72. "Review of drugs for overactive bladder," *Worst Pills, Best Pills*, Feb 2010.
73. "What is urinary incontinence?," *HealthNews*, March, 2001
74. "Two-drug combo improves overactive bladder," *Focus on Healthy Aging*, Feb 2001. (*JAMA*, Nov 2006)
75. *Cochrane Database of Systematc Reviews*, CD001405. (*JHML*, March 2010)
76. *More*, Nov 2009.
77. "Controlling incontinence," *Better Bladder and Bowel Control*, Harvard College Special Report, 2007.
78. "Give your bladder a break," *More*, Nov 2008.
79. "Questions & answers," *Health News*, May 2005.

80. TM Johnson et al., *Journal of Urology,* Nov 2007, 178:2045.
81. "Shy bladder," Miller MD, *Harvard Mental Health Letter,* Jan 2004.
82. Private correspondence, June 2008.
83. *Shy Bladder Syndrome,* Soifer, Zgourides, et al., New Harbinger, 2001.
84. Private correspondence, June 2008.
85. "Shy bladder," *Harvard Mental Health Letter,* Jan 2004.

LUTS

86. *Herbal Medicine,* Weiss, page 254.
87. "Combined extracts of *Urtica dioica* and *Pygeum africanum* in the treat ment of benign prostatic hyperplasia, a double-blind comparison," Krzeski et al., *Clinical Therapeutics,* 15(6):1011-20.
88. "A wee problem," *AARP,* Jan/Feb 2005. (quoted: Charles Napier, 68)
89. *Nutrition Guide,* page 28.
90. *Ibid.*
90A. Study by the Boston Area Community Health Services, *Journal of Nutrition,* 141:267, 2011.
91. "A wee problem," *AARP,* Jan/Feb 2005.
92. "12 Surgeries," *Consumer Reports on Health,* Oct 2005.
93. "Microwaves help restore urine flow," *HealthNews,* 10 Sept 1999.
94. Personal correspondence, Jan 2009.

Urinary Tract Infections

95. "Risk factors for recurrent urinary tract infection in young women," *Journal of Infectious Diseases,* Oct. 2000; 182:1177-82.
96. "Urinary tract infections," *Life Extension,* April 2010. (*Am J Med,* 8 July 2002, 113 Suppl 1A:5S-13S.)
97. David Staskin MD, professor of urology, quoted in *The Doctor's Book of Home Remedies,* Bantam, 1991.
98. "Treatment of uncomplicated cystitis," Hooton et al., *JAMA,* 293:949-55, 23 Feb 2005.
99. *Our Bodies, Ourselves for the New Century,* page 650.
100. "Banishing urinary tract infections," *HWHW,* Dec 2002.
101. "Cranberries," *Nutrition Action Healthletter,* June 2005.
102. *Canada Journal of Urology,* 2002; 9:1558.
103. *British Medical Journal,* 322:1571, 30 June 2001.
104. *JAMA,* 1994; 271:751-754.
105. "Research backs cranberries for preventing urinary tract infections," *Harvard Women's Health,* April 2008. (*Cochrane Reviews,* 23 Jan 2008)
106. "Cranberry juice and UTIs: maybe grandma was right," Beth Fontenot, *Nutrition Forum,* Sept/Oct 1998.
107. "Cranberry or trimethoprim for the prevention of recurrent urinary tract infections? A randomized controlled trial in older women. *Journal of Antimicrobial Chemotherapy,* 63(2):389-95, Feb 2009.
108. "Ask Dr. Etingin: Cranberries," *WHAd,* Aug 2005.

109. "Antibacterial activity of gossypetin isolated from *Hibiscus sabdariffa*," *The Antiseptic*, 99(3):81-2, Mar 2002.
110. "Double-blind, placebo-controlled study of *Hibiscus sabdariffa* extract in the prevention of recurrent cystitis in women," presented at Convergences in Pelviperineal Pain, 16-19 Dec 2009, Nantes, France.
111. *Herbal Healing for Women*, Gladstar, page 190.
112. *Science News*, Vol 169, page 355.
113. "Coping with persistent bladder infections," *Spa Life,* Fall 2004.
114. *Ibid.*
115. *International Journal of Epidemiology*, April 2001.
116. *Women's Encyclopedia of Health and Emotional Healing*, Denise Foley, editor, Rodale Press, 1993.
117. "Banishing UTIs," *HWHW*, Dec 2002.
118. "Improper antibiotic treatment for bladder infections," *Worst Pills, Best Pills,* June 2004.
119. *HWHW*, Oct 2007.
120. "Increasing prevalence of antimicrobial resistance among uropathogens causing acute cystitis," Gupta et al., *JAMA*, 281:736-8, Feb 1999.
121. "Banishing UTIs," *HWHW*, Dec 2002.
122. *Ibid.*
123. "Vaccine curbs urinary tract infections," *WHAd*, Dec 2003. (*Journal of Urology*, Sept 2003.)
124. "Urinary catheters, a major source of infection," *HealthFacts,* Sept 2005.
125. "Antimicrobial resistance . . . uropathogens," *Journal Watch*, 19(7).

Interstitial Cystitis

- Interstitial Cystitis Ass'n: 800-435-7422, www.ichelp.org
- American Academy of Pain Management, www.aapainmanage.org
- *Headache in the Pelvis*, Rodney Anderson, National Center for Pelvic Pain, 2002.
- *Interstitial Cystitis Guide*, Robert Moldwin MD, New Harbinger, 2000.

126. Vicki Ratner MD, founder, Interstitial Cystitis Association.
127. "Interstitial cystitis," *JHML,* June 2003.
128. "Living with interstitial cystitis," Anne Rochon Ford, *A Friend Indeed*, March/April 1999.
129. "Randomized double-blind trial of oral L-arginine for treatment of interstitial cystitis," *Journal of Urology*, Feb 1999.
130. Tufts University study reported on by Susan Lark MD, May 2008.
131. *WHAct*, March 2009, www.cystitispatientsurvey.com
132. *Ibid.*
133. *Ibid.*
134. "The treatment and mistreatment of chronic urgency and frequency," Kay Zakariasen MA & Jennifer Hill MD, *WHAct*, March/April 2009.
135. *WHAct*, April 2009. Survey results at: www.cystitispatientssurvey.com

136. "The Hidden Pain of Interstitial Cystitis," *WHAd*, Feb 2004.
137. *Ibid.*
138. *International Urogynecology Journal*, Nov 2003.

Bladder Cancer

139. "What you need to know about bladder cancer," Mark Schoenberg MD, *Bottom Line Health*, Sept. 2004.
140. "Treatments for early-stage bladder cancer . . . ," *HealthFacts*, May 2009.
141. "What . . . bladder cancer," Schoenberg, *Bottom Line Health*, Sept 2004.
142. *Ibid.*
143. *Choices*, Marion Morra & Eve Potts, Avon Books, 1994.
144. "What . . . bladder cancer," Schoenberg, *Bottom Line Health*, Sept 2004.
145. *American Journal of Clinical Nutrition*, Oct 2008.
146. "Hair dye and cancer," C Robb-Nicholson MD, *HWHW*, Aug 2001.
147. "Hair dye increases bladder cancer risk," Manuela Gago-Dominguez MD, *Bottom Line Health*, Aug 2001.
148. "Hair dye and cancer," C Robb-Nicholson MD, *HWHW*, Aug 2001.
149. *Ibid.*
150. "Treatments for early-stage bladder cancer . . . ," *HealthFacts*, May 2009.
151. "Detection of bladder cancer using a point-of-care proteomic assay," *JAMA*, 293: 810-6, 16 Feb 2005.
152. "Can blood tests detect cancer early?," *HealthNews*, May 2002.
153. "Screening for bladder cancer," *HealthNews*, Oct 2009.
154. From Anderson Cancer Center, *BottomLine Health*, April 2006.
155. "What . . . about bladder cancer,"*Bottom Line Health*, Sept 2004.
156. *NEJM*, 340: 1390, 1424, 1999.

Trauma

- *Quest for Respect*, Linda Braswell, Pathfinder, 1996.
- *Ressurection After Rape*, Matt Aktinson, RAR Publishing, 2008.
  "This is the best book, even if it is written by a man."
- *Rebuilding the Garden: Healing the Spiritual Wounds of Childhood Sexual Assault*, Karla McLaren, Laughing Tree Press, 1997.
- *The Rape Recovery Handbook*, Aphrodite Matsakis, New Harbinger, 2003
- Men's organizations aimed at preventing sexual assault:
  www.mencanstoprape.org
  www.nomas.org
  www.menstoppingviolence.org
- For men who have been abused or assaulted: www.mrcforchange.org

1. Shantideva, quoted in *Boundless Healings*, page 18.
2. *Emotional Genius*, Karla McLaren, Laughing Tree, 2001, page 111.
3. This knowledge has led me to devote my life to countering the trauma wo/men experience in modern medical settings.

4. George Mason University, Worldwide Sexual Assault Statistics, 2005.
5. I have been sexually assaulted four times: an attempted gang rape in Manhattan; a rapist who fled my blood-curdling scream; a doctor who blythely told me my cervix had no nerves while I cried in pain; and the obstetrician who shoved my baby's head back in to do an episiotomy. I repelled the rapists, but not the medical professionals.
6. Finkelhor et al., 1990.
7. "Rape statistics," John Hamlin, University of Minn., 3 March 2005.
8. *Ibid.*
9. *Mindfulness in Plain English*, Bhante Gunaratana, Wisdom, 2010.
10. *Mindful Therapy*, Thomas Bien, Wisdom, 2010.
11. *One Again*, Linda Jean McNabb, Hampton Roads, 2009.
12. *Soul Retrieval*, Sandra Ingerman, Harper Collins, 2006.
13. www.tir.org
14. *Emotional Genius*, Karla McLaren, Laughing Tree, 2001, page 139.
15. *Ibid.*, page 108.
16. *Ibid.*, page 138.

Vulva

• www.yoni.com
• *Cunt*, Inga Muscio, Seal Press, 2009. www.ingalagringa.com
• *Heart of the Flower: The Book of Yonis*, Andrew Barnes & Yvonne Lumsden, Pangia, 2010. www.heartoftheflower.com
• *The Yoni: Sacred Symbol of Female Creative Power*, Rufus Camphausen, Inner Traditions, 1996.

1. Betty Dodson, *Sex for One, The Joy of Selfloving*, Crown, 1974
2. Tee Corrine, *The Cunt Coloring Book*, Last Gasp, 1989 (orig. 1975).
3. Max Dashu's Sacred Vulva poster from www.suppressedhistories.net
4. Judy Chicago, *The Dinner Party*, Viking Penguin, 1996.
5. Morgan Hastings, *The Big Coloring Book of Vaginas*, 2007. Available from www.bigbookaltpress.com
6. *The V Book*, page 19.
7. "Clinical Tips: Vulvar Vestibulitis," *Natural Health Associates*, no date.
8. *The V Book*, page 35.

Vulvodynia

• www.med.umich.edu/obgyn/vulva/vulvedu.html
• www.vulvarpainfoundation.org
• www.vulvarhealth.org
• www.nva.org (National Vulvodynia Association)
• *Vulvodynia Survival Guide*, Howard Glazer, Harbringer, 2002.

9. "A painful women's problem isn't in the mind," Jane E. Brody, *New York Times*, 27 Oct 1993.

10. "News from the society for women's health research," *WHAd*, Oct 2004.
11. "From obscurity to Oprah," Leah Thayer, *Nat'l Women's Health Network News*, May/June 2003.
12. "Genital problems and natural solutions," Bonnie C. Minsky, *Conscious Choice Magazine*, Jan 2004.
13. "Genital pain more common than previously thought," *WHAd,* March 2004.
14. "No sex in the city," C. Von Hoffman, *Health*, Nov. 2001.
15. "Conquering vulvar pain," *Center for Women's Healthcare*, April 2002.
16. *Women's Bodies, Women's Wisdom*, Northrup, page 245.
17. *Prescriber and Clinical Repertory of Medicinal Herbs*, Lt. Col. F. Harper-Shove, Health Science Press, 1938, 1972.
18. *Integrative Herb Guide for Nurses*, page 716.
19. "Genital problems and natural solutions," Bonnie Minsky, *Conscious Choice Magazine*, Jan 2004.
20. *Vulvodynia Survival Guide*, Glazer, New Harbinger, 2002, page 106.
21. *Treatment of Vulvodynia with Calcium Citrate*, C. Solomons, 1994.
22. "A painful. . . ," Jane Brody, *NY Times*, Oct 1993.
23. "Oxalate content by food group," handout from Vulvodynia Self-Help Group, 2002.
24. *Natural Choices for Women's Health*, Laurie Steelsmith, Three Rivers Press, 2005.
25. *Herbalgram,* number 58, page 43.
26. *Treatment of Vulvodynia with Calcium Citrate*, C Solomons, 1994.
27. "Chronic Vulvar Pain," *Women's Health Network News*, Nov/Dec1993.
28. "Antibiotic use increases symptomatic vulvovaginal candidiasis," *American Journal of Obstetrics & Gynecology*, 180:14-7, Jan 1999.
29. Personal correspondence from Susan Klein, 1994.
30. *Vulvodynia Survival Guide*, Glazer, New Harbinger, 2002, page 90.
31. *Ibid.*, page 91.
32. *Women's Encyclopedia of Natural Medicine,* Tori Hudson, page 30.

Clitoris

- *The Clitoral Truth, The Secret World at Your Fingertips*, Rebecca Chalker, Seven Stories Press, 2000. www.clitoraltruth.com
- *The Nature and Evolution of Female Sexuality*, Mary Jane Sherfey, Random House, 1966.

Meet Your Clitoris

1. *Woman*, Natalie Angier, page 58.
2. *Ibid.*, page 60.
3. *Ibid.*, pages 68, 69, 70, 72.
4. Ultrasound scans show that women who orgasm during intercourse have an unusually thick urethrovaginal space; this is the G-spot. It is found in about 25 percent of women. (*The Week*, 14 March 2008.)

5. Jacques Duval, 1612, quoted in *Woman*, Natalie Angier, page 62.
6. *Woman*, Natalie Angier, page 70.

How to Have An Orgasm

7. *Women's Anatomy of Arousal,* page 35.
8. Annie Sprinkle, PhD sex educator: www.anniesprinkle.org
9. Barbara Carrellas: urbantantra.org
10. Sheri Winston: www.intimateartscenter.com
11. *New View of A Woman's Body*, page 47.
12. *Woman*, Natalie Angier, page 70.
13. "Enliven your sex life," *Women's HealthAdvisor*, Jan 2005.
14. *Ibid.*
15. "Boosting desire: What works for women," JHML, March 2007.
16. *Woman*, Natalie Angier, page 73.
17. *Ibid.*, page 70.
18. *WHAct*, Feb 2009. (*American J. Pub Health*, Oct 2008)
19. *Woman*, Natalie Angier, page 72.
20. *Ibid.*, page 71.
21. *The Functions of the Orgasms*, Michel Odent, Pinter & Martin, 2009.
22. *Don Juan and the Art of Sexual Energy*, Tunneshende, Bear, 2001, page 136.
23. "Enliven your sex life," *WHAd*, Jan 2005.
24. *What Your Doctor May Not Tell You About Fibroids*, page 112.
25. *Woman*, Angier, page 71.
26. *The Perfect Fit*, Edward Eichel, Signet, 1992.
27. "Sex & Drugs," Beth Howard, *More*, May 2009.
28. "The vibrator," *Scientific American*, Dec 2008.
29. *Ibid.*
30. *Journal of Sexual Medicine*, June 2009. (internet-based survey completed by over two thousand 18–60-year-old women; a companion survey found nearly half of 18–60-year-old men use vibrators.)
31. "How to have great sex," Beth Howard, *More*, May 2009. (quote: Gail Saltz, *The Ripple Effect: How Better Sex Can Lead to a Better Life*)
32. "How to have great sex," Beth Howard, *More*, May 2009. (quote: Christiane Northrup, *The Secret Pleasues of Menopause*)
33. "Boosting desire," *JHML*, March 2007.
34. "Enliven your sex life," *Women's HealthAdvisor*, Jan 2005.
35. *The Secret Pleasues of Menopause*, Christiane Northrup. (*More*, May 2009)
36. *Archives of Sexual Behavior*, Barry Komisarul, 1992. (*More*, Feb 2011)
37. *More*, Feb 2011. (*Journal of Sexual Medicine*)
38. "Orgasm and migraine," RW Evans et al., *Headache*, 41;512-14, 2001.
39. *NEJM*, page 1647, 19 Oct 2006.
40. "Boosting desire," *JHML*, March 2007.
41. "Enliven your sex life," *WHAd*, Jan 2005.

42. *WHAd*, Dec 2004. (randomized, placebo-controlled multi-center clinical trials presented at the meeting of the North American Menopause Society)
43. "Enliven your sex life," *Women's HealthAdvisor*, Jan 2005.
44. *Ibid.*
45. *WHAct*, July/Aug 2009.
46. "Boosting desire: What works for women," JHML, March 2007.
47. *Ibid.*

Clitorectomy

- *Warrior Marks,* Alice Walker, Harcourt+Brace & Company, 1993.

48. *Woman*, Angier, page 81.
49. *Women's Encyclopedia of Myths and Secrets*, Barbara Walker, Harper, 1983.
50. *Woman*, Angier, page 76.
51. *The Vagina Monologues*, Eve Ensler, Villard, 1998.
52. *Woman*, Angier, page 80.
53. *Ibid.*, page 79.
54. *Ibid.*
55. *Ibid.*, page 64.
56. *Ibid.*
57. The Federal Prohibition of Female Genital Mutilation Act of 1995 makes it illegal to cut the labia minora, labia majora, and/or clitoirs of any girl under the age of 18 except for medical reasons.
58. *Woman*, Angier, page 78.
59. Adapted and quoted from *Woman*, Angier, page 77.
60. *Ibid.*

Vagina

1. www.badmimi.com
2. *The Vagina Monologues*, Eve Ensler, Villard, 1998.
3. "Antibiotics and vaginal infections," *NEJM Health News*, 2001.
4. *Taking Charge of Your Fertility,* Toni Weschler, HarperCollins, 2002.
5. *Honoring Our Cycles*, Katie Singer, New Trends, 2006, and *The Garden of Fertility*, Avery, 2004.
6. "Antibiotics and vaginal infections," *NEJM Health News*, 2001.

Vaginal Dryness

7. "Is vaginal estrogen safe?," *Harvard Women's Health*, Nov 2007.
8. *What Your Doctor May Not Tell You About Fibroids*, page 59.
9. "Sexual activity. . . ," *HWHW*, March 2010.
10. *WHAd*, July 2006.
11. "Is vaginal estrogen safe?," *Harvard Women's Health*, Nov 2007.
12. *Ibid.*
13. "Soft, pink comforting mallow, hollyhock flowers, my grandmother's cheeks, safety among the flowers," writes Dana Woodruff, 2010.

Don't Douche

14.“ Dangerous Hygiene,” *Health*, July/Aug 1992.
15. *Ibid.*
16. *Ibid.*

Non-specific vaginitis

17. Communication from anonymous student, 2008.
18. Personal conversation with herbalist Rina Nissim, in Switzerland, 1998.

Vestibular Cysts/Ulcers

19. *How to Stay Out of the Gynecologist's Office,* page 23.
20. *The Goddess Oracle*, Amy Sophia Marashinsky, HarperCollins, 2003.
21. “DES may be forgotten, but it's not gone,” *Health News,* May 2003.

Vaginal Cancer

22. “DES may be forgotten, but it's not gone,” *Health News,* May 2003.
23. *Ibid.*
24. *Ibid.*
25. “Cervical cancer vaccine also prevents vaginal, vulvar cancers,” *WHAd*, Aug 2006.
26. Some young women say Gardasil ruined their health. As with all drugs, there is a risk-to-reward ratio. Consider them both before using.

Vaginal Infections & STDs

- www.PlannedParenthood.org
- www.cdc.gov/std
- *Sexually Transmitted Diseases*, Montreal Health Press, Canada, 1987.

1. *Houston Chronicle*, 12 March 2008.
2. *WHAct*, July/Aug 2004.

STDs

3. “Sexually Transmitted Diseases,” Planned Parenthood, 1999, page 6.
4. *Ibid.*, page 13.
5. *Ibid.*, page 18.
6. Center for Disease Control: STD surveillance website

Yeast (*Candida*)

7. “Big Love,” *Discover*, May 2007.
8. “Yeast Infections,” *Environmental Nutrition*, Dec 1998.
9. *Wellness Letter*, Sept 2004.
10. “Mushroom remedy for chronic yeast infections: maitake may reduce itching and soreness,” *Prevention*, Nov 2001.
11. *Encyclopedia of Natural Medicine*, Murray & Pizzorno, page 186.
12. *Herbs for Health and Healing,* page 81.
13. *The Green Pharmacy*, page 463.
14. *Encyclopedia of Natural Medicine*, Murray & Pizzorno, page 187.
15. *The Family Herbal*, page 212.

16. *The Green Pharmacy*, page 463. *(Encyc. Nat. Med.*, page 186)
17. *University of CA Berkeley Wellness Letter*, Sept 2004.
18. *Worst Pills, Best Pills*, Nov 2004. (*British Medical Journal*, 27 Aug 2004)

Trich

19. *Natural Healing in Gynecology*, page 75.
20. "Big love," *Discover*, May 2007.
21. S. Gupre, *Am J Des Child*, 129(866), 1975. ("Antimicrobial actions of berberine sulfate," D. Hoffman, *Townsend Letter*, no date)
22. "In vitro effects of berberine sulfate on the growth of *Entamoeba histolytica, Giardia lamblia, Trichomonas vaginalis*," M. Torii, et al., *Annals of Tropical Medical Parasitology*, 85(417-25), 1991.
23. S. Gupre, *Am J Des Child*, 129(866), 1975
24. "In vitro effects of berberine sulfate. . . ," M Torii, et al., *Annals of Tropical Medical Parasitology*, 85(417-25), 1991.
25. *The Complete Book of Essential Oils*, page 267.

Bacterial Vaginosis

26. "Bacterial vaginosis: diagnosis, prevention, and treatment," Susanne Hendrick, 1993.
27. *The V Book*, page 219.
28. *Ibid.*
29. *Ibid.*
30. "All infections aren't yeast based," *Prevention*, Oct 2001.
31. "Bacterial vaginosis often comes back," Paul Donohue MD, 1998.
32. "More than a gut feeling," *Science News*, 161(72-3).
33. *Textbook of Modern Herbology*, page 111.
34. "Bacterial vaginosis often comes back," Paul Donohue MD, 1998.

Chlamydia

35. "Chlamydia: cloak and dagger," *Harvard Medical School*, Oct 1988.
36. "Can *Chlamydia* be stopped?" *Scientific American*, May 2005.
37. "Chlamydia - reported cases among women. . . ," *NIH Morbiditiy and Mortality Weekly*, 48(53):30, 6 April 2001.
38. "Testing for *Chlamydia* in adolescent females," *Journal Watch* (*NEJM*), 1 Nov 2000.
39. "Can *Chlamydia* be stopped?" *Scientific American*, May 2005.
40. "Sexually Transmitted Diseases," Planned Parenthood, 1999.
41. "Another infection rages silently in young adults," K. Fackelmann, *Science News,* 154(204), 26 Sept 1998.
42. "Can *Chlamydia* be stopped?" *Scientific American*, May 2005.
43. *Ibid.*
44. http://www.cdc.gov/std/stats/womenandinf.htm, June 2007.
45. "Can *Chlamydia* be stopped?" *Scientific American*, May 2005.
46. *Ibid.*

47. "Chlamydia: cloak and dagger," *Harvard Health Letter*, Oct 1988
48. *Science News,* 154(204), 26 Sept 1998.
49. *Ibid.*
50. "Effect of nonoxynol-9 gel on . . . gonorrhea and chlamydial infection," RE Roddy, *JAMA*, 287:1117-22, 6 March 2002.
51. "Can *Chlamydia* be stopped?" *Scientific American*, May 2005.
52. "Effectiveness of . . . nonoxynol-9 vaginal gel . . . in female sex workers," Van Damme et al., *Lancet*, 360:971-7, 28 Sept 2002.
53. "Effect of nonoxynol-9 gel on . . . ," RE Roddy, *JAMA*, 2002.

Herpes
54. *Our Bodies, Ourselves*, page 351.
55. "Genital herpes: common but misunderstood," *HWHW*, Dec 2005.
56. "Antiviral suppresses genital herpes," *Science News,* 19 Sept 1998.
57. "By the numbers," *Discover*, Sept 2001.
58. "Genital herpes. . . .," *HWHW*, 2005.
59. ". . . new infections with herpes simplex virus . . .," Langenberg AGM et al., *NEJM*, 341:1432-8, 4 Nov 1999.
60. "Herpes marchs on," *The Week*, 26 March 2010.
61. "Genital herpes: tincture of time," *HealthNews*, August, date missing.
62. *JAMA*, April 1999, pp. 210-212.
63. "Herpes marchs on," *The Week*, 26 March 2010.
64. "Genital herpes. . . .," *HWHW*, 2005.
65. *Herbal Remedies for Women,* page 218.
66. *Ibid.*
67. "Antiviral suppresses genital herpes," *Science News,* 1998.

Gonorrhea
68. *PDR Family Guide to Women's Health*, page 118.
69. "Tenacious STD," *Science News*, 171:245, 21 April 2007.
70. *PDR Family Guide to Women's Health*, page 118.
71. "Sexually Transmitted Diseases," Planned Parenthood, 1999.
72. *PDR Family Guide to Women's Health*, page 119.
73. *Encyclopedia of Natural Medicine*, Murray & Pizzorno, page 529.
74. "Tenacious STD," *Science News*, 171:245, 21 April 2007.
75. *Ibid.*

Syphillis
76. CDC Syphilis Report, 2007.
77. NDRI.com (as of 1/1/11)
78. *Nature*, 433: 417-421, 27 Jan 2005.
79. *PDR Family Guide to Women's Health,* pages113-115.
80. *Ibid.*

Cervix

• www.cervicalcancercampaign.org

1. *A New View of a Woman's Body*, Fed. of Feminist Health Centers, 1981.
2. Personal correspondence, 2009.
3. *How to Stay Out of the Gynecologist's Office*, page 30.

Genital Warts/HPV

4. "The cervical dilemma: Some warts better left untreated," Kathy Fackelmann, *Science News*, 139: 362-3, 8 June 1991.
5. "HPV doesn't have to spell cancer," C Aschwanden, *Health*, Jan 2002.
6. "Cervical cancer vaccines in context," A Fugh-Berman, *WHAd*, 2007.
7. "HPV doesn't . . . cancer, "Aschwanden, *Health*, Jan 2002.
8. "Contagion: A sometimes lethal sexual epidemic that condoms can't stop," Jerome Groopman, *New Yorker*, 13 Sept 1999.
9. *The No-Hysterectomy Option*, H Goldfarb MD, John Wiley & Sons, 1990.
10. "Cervical cancer vaccines in context," A Fugh-Berman, *WHAd*, 2007.
11. "Contagion. . . ," Jerome Groopman, *New Yorker*, 13 Sept 1999.
12. "Non-AIDS sexually transmitted diseases remain a serious and sizeable threat," Deborah Narrigan, *Network News*, Nov 1989.
13. "Contagion. . .,"*New Yorker*, 1999.
14. "FDA licenses new vaccine. . . .," FDA news release, June 2006.
15. "Contagion. . . ," Jerome Groopman, *New Yorker*, 13 Sept 1999.
16. *Ibid.*
17. "Infections tied to head and neck cancers," L. Wang, *Sci. News, 159:229.*
18. *Natural Healing in Gynecology*, page 43.
19. C*omplete Woman's Herbal*, Anne McIntyre, page 240.
20. "Treatment of skin papillomas with topical alpha-lactalbumin-oleic acid," Catharina Svanborh MD, *NEJM*, 350:2663-2672, 2004.
21. "Papilloma virus infections spike in sunny months," *Sci. News, 165:237.*
22. *Our Bodies, Ourselves*, page 357.
23. "Do-it-yourself treatment for genital warts," *Health Facts,* Feb 1998.
24. "Screening for cervical cancer," *HealthFacts,* XV (136), Sept 1990.
25. "Adding an HPV," *WHAd*, July 2002.
26. "One way to avoid unnecessary testing after ambiguous pap results," *HealthFacts,* May 2001.
27. *PDR Family Guide to Women's Health,* page 107.

Pap Smear

28. "Accuracy of the Papanicolaou test in screening for and follow-up of cytologic abnormalities: a systematic review," K.Nanda MD et al., *Annals of Internal Medicine,* 132:810-819, 2000.
29. "The New pap test report: revised guidelines . . . ," *WHAd*, Aug 2002.
30. "Pap test standardization causing unnecessary biopsies," *HealthFacts,* March 1994.
31. "One way to avoid unnecessary testing," *HealthFacts,* 2001.

32. "Cancers that do not kill, prevalent and usually treated aggressively," *Health Facts*, Aug 2006.
33. "2001 Consensus guidelines for management of women with cervical cytological abnormalities," *JAMA*, Vol 287:2120-2129.
34. "HPV test clarifies ambiguous Pap results," *Health News*, 2001.
35. *Medical Self Care Book of Women's Health*, page 5.
36. *Lancet Oncology*, Oct 2008.
37. "One Way to Avoid Unnecessary Testing," *HealthFacts,* 2001.
38. National Cancer Institute website, 2006.
39. "Vinegar swab reveals cervical problems," *Science News,* 155(219).
40. "Pap smears still necessary after menopause," *Focus on Healthy Aging,* May 2001.
41. "Interpretive variability is substantial for all types of cervical specimens," M. Stoler MD and M. Schiffman MD, *JAMA*, 21 March 2001.

Dysplasia

42. "Abnormal Pap smears: is treatment needed?," A. K. Kirby et al., *Lancet,* 339:828, April 1992.
43. "Dysplasia study supports 'wait and see' approach," *The Women's Letter,* 3(2).
44. "Making sense of PAP tests," Michele Turk, *Am. Health,* March 1994.
45. Philippa Holowaty, *Journal of the Nat'l Cancer Inst.*, 1999.
46. "Nutrients and cervical cancer prevention," C Massion MD, *Alternative Therapies in Women's Health,* 2(8):57-60, Aug 2000.
47. Mark Schiffman, National Cancer Institute, quoted in "Making sense of PAP," M. Turk, 1994.
48. "Women in healthcare talk about cervical dysplasia, HPV, and fibroids," *East West*, Nov 1990.
49. "Keep off the grass," *UCBW*, June 2009.
50. "Summary of data for indole-3-carbinol," *National Institute of Environmental Health Sciences*, 1998.
51. MC Bell et al., "Placebo-controlled trial of indole-3-carbinol in the treatment of cervical dysplasia," presented at 30th Annual Meeting of the Society of Gynecological Oncologists, 20-24 March 1999.
52. "Indole-3-carbinol for cancer prevention," Judith Balk MD, *Alternative Medicine Alert,* 105-107, Sept 2000.
53. "Dietary intake and blood levels of lycopene: association with cervical dysplasia," Kanetshy, et al., *Nutr Cancer* 31:31-40, 1998.
54. CE Butterworth MD et al., *JAMA*, 1992.
55. *Women's Encyclopedia of Natural Medicine*, Hudson, page 53.
56. "Retin-A fights cancer," LD Peden, *American Health,* Oct 1993.
57. "Abnormal cells in the uterine cervix," Ray Peat, *Townsend Letter for Doctors,* Jan 1988.
58. *British Journal of Cancer*, Oct 2009. www.nature.com/bjc/journal/v101/n1/full/6605098a.html

60. "Women in health-care talk about. . . ," *East West*, Nov 1990.
61. *Herbal Healing for Women*, Gladstar, page 164.
62. Available from www.eclecticherb.com
63. "Women in health-care talk about. . . ," *East West*, Nov 1990.
64. *Women's Encyclopedia*, Tori Hudson ND, pages 55, 65.
65. *British Journal of Cancer*, 79:1448, 1999.
66. "Laser surgery outclassed by new. . . ," *Health Facts*, Aug 1992.
67. FL Meyskens, et al., *Journal of the Nat'l Cancer Ins.*, 6 April 1994.
68. "Vitamin A derivative applied to cervix can cause regression of abnormalities," *Health Facts*, May 1994.
69. *How to Stay Out of the Gynecologist's Office*, page 86.
70. "Making sense of PAP tests," Michele Turk, *Amer. Health*, 1994.
71. *The No-Hysterectomy Option*, H. Goldfarb, MD, with Judith Greif, MS, RNC, John Wiley & Sons, 1990.

Cervical Cancer

• www.hvpandcervicalcancercampaign.org
72. "Ovarian cysts," *HealthFacts*, July 1991. (*JAMA*, Feb. 1989)
73. "Amount of virus sets cancer risk," *Science News*, 23 Sept 1995.
74. "A cervical cancer breakthrough," *The Week*, 21 Oct 2005.
75. "Special report: gynecologic cancers," *Weill Medical College Women's Health Advisor*, June 2006.
76. "One way to avoid unnecessary testing after ambiguous Pap results," *HealthFacts*, May 2001.
77. "Screening for cervical cancer," *HealthFacts*, XV (136), Sept 1990.
78. "Differences in cervical cancer mortality among black and white women," EA Howell, *Obstet Gynecol*, 94(509-15), Oct 1999.
79. "Does his circumcision lower her risk for cervical cancer?," Andrew Kaunitz MD, *Journal Watch*, 7(6):41.
80. "Screening for cervical cancer," *HealthFacts*, Sept 1990.
81. *Encyclopedia of Natural Medicine*, Murray & Pizzorno, page 278.
82. "Co-conspirator? Genital herpes linked to cervical cancer," N. Sepa, *Science News*, 162:292-3, 9 Nov 2002.
83. "Pap smears: do older women really need them?," Linda Wilton RN, *A Friend Indeed*, XVII(3), July/Aug 2000.
84. "Underdiagnosis of HIV and AIDS in women," Tori Hudson ND, *Townsend Letter for Doctors*, July 1992.
85. "Study links chlamydia to cancer," *JAMA*, 2001.
86. "Personality patterns in patients with malignant tumors of the breast and cervix," Tarlau and Smalheiser, *Psychosomatic Medicine*, vol 13(117), 1951.
87. "Psychological setting of uterine cervical cancer," LG Koss, *Annals of the New York Academy of Sciences*, vol 125(807-13), 1966.
88. *Women's Bodies, Women's Wisdom*, Christiane Northrup, page 243.

89. Study by CE Butterworth, MD at U of Alabama Med School (*Encyclopedia of Natural Medicine*).
90. "Douching: new dangers identified," Cynthia Pearson, *The Network News,* March 1991. (*Am.J. of Epid*, 15 Feb 1991)
91. Directions for making decocted tincture: *Herbal Emissaries*, page 294.
92. Products available from www.edgarcayce.com
93. *Desk Reference to Nature's Medicine*, Foster, page 117.
94. *Ibid.*
95. "Nutrients and Cervical Cancer Prevention," C. Massion MD, *Alternative Therapies in Women's Health,* 2(8):57-60, Aug 2000.
96. "Physician's perspective: alternative cancer therapies can be dangerous," Carolyn Runowicz MD, *Health News (NEJM)*, Feb 2003.
97. "The effect of beta-carotene and the regression and progression of cervical dysplasia," *Journal of Clinical Epidemiology*, 44(273-283), 1991.
98. "Effects of beta-carotene and other factors on the outcome of cervical dysplasia," *Gynecology Oncology*, 65(483-492), 1997.
99. Randomized double-blind trial of beta carotene and vitamin C in women with minor cervical abnormalities," *British Journal of Cancer*, 79(1448-1453), 1999.
100. Ad from a 1957 medical journal, reprinted in *Science News*.
101. "DES – Forgotten by many but still an important women's health issue," Ann Mulligan, *The Network News,* Nov/Dec 1998.
102. "DES," Susan Ince, *Women's Health and Fitness News,* Dec 1988.
103. "Effects of beta-carotene . . . dysplasia," *Gyne Onc*, 65(483-492), 1997.
104. *The Complete Book of Essential Oils and Aromatherapy,* page 251.
105. "FHIT gene, smoking, and cervical cancer," Christine Holschneider et al., Society for Gynecological Oncologists, 1 March 2000.
106. "Tobacco in semen," www.ncbi.nlm.nih.gov/pubmed/16169398
107. "Chemoradiation boosts cervical cancer survival," *Lancet,* 8 Sept 2001.
108. *Herbal Medicine, Healing & Cancer*, Donald Yance page 15.
109. *The Complete Woman's Herbal*, Anne McIntyre, page XXX.
110. *For Women of All Ages*, Sheldon Cherry MD, page 189.
111. "From abnormal Pap to hysterectomy," *Health Facts,* Aug. 1992.

Uterus

Menstruation

Some euphemisms for menstruation: Auntie Flo; the Red Sox have a home game; riding the crimson tide; the English are coming; saddling up old rusty; wearing the red badge of courage; having ketchup with your steak; are there communists in the fun house?

- Cloth menstrual pads and keeper cups available from: www.lunapads.com; www.gladrags
- Menstrual sea sponges from: www.jadeandpearl.com

- "Temple of the Blood" CD, meditation by Katherine Cunningham from www.lulu.com
- The Museum of Menstruation: www.mum.org
- Society for Menstrual Cycle Research: www.menstruationresearch.org
- Center for Menstrual Cycle/Ovulation Research: www.cemcor.ubc.ca
- *Blood Magic, The Anthropology of Menstruation*, Thomas Buckley & Alma Gottlieb, University of California Press, 1988.
- *Dragontime: Magic & Mystery of Menstruation*, Luisa Francia, Ash Tree Publishing, 1991.
- *Bloodtime, Moontime, Dreamtime* DVD by Roberta Cantow. www.originaldigital.net/bmd/
- *Her Blood Is Gold,* Lara Owen, HarperSanFrancisco, 1993.
- *Moon Days*, Cassie Premo Steele, PhD, Ash Tree Publishing, 1999.
- *Red Moon*, Miranda Gray, Element, 1994.
- *Songs of Bleeding*, Spider, Black Thistle, 1992.
- *105 Ways to Celebrate Menstruation*, Kami McBride, Living Awareness, 2004.

1. *What Your Doctor May Not Tell You About Fibroids*, page 53.
2. "Tampon safety, revisited," Yoland Lenzy and Amy Allina, *National Women's Health Network News*, July/Aug 1999.
3. *Ibid.*
4. *Ibid.*
5. *Ibid.*
6. *Ibid.*
7. *Ibid.*

Menstrual Pain

8. "Cured with cod liver oil," *Wise Traditions*, Dec 2003.
9. *What Your Doctor May Not Tell You About Fibroids*, page 128.
10. "Dong Quai a versatile Oriental herb for women's health problems," Brigitte Mars, *East West*, Nov 1990.
11. *What Your Doctor May Not Tell You About Fibroids*, page 57.
12. "Tubal ligation: link to menstrual problems," *American Journal of Obstetrics and Gynecology*, 166:1698, June 1992.

Heavy Bleeding

13. *Acta Obstetric Gynecology Scandanavia*, 45: 320-351, 1966.
14. *Our Bodies, Ourselves*, page 657.
15. *What Your Doctor May Not Tell You About Fibroids*, page 51.
16. *HWHW*, May 2002.
17. "Do endometrial polyps need to be removed?" *HWHW*, May 2002.
18. *Science News*, 165:335, 22 May 2004.
19. *What Your Doctor May Not Tell You About Fibroids*, page 99.
20. *Women's Wellness Today*, Special Report, Susan Lark, 2006.
21. "Anemia," *Women's Health Today*, Susan Lark, 2006.

22. *HealthFacts*, March 2000.
23. *Delmar's Integrative Herb Guide for Nurses*, page 647.
24. "Cured with cod liver oil," *Wise Traditions*, Dec. 2003.
25. *What Your Doctor May Not Tell You About Fibroids*, page 101.
26. "Vitamin A is bone poison," *NEJM*, 23 Jan 2003. (www.webmd.com)
27. *What Your Doctor May Not Tell You About Fibroids*,, page 111.
28. *Fibroid Tumors & Endometriosis*, Dr. Susan Lark.
29. *What Your Doctor May Not Tell You About Fibroids*, page 143.
30. *Ibid.*, page 144.
31. *Ibid.*, page 145.
32. "Surgical options for women with heavy menses," *Science News*, 165:197, March 24, 2004. (*JAMA*, 24/31 March 2004)
33. *What Your Doctor May Not Tell You About Fibroids*, page 148.
34. "Mirror-Image Molecules," *Science News*, 29 May 1993.
35. *Science News*, 3 Feb 2007.

Fibroids

• HERS (Hysterectomy Education and Resource Services): free counseling at 1-888-750-HERS or 610-667-7757 www.hersfoundation.com
• National Uterine Fibroids Foundation: 800-874-7247; www.nuff.org
• Center for Uterine Fibroids: 800-722-5520; www.fibroids.net
• http://nwhn.org/fibroid-treatment-options

36. "Pelvic organ prolapse & ending the epidemic of unnecessary hysterectomies," Pam Geyer, *Women's Halth Activist*, Nov/Dec 2009.
37. "Zapping fibroids without surgery," *WHAd*, July 2005.
38. *What Your Doctor May Not Tell You About Fibroids*, page 17.
39. "Women and fibroids: making the best decisions," *Women's Health Activist*, Nov/Dec 2006.
40. Statement by Elizabeth Stewart MD, clinical director of the Center for Uterine Fibroids at Brigham and Women's Hospital, Boston.
41. "Take tea and see: treating fibroid tumors without surgery," Sarah Arsone, *Ms*, Dec 1988.
42. *What Your Doctor May Not Tell You About Fibroids*, page 26.
43. "Zapping fibroids without surgery," *WHAd*, July 2005.
44. Sadja Greenwood MD, "Uterine fibroids," *Medical Selfcare*, July 1988.
45. "Genetic culprit: mutation increases risk for uterine fibroids," Nathan Seppa, *Science News* 161:149, 9 March 2002.
46. "Fibroids: new options, not enough answers," *The Women's Health Activist* (National Women's Health Network), July 2010.
47. "What to do about fibroids," *HWHW*, July 2008.
48. *What Your Doctor May Not Tell You About Fibroids*, page 15.
49. *Ibid.*, page 17.
50. *Ibid.*
51. "Genetic culprit . . . ," Nathan Seppa, *Science News*, 9 March 2002.

52. *What Your Doctor May Not Tell You About Fibroids*, page 23.
53. *Ibid.*, pages 24 and 138. (*Amer. J. of Obst. and Gynec.*, 1995)
54. *HealthFacts*, March 2000.
55. *What Your Doctor May Not Tell You About Fibroids*, page 10.
56. *Ibid.*
57. *Ibid.*, page 21.
58. *Ibid.*
59. *Ibid.*, page 19.
60. *Ibid.*, page 17.
61. *HealthFacts*, March 2000.
62. *What Your Doctor May Not Tell You About Fibroids*, page 20.
63. *Ibid.*, page 29.
64. *Natural Choices for Women's Health*, Laurie Steelsmith, Three Rivers Press, 2005.
65. *Ayurvedic Healing for Women*, Atreya, page 156.
66. *Women's Bodies, Women's Wisdom*, Chris Northrup, page 187.
67. *What Your Doctor May Not Tell You About Fibroids*, page 88.
68. "Uterine fibroids may have a dietary links," *Journal of Obstetrics and Gynecology*, Sept 1999. (*Network News*, Sept/Oct 1999)
69. *What Your Doctor May Not Tell You About Fibroids*,, page 24.
70. "Fending off fibroids," Susan Lark MD, *Vegetarian Times*, Sept 1993.
71. *Journal of Obstetrics and Gynecology*, Sept 1999. (*HealthFacts*, Nov. 1999)
72. *Journal of Obstetrics and Gynecology*, Sept 1999.
73. *Ayurvedic Healing for Women*, Atreya, Weiser, 1999.
74. *What Your Doctor May Not Tell You About Fibroids*, page 111.
75. *Ibid.*, page 71.
76. *Ibid.*, page 72.
77. *Ibid.*, page 69.
78. *Ibid.*
79. Personal correspondence from Chinmayo Forro, CDM, midwife.
80. *What Your Doctor May Not Tell You About Fibroids*, page 65.
81. *Ibid.*, page 70.
82. *Delmar's Integrative Herb Guide for Nurses*, page 726.
83. *Alternative Medicine Digest*, March 1998.
84. "Fighting fibroids naturally," Meg Lundstrom, *Country Living*, 2001.
85. *Fibroid Tumors & Endometriosis: Self Help*, Dr. Susan Lark, page 201.
86. *American Journal of Obstetrics and Gynecology*, 1995. (*Fibroids*, page 138)
87. *HealthFacts*, March 2000.
88. "New fix for fibroids?," *More*, Jan 2011. (NIH studies)
89. *Obstetrics & Gynecology*, Feb 2003. (*HealthNews*, April 2003)
90. *Fertility and Sterility*, Stefano Palomba MD. (*Fibroids*, page 159)
91. "Uterine leiomyomata: A review," Tori Hudson ND, *Townsend Letter for Doctors*, Oct 1993.

92. *What Your Doctor May Not Tell You About Fibroids*, page 42.
93. *Ibid.*, page 84. (Study by R. Reiter MD, U of Iowa Coll Med.)
94. "Fibroids: New treatments will prevent hysterectomy for millions of women" *American Health*, Sept 1993.
95. "Saying good-bye to fibroids: Now you can shrink these tumors and skip major surgery," *Health*, March 2000.
96. Phyllis Gee MD, director, North Texas Fibroid Inst., Plano, TX.
97. "Ultrasound option to messy surgery," www.insightec.com.
98. *Hysterectomy, Exploring Your Options*," Esher Eisenberg MD, Johns Hopkins, 2003, page 35.
99. "Lasers Help Shrink Uterine Fibroids," *New York Times*, 12 Dec 2000.
100. "New technique offers less-invasive treatment for fibroids," *Women's Health Advisor*, July 2002.
101. *HealthFacts*, March 2000.
102. "Trade-offs in fibroids treatments," *Science News*, 3 Feb 2007.
103. "New Hope for Fibroids?," Mary J Minkin, MD, *Prevention*, Jan 2002.
104. "Trade-offs in fibroids treatments," *Science News*, 3 Feb 2007.
105. "Zapping fibroids without surgery," *WHAd*, July 2005.
106. *Ibid.*
107. "New hope for fibroids?," Minkin, MD, *Prevention*, Jan 2002.
108. "Fibroid embolization warning," *HealthNews*, 10 Sept. 1999.
109. "Zapping fibroids . . . ," *WHAd*, July 2005.
110. "Common uterine conditions," US Dept. of Health and Human Services, 2009. www.ahrq.gov/consumer/uterine1.htm
111. *A Woman's Guide to Sexual Health*, Minkin & Wright, page 205.
112. *Fibroids: The Complete Guide*, Johanna Skilling.
113. *A Woman's Guide to Sexual Health*, page 206.
114. *A Woman's Guide to Sexual Health*, page 205.
115. *What Your Doctor May Not Tell You About Fibroids*, page 68.
116. *Hysterectomy, Exploring Your Options*," Esher Eisenberg MD, Johns Hopkins, 2003.
117. *The Center for Women's Health Care*, July 2005.
118. "Zapping fibroids," *WHAd*, July 2005.

Adenomyosis

119. "Adenomyosis, understanding the basics," David Redwine, handout, 2010.
120. "Adenomyosis and risk of pre-term delivery," *British Journal of Gynecology*, 114;165-169, Feb 2007.
121. "Adenomyosis: the forgotten diagnosis," Tori Hudson ND, *Townsend Letter for Doctors*, April 1994.
122. *What Your Doctor May Not Tell You About Fibroids*, page 39.

Endometriosis

- Endometriosis Ass'n 800-992-3636 (in Canada: 800-426-2363) www.endometriosisassn.org
- Endo. Research Center (800-239-7280) www.endocenter.org
- M. Ballweg, *The Endometriosis Sourcebook*, Contemporary, 1995.
- *Coping with Endometriosis*, Putnam, 2000.

123. "Endometriosis: the hidden epidemic," Joseph Anthony, *American Health*, May 1996.
124. "Endometriosis linked to other diseases," *HealthFacts*, Dec 2002. (*Human Reproduction*, Oct 2002)
125. Dr. Martha Richardson, *HWHW*, Feb 2006.
126. "Endometriosis," Tori Hudson, *Townsend Letter*, Aug/Sept 1994.
127. Joseph Anthony, *American Health*, May 1996.
128. *Ibid.*
129. ". . . to lower endometriosis risk," *Health*, Dec 2004.
130. "Endometriosis linked to other diseases," *HealthFacts*, Dec 2002.
131. Sharon Lerner, "Dioxin-endometriosis link," *Ms.*, July/Aug 1995.
132. *Ibid.*
133. Dr. Sherry Rier, immunologist at Dartmouth Medical School, lead author of study, quoted in "Endometriosis," *American Health*, May 1996.
134. "Endometriosis: a review," Tori Hudson ND., *Townsend Letter for Doctors*, Aug 1994. (Dr. David Redwine's book: *Fertility & Sterility.*)
135. "... to lower endometriosis risk," *Health*, Dec 2004.
136. *Ibid.*
137. *Ibid.*
138. *Nutrition Action Healthletter*, June 2010. (*Human Reproduction*, online)
139. *Ibid.*
140. "Vegetarians get estrogen boost," *Harvard Medical School Health Letter*, Feb 1991.
141. "Dong Quai is a versatile Oriental herb for women's health problems," Brigitte Mars, *EastWest*, Nov 1990.
142. "Herbal relief for endometriosis," *Body + Soul*, Nov 2009.
143. Andrea DuBrow, "Endometriosis: new developments," *Women's Health Network News*, Sept/Oct 1999.
144. "Mirror-image molecules," *Science News*, 29 May 1993.
145. "Endometriosis at midlife and beyond," *HWHW*, Feb 2006.
146. "Where women's care falls short," *Consumer Reports*, Dec 2003.
147. "Lupron: if it kills prostate cancer, what does it do to women's health?," *WHAct*, Nov/Dec 2008.
148. *Ibid.*
149. "Putting homeopathy to the test," Barbara Bornmann, 1993.
150. *WHAct*, Nov/Dec 2008.

Hysterectomy

- "Common Uterine Conditions: Options for Treatment" includes information on drugs, hormones, life-style changes, and watchful waiting. 800-358-9295 or www.ahrq.gov/consumer/uterine1.htm
- HERS (Hysterectomy Education and Resource Services): free counseling to determine if you need surgery. 1-888-750-HERS or 610-667-7757 www.hersfoundation.com

151. "Pelvic organ prolapse & ending the epidemic of unnecessary hysterectomies," Pam Geyer, *Women's Halth Activist*, Nov/Dec 2009.
152. "Surgical options for women with heavy menses," *Science News*, 165:197, 24 March 2004.
153. Center for Disease Control statistics, 2008.
154. "Abnormal uterine bleeding," *Health News*, June 2004.
155. *HealthFacts*, March 2000. (*Obstetrics and Gynecology*, Feb 2000.)
156. "The endangered uterus," *More*, Jan 2009.
157. "Raise hell about hysterectomies," *Health*, May 2000.
158. Carla Dionne, National Uterine Fibroids Foundation. (*More*, Jan 2009.)
159. *Women Talk About Gynecological Surgery*, Amy Gross & Dee Ito, Harper Perennial, 1991.
160. Winnifred Cutler, study presented to the American College of Obstetrics and Gynecology in 2000. (*More*, Jan 2009.)
161. "Hysterectomy often improves sex life," *Science News*, 8 Jan 2000. (*JAMA*, 24 Nov 1999.)
162. Beth Battaglino, The National Women's Health Resource Center. (*More*, Jan 2009.)
163. "No difference in functioning linked to type of hysterectomy," *Women's Health Advisor*, July 2006. (*Cochrane Collab*, May 2006.)
164. "The endangered uterus," *More*, Jan 2009.
165. *Ibid.*
166. "Hysterectomy and the heart," *Harvard Heart Letter*, June 2006.
167. *Obstetrics and Gynecology*, 241-6, Feb 1998.

Preventing Endometrial Cancer

168. *What Your Doctor May Not Tell You About Fibroids*, page 40.
169. "Preventing Uterine Cancer," *HealthNews*, 1999.
170. "Cancer," *Nutrition Action Healthletter*, Nov 2008.
171. "Cancer Prevention," Mitchell Gaynor MD, *Natural Pharmacy*, April 1999.
172. "Women who get most fiber at 29% less risk of uterine cancer," *Tuft's Uni. Health & Nutrition News*, March 2008. (*Am J Clin Nut*, Dec 2007)
173. *Ibid.*
174. "Alternative cancer therapies . . . dangerous," *HealthNews*, Feb 2003.

175. "Association of soy and fiber consumption with endometrial cancer risk," Goodman, et al., *Am J Epidemiology*, 146:294-306, 1997.
176. "Foods rich in plant estrogens may cut uterine cancer risk," *Women's Health Advisor*
177. *Journal of the National Cancer Institute*, 6 Aug 2003.
178. *Cancer Epidemiological Biomarkers Preview*, 16:723, 2007.
179. *International Journal of Cancer*, 2 July 1999.
180. *International Journal of Cancer*, 123:1877, 2008.
180A. "Regular workouts reduce uterus cancer risk by 30%," *Tufts Uni. Health & Nutrition Letter*, Jan 2011.
181. "High daily alcohol intake may raise endometrial cancer risk," *WHAd*, Nov 2007.
182. "Coffee could cut cancer risk," *Tufts Health Letter*, March 2010.
183. "UVB rays decrease cancer risk," *HealthNews*, Oct 2006.
184. *What You Need to Know About Cancer of the Uterus,* National Institutes of Health Publication #88-1562.
185. "Oral contraceptives? Low-dose version reduces risk of uterine and ovarian cancer," Nancy Cetel MD, *Lear's*, Aug 1993.
186. *Our Bodies, Ourselves*, page 314.
187. "Tamoxifen linked to rare form of uterine cancer," Cindy Pearson, *The Women's Health Network News*, Nov/Dec 2002.
188. "Tamoxifen update: overhyped for healthy women?," Ann Pappert, *Ms.*, Dec 2000.
189. *The Week*, 23 May 2008.

Endometrial Hyperplasia

190. *What Your Doctor May Not Tell You About Fibroids*, page 27.
191. *Ibid.*, page 28.
192. "Uterine hyperplasia," Marcy Holmes, 2009.

Uterine/Endometrial Cancer

- National Women's Health Network information packet on uterine cancer: www.womenshealthnetwork.org.
- *Healing Cancer Peacefully*, Nancy Offenhauser, Round House Press, 2009.

193. "Is the D & C becoming obsolete?," *WHAd*, March 2002.
194. "Answers," NWHN Women's Health Clearinghouse, June 2001.
195. "Women who get the most fiber at 29% less risk of uterine cancer," *Tuft's Uni. Health & Nutrition Newsletter*, March 2008.
196. "Endometrial cancer deaths rise sharply," *Good Medicine*, 2002.
197. Probably due to DES, a drug given to pregnant women, which gives rise to difficult-to-treat reproductive organ cancers in their offspring.
198. "Endometrial cancer . . . additional treatment," *Health News*, May 2005.
199. "Uterine cancer could be harbinger of other cancers," *Health News*, Nov 2006. (*Cancer Research*)
200. *A Homepathic Approach to Cancer*, Ramakrishnan.

201. *What Your Doctor May Not Tell You About Fibroids*, page 28.
202. *WHAct*, July/Aug 2005. (*Amer. J. Epidem.*, April 2005)
203. *Ibid.*
204. "Chemo or radiation for high-risk endometrial cancers? " *HealthNews*, Dec 2006. (*Brit J of Cancer*)
205. "Is the D&C becoming obsolete? " *WHAd*, March 2002.

Pelvic Inflammatory Disease/PID

206. www.cdc.gov/std/pid/stdfact-pid/.htm
207. *Women's Encyclopedia of Natural Medicine*, Tori Hudson, page 217.
208. *Ibid.*
209. *Ibid.*
210. *Ibid.*
211. *Our Bodies, Ourselves*, page 658.
212. "Echinacea species as potential immunostimulatory drugs," *Economic and Medical Plant Research*, 5:253-321, 1991. (cited by Tori Hudson)
213. *Women's Encyclopedia of Natural Medicine*, Tori Hudson, page 218.
214. *Ibid.*, page 74.
215. *A Woman's Guide to Sexual Health*, Minkin & Wright, page 96.
216. *Our Bodies, Ourselves*, page 660.
217. *Ibid.*, page 659.

Endometrial Polyps

218. "Do endometrial polyps need to be removed?" *HWHW*, May 2002.

Ovaries

Ovarian Cysts/PCOS

• *Positive Options for Polycystic Ovary Syndrome*, Christine Craffs-Hinton and Adam Dalen MD, Hunter House, 2004.

1. "Relative frequency of primary ovarian neoplasms: A 10-Year Re view," Koonings, et al., *Obstet Gynecology*, 74:921-26, 1989.
2. "Ovary removal contributes to heart disease," *HealthNews*, Dec 2005. (*Obstetrics & Gynecology*, 2005)
3. Mayo clinic, abstract presented at the American Academy of Neurology conference, April 2005. (*WHAct*, July 2005)
4. *WHAct*, July 2005.
5. *Ibid.*
6. "Ovarian tumor options," *HealthNews*, June 25, 1998. (*Journal of Gynecologic Oncology*, April 1998)
7. National Institutes of Health, "Ovarian cancer: screening, treatment, and follow-up consensus statement," April 1994.
8. *No More Hysterectomies*, Vicki Hufnagel MD, NAL, 1988.
9. "Ovarian cysts: what doctors don't know," Maggy Brown, *HealthFacts*, July 1991.

10. "How common are adnexal cysts in postmenopausal women?" Robert Tebar MD, *Journal Watch*, vol 25/6, 15 March 2005.
11. "Unearthing true desires keeps your ovaries healthy," Mona Lisa Schultz MD, *Body Wisdom*, 2000.
12. *The Hysterectomy Hoax*, Stanley West MD, Doubleday, 1994.
13. "Ovarian cysts," Maggy Brown, *HealthFacts*, July 1991.
14. *Society for Gynecological Oncologists*
15. "Common uterine conditions," US Dept. of Health and Human Services, 2009. www.ahrq.gov/consumer/uterine1.htm
16. "Ovarian cysts," Maggy Brown, *HealthFacts*, July 1991.
17. *The Hysterectomy Hoax*, Stanley West MD, Doubleday, 1994.
18. "iThe nfertility syndrome that can shorten your life," Ingfei Chen, *Health*, April 2000.
19. *The Hysterectomy Hoax*, Stanley West MD, Doubleday, 1994.
20. "Polycystic ovary syndrome," *WHAct*, Jan/Feb 2008.
21. News Notes, *Wise Traditions*, Winter 2003.
22. "Polycystic ovary syndrome," *HWHW*, Nov 1996.
23. *Ibid.*
24. "What is PCOS?," *Nat'l Women's Health Network*, May/June 2001.
25. "Polycystic ovary syndrome," *Tufts Health Letter*, Vol 19, No 5, July 2001.
26. "PCOS," Andrea Dunaif MD, *HealthNews*, July 25, 1998.
27. *HWHW*, Nov 1996.
28. "The infertility syndrome. . . ," Ingfei Chen, *Health*, April 2000.
29. "PCOS may raise heart disease risk," *HealthNews*, April 2002.
30. "The infertility syndrome. . .," Ingfei Chen, *Health*, April 2000.
31. *Ibid.*
32. "Polycystic ovary syndrome," *Tufts University Health and Nutrition Letter*, Vol 19, No 5, July 2001.
33. "Experts dispute soy infant formula safety," Sally Fallon, *Weston A. Price Foundation*, 2002.
34. "Polycystic ovary syndrome," *Harvard Women's Health*, Nov 1996.
35. "Vegan diet helps treat type-2 diabetes," *Envi. Nutr.*, Oct 2006.
36. "Experts dispute soy . . . ," Sally Fallon, *WA Price Foundation*, 2002.
37. *Ibid.*
38. "Polycystic ovary syndrome," *Harvard Women's Health*, Nov 1996.
39. "Help for polycystic ovaries," T Willard, *Herbs for Health*, April 2006.
40. News Notes, *Wise Traditions*, Winter 2003.
41. "PCOS," Andrea Dunaif MD, *HealthNews*, 25 July 1998.
42. "What is PCOS?," *National Women's Health Network*, May/June 2001.
43. Private correspondence from Holly Guzman, Feb 2009.
44. *No More Hysterectomies*, Vicki Hufnagel MD, NAL, 1988.
45. "Healthy ovaries should not be removed," *HealthFacts*, May 2009.
46. *A Woman's Guide to Sexual Health*, Minkin & Wright, page 301.
47. *Ibid.*, page 356.

48. Private correspondence from Ingrid Gordon, RN-BC, April 2009. She has had three ectopic pregnancies.
49. *A Woman's Guide to Sexual Health*, Minkin & Wright, page 357.
50. *Ibid.*, page 359.

Ovarian Cancer

- Gilda Radner Ovarian Cancer site: http:/ovariancancer.com/app/index.php
- Nat'l Ovarian Cancer Coalition, www.ovarian.org 1-800-OVARIAN
- Ovarian Cancer National Alliance, www.ovariancancer.org

51. "Progress report on ovarian cancer screening," *Harvard Women's Health Watch*, April 2010.
52. "Screening test for ovarian cancer," *WHAd*, March 2002.
53. "Progress report on ovarian cancer screening," *Harvard Women's Health Watch*, April 2010.
54. "The math on false positives," *Scientific American*, Oct 2002.
55. "Ovarian cancer: screening, treatment, and follow-up consensus statement," National Institutes of Health, April 1994.
56. "About your health: CA-125," *Nat'l Women's Health Network News*, Jan/Feb 2003.
57. "Ovarian cancer tests," *Health Facts*, Dec 1991.
58. "Progress report on ovarian cancer screening," *Harvard Women's Health Watch*, April 2010.
59. "Proteins' promise," *ScienceNews*, May 2005.
60. "Screening test for ovarian cancer," *WHAd*, March 2002.
61. "Finding ovarian cancer earlier," *Reader's Digest*, March 2008.
62. "Proteomics test for ovarian cancer," *OCNA*, Jan 2004.
63. "Early chemotherapy to prevent ovarian cancer recurrence is unnecessary," *HealthNews*, Aug 2009.
64. *Ibid.*
65. "Who is at increased risk for ovarian cancer?" National Ovarian Cancer Association.
66. "Ovarian cancer and talc," *Cancer*, 50:372-376, 1982.
67. "Talc in normal and malignant ovarian tissue," *Lancet*, 1:499, 1979.
68. *Women's Bodies, Women's Wisdom*, Christiane Northrup, page 218.
69. *American Journal of Epidemiology*, 132:871-876, 1990; and 134(5):457-59, 1991.
70. "Dietary animal fat and relationship to ovarian cancer risk," *Obstetrics & Gynecology*, 63(6):833-838, 1984.
71. "New hope for ovarian cancer," *The Center for Women's Health Care*, Dec 2006.
72. *Journal of the American Dietetic Association*, March 2010.
73. *Ibid.*
74. *Women's Bodies, Women's Wisdom*, Christiane Northrup, page 216.

75. *Ibid.*, page 215.
76. "Birthing age and ovarian cancer risk," Nathan Seppa, *Science News*, 31 July 2004.
77. *Women's Bodies, Women's Wisdom*, Christiane Northrup, page 216.
78. "New evidence of tea benefits," *Environmental Nutrition*, Oct 2006.
79. *JHML*, Vol 18/7. (*Archives of Internal Medicine*, Dec 2005)
80. "New evidence of tea benefits," *Environmental Nutrition*, Oct 2006.
81. "Onions and garlic reduce cancer risks," *Am J Clin Nutr*, Nov 2006. (*Center for Women's Healthcare*, Feb 2007)
82. "Tomatoes, carrots help thwart ovarian cancer," *In'l J Can*, 1 Oct 2002.
83. *A Maverick of Medicine Speaks to Women*, Duane Townsend MD, Woodland, 2003.
84. "High levels of saturated fat promote ovarian cancer," *Journal of the National Cancer Institute.* (*New York Times*, 21 Sept 1994)
85. *Saturday Evening Post*, Sept/Oct 2007.
86. *Ibid.*
87. *Environmental Nutrition*, April 2005. *(Eur J Can Prev*, Feb 2005)
88. *Cancer Epidemiology Biomarkers Review*, 15:364, 2006.
89. *Nutrition Action Healthletter*, Nov 2008.
90. "Drinking more milk may reduce ovarian cancer risk," *Am J Epide*, Sept 2002.
91. *Ibid.*
92. *American Journal of Clinical Nutrition*, Jan 2009.
93. *Tufts Health & Nutrition Letter*, Jan 2008.
94. "High levels of saturated fat promote ovarian cancer," *Journal of the National Cancer Institute.* (*New York Times*, 21 Sept 1994)
95. *Tufts Health & Nutrition Letter*, Jan 2008.
96. Hartge, Schiffman, Hoover, et al., "A case control study of epithelial ovarian cancer," *Am J Ob/Gyn,* 161:10-16, 1989.
97. "Being overweight may raise ovarian cancer risk," *Women's Health Advisor*, Aug 2006. (*Cancer*, 15 May 2006.)
98. *A Maverick . . . Speaks to Women*, D Townsend MD, Woodland, 2003.
99. Presentation at the *American Association for Cancer Research*, Baltimore, 30 Oct - 2 Nov 2005.
100. *Wise Traditions*, Winter 2003.
101. "Ovary-boosting pain reliever," *Health*, March 2007.
102. "Possible liver damage with low doses of acetaminophen," *JAMA*, 1 July 2006.
103. "Reducing the risk of ovarian cancer," *NEJM*, 13 Aug 1998.
104. "Birth control myths – debunked," *Health*, March 2007.
105. "Progestin enhances an anticancer process," *Sci. News*, 26 Sept 1998.
106. "The pill: not just a contraceptive," *Consumer Reports*, April 1999.
107. "Hair dye and cancer," *HWHW*, Aug 2001. (1993 study)
108. "Possible cancer link?," *Alternative Medical Advisor,* Aug 1999.

109. "Progress report on ovarian cancer," *HWHW*, May 2000.
110. "Tubal ligation cuts ovarian cancer risk," *Lancet*, 12 May 2001.
111. "Salpingo-oophorectomy and the risk of . . . cancer in women with BRCA mutation," Finch et al., *JAMA*, 296:185-192, 12 July 2006.
112. "Ovary removal reduces risk for carriers of BRCA mutations," *JAMA*, 12 July 2006. (*WHAd*, Oct 2006.)
113. "Progress report on ovarian cancer," *HWHW*, May 2000.
114. *Women's Bodies, Women's Wisdom*, Northrup, page 216.
115. "The math on false positives," *Scientific American*, Oct 2002.
116. *Cancer*, Aug 2005.
117. "Ovarian cancer: should you be tested?," Leslie Vreeland, *Lear's*, Feb 1994.
118. "Three tests that could save your life," *More*, Jan 2011. (miradx.com)
119. "Ovarian cancer prevention," *WHAct*, Jan/Feb 2008.
120. "Preventing inherited ovarian cancer," *HealthNews,* 10 Sept 1998.
121. "Ovarian cancer: women break the silence," *Ms,* March/April, 1998.
122. *Obstetrics & Gynecology*, May 2009.
123. *Women's Bodies, Women's Wisdom*, Christiane Northrup, page 222. [She says, in 1994, rates have not changed in the past 40 years.]
124. "4 symptoms of ovarian cancer identified," *WHAd*, Nov 2007.
125. "Rectosigmoid obstruction caused by ovarian cancer," Taal, Steinmetz, & Jager, *Clinical Radiology*, 41:170-74, 1990.
126. "Ovarian cancer revealed?," *WHAd*, Oct 2004.
127. "Molecule reveals ovarian cancer," *Science News*, 10 Nov 2001.
128. *Nutrition Action Healthletter*, Nov 2008.
129. "Special report: gynecologic cancers," *WHAd*, June 2006.
130. *American Journal of Epidemiology*, May 2001.
131. "Ovulation cycle linked to ovarian cancer," *Science News*, 5 July 1997.
132. "New hope for ovarian cancer," *The Center for Women's Health Care*, Dec 2006.
133. "Tubal fimbria emerges as an origin for pelvic serious cancer," CP Crum et al., *Clinical Med. Research*, March 2007, 5(1): 35-44.
134. "Being obese or overweight reduces survival rate from ovarian cancer," *Cancer*, 1 Oct 2006. (*Envir. Nutrition.*, Dec 2006.)
135. News report forwarded to me by way of Beijing, 2010.
136. "Estrogen linked to ovarian cancer," *Physician's Committee for Responsible Medicine*, Nov 2001
137. "Windows of time," *Breast Cancer Action*, Sept/Oct 2000.
138. "Body clock vs cancer, " *Bottom Line Health,* 15 December 2000.
139. "Progress report on ovarian cancer," *HWHW*, May 2000.
140. "Chemo update for ovarian cancer," *JHML*, Aug 2006.
141. "Risk of leukemia after platinum-based chemotherapy for ovarian cancer," Travis, et al., *NEJM,* 340:351-57, 1999.

142. "Keep those ovaries," *A Friend Indeed*, Nov 1989.
143. *Hysterectomy: Before and After*, Winnifred Cutler, Harper, 1990.
144. *The Medical Self-Care Book of Women's Health*, page 63.
145. "Chemo update for ovarian cancer," *JHML*, Aug 2006.
146. *HealthNews*, March 2008.
147. Available at the Pittsburgh Medical Center (www.upmc.com)
148. *HealthNews,* Jan 2007. (*American Journal of Roentgenology*)

Penis

- Circumcision Information: www.nocirc.org
- *Marked in the Flesh: Circumcision from ancient Judea to Modern America*, Leonard B. Glick, Oxford University Press, 2005.

"With regard to circumcision, one of the reasons for it is, in my opinion, the wish to bring about a decrease in sexual intercourse and a weakening of the organ in question, so that . . . the organ be in as quiet a state as possible. . . . if at birth this member has been made to bleed and has had its covering taken away from it, it must indubitably be weakened." Maimonides, *Guide to the Perplexed* (Quoted in *God is Not Great*, Christopher Hitchens, Twelve, 2007.)

1. *The Male Herbal*, Green, page 102.
2. The current incidence is one out of one hundred thousand (1/100,000).
3. *The Sexual Herbal*, Mars, page 322.
4. *The Male Herbal*, Green, page 109.
5. "Balloons, condoms release likely carcinogens," *Sci.News,* 23 April 2005.
6. *Ibid.*
7. *Science News*, 25 April 2009.
8. "Effect of nonoxynol-9 gel on . . . gonorrhea and chlamydial infection," RE Roddy, *JAMA*, 287:1117-22, 6 March 2002.
9. *Sexually Transmitted Diseases*, Planned Parenthood, 1999, page 5.
10. *The New Healing Yourself*, Joy Gardner, Crossing Press, 1989, page 212. She says trich is killed if you don't ejaculate for 10 days.
11. *Science News*, 25 April 2009.
12. *Science News*, 18 Nov 2006.
13. *Science News*, 30 Dec 2006.
14. Personal correspondence from James Green.
15. *The Male Herbal*, Green, page 104.
16. *Ibid.*, page 106.
17. "Demand for circumcision exceeds availability in sub-Saharan Africa," *Science News*, 3 Jan 2009.
18. *The Male Herbal*, Green, page 106.
19. *Ibid.*, page 107.
20. *Vital Man*, Buhner, page 72.
21. *The Healing Power of Ginseng*, Paul Bergner, Prima, 1996, page102.

22. "Ginkgo biloba extract in the therapy of erectile dysfunction," R Sikora et al., *Journal of Urology*, 141:188A, 1989.
23. *Vital Man*, Buhner, page 73.
24. *Dr. Duke's Essential Herbs*, page 137.
25. *Vital Man*, Buhner, page 75.
26. *Complete Guide to Herbal Medicines*, page 597.
27. "Man to Man," *Natural Health*, Jan 1998.
28. *Ibid.*
29. *Vital Man*, Buhner, page 76.
30. *The Sexual Herbal*, Mars, page 322.
31. *Vital Man*, Buhner, page 74.
32. "Effect of large doses of nitric oxide precursor, L-arginine, on erectile dysfunction," Zorgniotti et al., Int J Impot Rev, 1:33-5, 1994.
33. *Vital Man*, Buhner, page 77.
34. *Ibid.*, page 78.
35. *Ibid.*

Testicles

- Chinese/Japanese dogwood fruits from www.nl-suplies.com or www.1stchineseherbs.com or www.theherbcupboard.com
- Rye pollen available from www.cernelle.se.com

1. *HealthNews*, May 2004.
2. *The Sexual Herbal*, Mars, page 316.
3. *Our Bodies, Ourselves, for the New Century*, page 637.
4. *Medicinal Plants of the Mountain West*, Michael Moore, Museum of New Mexico Press, 1979, page 124.

Fertility/Infertility

5. Jan Blancato, "Male infertility and reproduction," *Integrative Medicine Consult*, May 2000.
6. *Vital Man*, Buhner, page 71.
7. Blancato, "Male infertility. . . ," *Integrative Medicine Consult*, May 2000.
8. *Vital Man*, Buhner, page 65.
9. *Ibid.*, page 65.
10. *Ibid.*, page 63.
11. *Ibid.*
12. *The Healing Power of Ginseng*, Paul Bergner, Prima, 1996, page 102.
13. Blancato, *Integrative Medicine Consult*, May 2000.
14. "Semen abnormalities, treatment by Chinese medicine," S Becker, *Journal of Chinese Medicine*, 62:46-51, 2000.
15. *Home Herbal*, Penelope Ody, Dorling Kindersley, 1995, page 119.
16. *The Week*, 14 March 2008.
17. *Vital Man*, Buhner, page71.
18. Blancato, *Integrative Medicine Consult*, May 2000.

19. "Effect of ascorbic acid on male fertility," Dawson et al., *Annals of NY Academy of Science*, 498:312-33, 1987.
20. "Treatment of oligospermia with the amino acid arginine," Schacter et al., *Journal of Urology*, 110:311-13, 1973.
21. "Carnitine supplementation in human idiopathic asthenospermia," Vitali et al., *Drugs Exp Clin Res*, 21:157-9, 1995.
22. "Fluoride-induced disruption of reproductive hormones in men," Ortiz-Perez et al., *Environmental Research*, 93:20-30, 2003.

Testicular Cancer

23. "Manhood's cancer," Janet Raloff, *Science News*, 26 Feb 1994.
24. *Ibid.*
25. *Archives of Disease in Childhood*, Sept 2000.
26. "Manhood's cancer," Janet Raloff, *Science News*, 26 Feb 1994.
27. *Ibid.*
28. *Ibid.*
29. "Positively against pollutants," *Discover*, May 2000.
30. *Esquire*, January 2000.
31. *Journal of the National Cancer Institute,* 1 Oct 1997.
32. "Manhood's cancer," Janet Raloff, *Science News*, 26 Feb 1994.

Testosterone Supplementation?

33. "Hormones for men," Jerome Groopman, *New Yorker*, 29 July 2002.
34. *Ibid.*
35. *Ibid.*
36. *Ibid.*
37. "High testosterone linked to prostate cancer," *Science News,* 8 Oct 2005.
38. "Unproven Elixir," Ben Harper, *Science News,* 10 May 2003.
39. *Ibid.*
40. *Ibid.*
41. *Ibid.*

Pine pollen

42. *The Natural Testosterone Plan,* Buhner, page 27.
43. *Ibid.*, page 28.
44. *Ibid.*
45. *Ibid.*, page 26.
46. *Ibid.*, page 29.
47. *Ibid.*, page 30.
48. *Ibid.*, page 31.

Prostate

1. "Radical prostates: female hormones may play a pivotal role," Janet Roloff, *Science News,* 151:126-127 22 Feb 1997.

PSA Test

2. "The prostate predicament," Benedict Carey, *Health*, May/June 1994.
3. "Prostate test found to save few lives," *New York Times*, 9 March 2009. (*NEJMonline*)
4. Thomas Schwenk MD, *Journal Watch General Medicine*, 29 Oct 2009.
5. "World's best free prostate cure," M Laux MD, *Naturally Well Today*, 2006.
6. uhoh missing ref, for quote no less!!
7. "PSA testing in the spotlight," *UCBW*, Nov 2000.
8. *LA Times*, 19 March 2009. (*NEJM*)
9. *New York Times*, 9 March 2009.
10. *Science News*, 8 April 2000.
11. "What's a man to do? Four vital health-care decisions," *Consumer Reports on Health*, Dec 2003.
12. *University of California at Berkeley Wellness Letter*, Sept 2007.
13. "Making sense of PSA," *HealthNews*, April 2001.
14. *Ibid.*
15. "The prostate predicament," Benedict Carey, *Health*, May/June 1994.
16. "Making sense of PSA," *HealthNews*, April 2001.
17. "PSA testing," *UCBW*, Nov 2000.
18. *Science News*, 8 April 2000.
19. "Checking PSA speed . . . ," *Consumer Reports on Health*, June 2007.
20. "When medical tests steer you wrong," *Bottom Line Health*, Oct 2004.
21. "Checking PSA speed . . . ," *Consumer Reports on Health*, June 2007.
22. "New test detects early prostate cancer," *HealthNews*, Sept 2005.
23. *JAMA*, 3 April 2002. (*HealthNews*, June 2002)
24. "Prostate cancer test becomes more accurate," *HealthNews*, July 1998. (*JAMA*, 20 May 1998)
25. "Flaxseed supplementation (not dietary fat restriction) reduces pros tate cancer proliferation rates in men presurgery," Demark-Wahnfried et al., *Cancer Epidemiology, Biomarkers & Prevention*, Dec 2008, 17; 3577.
26. *Urology*, 63(5):900-904, 2004.
27. *Urology*, 58(1):47-52, 2001.
28. Dr. David Williams, *Library of Medical Lies*, 2007.
29. "What men need to know about prostate cancer and diet," *Environmental Nutrition*, Sept 2002.
30. "Health benefit of pomegranate juice on prostate cancer and the heart," *Harvard Health Publications*, 2008.
31. *Healing Foods*, Amanda Ursell, page 60.
32. JM Potts, "Prospective identification of NIH cat. IV prostatitis in men with elevated PSA," *Journal of Urology*, 164:1550-3, Nov 2000.
33. *NEJM*, 349: 215-224, 2003.
34. *UCBW*, March 2007. (*Lancet*)
35. *Cancer*, March 1, 2005.

36. "The prostate predicament," B Carey, *Health*, May/June 1994.
37. *Ibid.*

BPH

38. "World's best free prostate cure," M Laux MD, *Naturally Well Today*, 2006.
39. *JAMA*, 280(18):1604-9, 1998.
40. "World's best free prostate cure," M Laux MD, *Naturally Well Today*, 2006.
41. American Urological Association, 2005.
42. *John Hopkins White Paper on Prostate Disorders*, 2009.
43. "Herbal prostate remedies?," Gerber, *HealthNews*, 4(12):1-2, 1 Oct 1998.
44. Body-slant furniture resource: www.ageeasy.com (888-243-3279)
45. *American Journal of Clinical Nutrition*, Feb 2007.
46. "Dietary factors in prostate enlargement," *Am. J. Clin. Nut.* 85:523, 2007.
47. *Eur URol*, 46:182-187, 2004.
48. *The Prostate Cure*, Harry Preuss and Brenda Adderly, Crown, 1998.
49. *British Journal of Urology*, 71:433-438, 1993. ("Healthy prostate," Sarah Brewer, *Great Life*, March 1998.)
50. *British Journal of Urology*, 66:398-404, 1990. (*Great Life*, March 1998)
51. *Healing Foods*, Amanda Ursell, page 191.
52. *The Health Builder*, JI Rodale, Rodale Books, 1957.
53. *Diet & Health*, page 600.
54. "Exercise and BPH," *HealthNews*, Jan 1998. (*Arch. Int. Med.*, Nov 1997)
55. *Herbal Medicine*, Rudolf Fritz Weis, page 254.
56. *Ibid.*
57. "Preventing prostate cancer," *Nutrition Action* , July/Aug 2001.
58. *Planta Medicina*, 66(1):44-47, 2000.
59. *American Journal of Epidemiology*, 15 Jan 2003.
60. *UCBW*, Nov 2003.
61. *Diet & Health*, pages 371 and 514.
62. *Nutrition Guide* , Carlton Fredericks, page 28.
63. Marie-France Palin, et al., "Inhibitory effects of *Serenoa repens* on the kinetic of pig prostatic microsomal 5-alpha-reductase activity," *Endocrine*, 9(1):65-59, Aug 1998.
64. "Prostate drug: good and mostly bad news," *HealthFacts*, July 2003.
65. "Preventing prostate cancer with finasteride–a mixed blessing," *Harvard Men's Health Watch*, Oct 2003.
66. *NEJM*, 17 July 2003. (*HealthNews*, Aug 2003)
67. "Medications for enlarged prostate do not increase hip fracture risk," *JAMA*, 8 Oct 2008. (*UCLA Healthcare*, Dec 2008)
68. "Best free prostate cure," M. Laux MD, *Naturally Well Today*, 2006.
69. "Benign prostatic hyperplasia: current pharmacological treatment," Jonler et al., *Drugs*, 47:66-81, 1994.
70. "Drug therapy for prostate problems," *HealthNews*, 31 March 1998.

Pygeum

71. "Passing problems: prostate and *Prunus*," *HerbalGram*, No. 43, 1998.
72. *Ibid.*
73. "Antiproliferative effect of *Pygeum africanum* extract on rat prostatic fibroblasts," Yablonsky et al., *Journal of Urology*, 157:2381-2387, 1997.
74. "Efficacy and acceptability of Tadenan (*Pygeum africanum extract*) in the treatment of BPH: a multicentre trial in central Europe," Breza et al., *Current Medical Research and Opinion*, 14(3):127-139, 1998.
75. "Herbs for the prostate," *Northeast Herbalists Ass'n News*, Summer 1998.
76. *Ibid.*

Prostatitis

77. "Prostatitis predicament," *HealthNews*, May 1999.
78. "The other common prostate problem," *JHML*, April 1999.
79. "Prostatitis predicament," *HealthNews*, May 1999.
80. *JAMA*, 282:236, 1999.
81. "Prostatitis predicament," *HealthNews*, May 1999.
82. Dr. Ira Sharlip at the UCSF Med. Center, quoted in "Prostate: the misunderstood gland," Michael Castleman, *Ms*, Sept 1985.
83. *Herbal Medicine*, Weiss, page 255.
84. *HealthNews*, March 2000.
85. Shoskes et al., *Urology*, 54(6):960-963, Dec 1999.
86. "A wee problem," *AARP*, Jan/Feb 2005.
87. *Ibid.*
88. "Quercetin mysteries," *UCBW*, June 2008.
89. *School of Natural Healing*, Dr. Christopher, page 296.
90. *HealthNews*, March 2000.

Preventing prostate cancer

91. "Can dietary choices prevent prostate cancer?," EPBarrette MD, *Alternative Medicine Alert*, Jan 2001.
92. *Ibid.*
93. "Risky Legacy," *Science News*, 26 Aug 2006.
94. Thomas Schwenk MD, *Journal Watch General Medicine*, 29 Oct 2009.
95. *Environmental Nutrition*, Sept 2009.
96. "New nutrient shield found to protect prostate," Hiroshi Tazaki MD, *Journal of Longevity*, 5(6):7-9, 1999.
97. "Prostate cancer protection?" *HealthNews*, March, 2000.
98. "What men need to know about prostate cancer and diet," *Environmental Nutrition*, Sept 2002.
99. *Journal of Biological Chemistry*, 6 June 2003.
100. *Healing Foods*, Amanda Ursell, page 47.
101. "Can dietary choices prevent prostate cancer?," E-P Barrette MD, *Alternative Medicine Alert*, Jan 2001.

102. "Best free prostate cure," M. Laux MD, *Naturally Well Today*, 2006.
103. "Food, not pills, best Rx for lycopene's cancer protection," *Environmental Nutrition*, Feb 2004.
104. Ziegler et al., *Pharmaceutical Biology*, 40 (Supplement):59-69, 2002.
105. "Intake of carotenoids/retinol . . . risk of prostate cancer," Giovannucci et al., *Journal of the National Cancer Institute*, 87(23):1767-76.
106. "Veggies and the prostate, part 1," *Nutrition Action Healthletter*, April 2007. (*Cancer Res.*, 67:836, 2007.)
107. "Lycopenes in the prevention of prostate cancer," Diane Graves, *HerbalGram*, #58, 2003.
108. *Cancer Res.*, 67:836, 2007.
109. http://health.yahoo.net/galecontent/lycopene/2
110. "Food, not pills, best Rx. . .," *Environmental Nutrition*, Feb 2004.
111. *American Journal of Clinical Nutrition*, 86:672, 2007.
112. *Carcinogenesis*, May 2001.
113. *Ibid.*
114. *American Herb Ass'n Quarterly Newsletter*, Summer 2007.
115. *Clinical Cancer Research*, 12(13):4018-4026, 2006.
116. *American Herb Ass'n Quarterly Newsletter*, Summer 2007.
117. *American Journal of Epidemiology*, July 1996.
118. "Green tea for prostate health," *Alt Med Advisor*, Nov 1999.
119. Ann Hsing, *Journal of the National Cancer Institute*, 2007.
120. "Phytoestrogens and prostate cancer: possible preventative role," Frederick Stephens, *Medical Journal of Australia*, 167:138-30, 4 Aug 1997.
121. "Does high soy milk intake reduce prostate cancer incidence?," BK Jacobsen et al., *Cancer Causes Control*, Dec 1998, 9(6):553-7
122. "Selenium reduces prostate cancer risk," *Cancer Epidemiology, Biomarkers and Prevention*, 12:866-871, 2003.
123. *Journal of the National Cancer Institute*, 19 Aug 1998.
124. "Selenium & prostate cancer," *Am. J Clin. Nut.*, 85:209, 2007.
125. *Journal of the National Cancer Institute*, 19 Aug 1998.
126. "Effects of selenium supplementation for cancer prevention," LC Clark et al., *JAMA*, 276:1957-1963, 1996.
127. "Can selenium avert prostate cancer?," *Science News*, 19 Sept 1998.
128. *The Lancet*, 2 June 2001.
129. "Do Arctic diets protect prostates?," *Science News*, 18 Oct 2003.
130. *Healing Foods*, Amanda Ursell, page 191.
131. M.Laux MD, "Best free prostate cure," *Naturally Well Today*, 2006.
132. *Herbal Drugs and Phytopharmaceuticals*, Witchl, page 171.
133. "Update on calcium and prostate cancer," *Harvard Men's Health Watch*, Jan 2004.
134. "Just the Flax," *Nutrition Action Newsletter*, Dec 2005. (*American Journal of Clinical Nutrition*, 80:204, 2004)
135. *Proceedings: Nat'l Acad'y of Sci.*, 13 Dec 2004. (*HealthNews*, April 2005)

136. *Planta Med.*, 63(4):307-10, 1997. (*Integrative Breakthroughs*, May 2000)
137. "Meat and potatoes man?" *Nutrition Action Healthletter*, Dec 2009. (*Amer. Journal of Epidemiology*, 170:1165, 2009)
138. "Only well-done meat raises prostate cancer risk," Robert Finn, *Family Practice News*, 15 Jluy 2007.
139. "What men need to know about prostate cancer and diet," *Environmental Nutrition*, Sept 2002.
140. *Cancer Epidemiological Biomarkers Preview*, 16:1364, 2007.
141. *Nutrition Action,* Nov 2008.
142. "Can vitmain D save your life?" *Discover*, Jan 2008.
143. *Journal Nat'l Cancer*, 123;1877, 2008. (*Nutrition Action*, Nov 2008)
144. "Tough questions about a hard plastic," *Wellness Letter*, Feb 2009.
145. "Boosting boron could be healthful," *Science News*, 14 April 2001.
146. "Protecting the prostate," *Environmental Nutrition*, Sept 2006.
147. *Oncology*, 59(4):269-282, 2000.
148. *Journal of Urology*, Nov 2009.
149. "Vigorous exercise slows progress of prostate cancer," *Health News*, Sept 2005. (*Archives of Intenal Med*)
150. *British Journal of Urology Int.*, 92(3):211-216, 2003.
151. *American Journal of Epidemiology*, 1 May 2003.
152. *Ibid.*
153. "Farm harm: Ag chemicals may cause prostate cancer," *Science News*, 10 May 2003. (*Amer. Journal of Epidem.*, May 2003)
154. "Prostate cancer linked to rotating work schedule," *Science News,* 23 Sept 2004.
155. Peter Gann MD, quoted in *Wellness Letter*, Feb 2009.
156. "Antioxidant supplements may raise women's skin cancer risk," John Cartmell, www.dietadvisor.com
157. *Journal of the National Cancer Institute*, 99:754, 20 May 2007.
158. *Ibid.*
159. *UCBW*, Nov 2003.
160. *Environmental Nutrition*, Feb 2004.
161. *Journal of Urology* , Dec 2001.
162. "Selenium reduces prostate cancer risk," *Cancer Epidemiology, Biomarkers and Prevention*, 12:866-871, 2003.
163. *Ibid.*
164. "Prostate cancer: the diet angle," *Berkeley Wellness Letter,* Jan 2006.
165. *Journal of Clinical Oncology*, June 2009.
166. *Diet & Health*, page 319.
167. *Journal of Human Nutrition and Dietetics*, June 2009.
168. "Prostate cancer study stopped; vitamin E and selenium disappoint," *Wellness Letter*, Feb 2009. (*JAMA*, 7 Jan 2009)
169. "Preventing prostate cancer: No clear answers," *Nutrition Action Health Letter*, July/Aug 2001.

170. "Calcium and prostate cancer," *Consumer Report on Health,* Aug 2003.
171. Robert Anderson MD, "Is calcium bad for my prostate health?" *Natural Health,* Sept 2001.
172. *HealthNews,* Nov. 1998. (Marshall Goldberg MD, Jefferson Medical College, on research at McGill University.)
173. "Best free prostate cure," M Laux MD, *Naturally Well Today,* 2006.
174. "Can this drug prevent prostate cancer?" *Wellness Letter,* Sept 2008.
175. "Keep tabs on your prostate," Laux MD, *Natural Wellness,* April 2008.
176. *Ibid.*
177. *Lancet,* 20 Sept 2000.
178. "High cholesterol a risk for prostate cancer," *Envi. Nutr.,* June 2006.
179. *Ibid.*
180. *JAMA,* 19 June 2002.
endnotes 181, 182, 183, 184, 185 were removed

Prostate Cancer

- *Surviving Prostate Cancer: What You Need to Know to Make Informed Decisions,* E. Fuller Torrey, Yale University, 2006.
- *Prostate Tales: Men's Experiences with Prostate Cancer,* Ross Gray, Men's Studies Press, 2003.
- *Herbal Therapy for Prostate Cancer,* James Lewis, Health Ed, 1999.
- *Dr. Peter Scardino's Prostate Book,* Peter Scardino MD, Avery, 2005.
- *Seven Keys to Treating Prostate Cancer,* Johns Hopkins, 2009.

186. "Treatment for early prostate cancer not better than 'wait and see,'" *HealthFacts,* March 2009.
187. *Tufts Health & Nutrition Newsletter,* Dec 2004.
188. *Ibid.*
189. "New weapons against prostate cancer," Richard Saltus, *Popular Science,* Aug 2000.
190. *HealthFacts,* March 2009.
191. *British Journal of Cancer,* 30 Sept 2009. *(Duke Medicine,* Jan 2010)
192. "New prostate cancer study provides help with treatment decisions," *HealthFacts,* Oct 2002. (*JAMA,* 12 Sept 2002)
193. *Journal of the American Medical Association,* 9 June 2004.
194. "Treating prostate cancer," *HealthNews,* 5 Aug 1997.
195. "Beware of biased treatment advice," *Consumer Reports on Health,* June 2007.
196. "Prostate: misunderstood gland," Michael Castleman, *Ms,* Sept 1985.
197. "Intensity modulated radiation therapy safe, effective for prostate cancer," *HealthNews,* Jan 2007.
198. "Preventing prostate cancer: No clear answers," *Nutrition Action Health Letter,* July/Aug 2001.
199. "Blocking hormones to treat prostate cancer," *Health After 50,* Feb 2008.
200. "Protect your prostate," Harvey Simon MD, *Harvard Medical School Men's Health Watch,* 2001.

201. "Lycopenes in the prevention of prostate cancer," Diane Graves, *HerbalGram*, #58, 2003.
202. "Prostate paradox,"Jerome Groopman, *New Yorker*, 29 May 2000.
203. "Protect your prostate," Harvey Simon MD, *Harvard Medical School Men's Health Watch*, 2001.
204. "Latent carcinoma of prostate at autopsy in seven areas," Breslow et al., *Internat'l Journal of Cancer*, 20:680-688, 1977.
205. "Farm harm: Ag chemicals may cause prostate cancer," *Science News*, 10 May 2003. (*Amer. Journal of Epidem*., May 2003)
206. "Intake of carotenoids and retinol in relation to risk of prostate cancer," Giovannucci et al., *J. National Can. Inst.,* 87:1767-1776, 1995.
207. "Prostate cancer and lifestyle," *Nutrition Action,* Oct 2005. (*Journal of Urology*, 174:165, 2005.)
208. *Journal of the National Cancer Institute*, 93:1872, 2001.
209. "Flaxseed may stop prostate tumor growth," *HealthNews*, Nov 2007. (2007 meeting of American Society of Clinical Oncology)
210. "Just the Flax," *Nutrition Action News*, Dec 2005. (*Urology* 58:47, 2001)
211. *The Lancet*, June 2, 2001.
212. "Fish and the prostate," *Nutrition Action Healthletter*, Jan/Feb 2009. (*Amer. Journal of Clinical Nutrition*, 88:1297, 2008)
213. "Altering fatty acid levels in diet may reduce prostate cancer growth rate," William Aronson, *Clinical Cancer Research*, 1 Aug 2006.
214. *European Urology*, 35:388, 1999.
215. "Phytoestrogens," Mark Wahlqvist, *Medical Journal of Australia*, 167: 119, 4 Aug 1997.
216. "Phytoestrogens and prostate cancer: possible preventative role," Frederick Stephens, *Medical J. of Australia*, 167:138-30, 4 Aug 1997.
217. "Histopathological changes in androgen-deprived localised prostatic cancer," M. Hellstrom et al., *European Urology*, 24:461-465, 1993.
218. *University of California Wellness Letter*, Dec2007.
219. "Clues to prostate cancer," *Nutrition Action Healthletter*, March 1996.
220. "Soy phytochemicals and tea bioactive components synergistically inhibit androgen-sensitive human prostate tumors in mice," Zhou et al., *J. of Nutrition*, 133:516-521, 2003. (*Alt. Med. Research,* June 2003)
221. *Cancer*, 97(6):1442-1446, March 2003. (*Alt. Med. Research*, May 2003)
222. *Nutrition Action*, Nov 2008.
223. *Cancer Epi Biomarkers Prev*, 16:63, 2007.
224. "Is calcium bad for my prostate health?," R. Anderson MD, *Natural Health*, Sept 2001.
225. "Update on calcium and prostate cancer," *Harvard Men's Health Watch*, Jan 2004.
226. *Ibid.*
227. Paul Bergner, *Clinical Herbalism*, Spring 2002.
228. *Cancer Research,* 15 March 2006.

229. "Protecting the prostate," *Environmental Nutrition*, Sept 2006.
230. "Spice component vs cancer cells," *Science News*, 18 May 2002.
231. "Vitamin E protects prostate," *J. National Can. Inst.*, 18 March 1998.
232. "Prostate cancer and supplementation," Heinomem et al., *Journal of the National Cancer Instiitiute*, 90:440-446, 1998.
233."Supplemental vitamin E intake and prostate cancer risk. . . ," JM Chan et al., *Cancer Epidemiological Biomarkers Preview*, 8:893-899, 1999.
234. *Ibid.*
235. "Prostate cancer: the diet angle," *UC Berkeley Wellness Ltr*, Jan 2006.
236. *UCBW*, Nov 2003.
237. "Decreased incidence of prostate cancer with selenium supplementation," Clark et al., *British Jour.of Urology*, 81(5):730-734, 1998.
238. *Prostate Cancer and Prostatic Diseases Journal*, 2003.
239. "The prostate predicament," B. Carey, *Health*, May/June 1994.
240. "Blocking a key gene could reduce prostate cancer's deadliness," *HealthNews*, March 2005.
241. "Blocking hormones treats prostate cancer," *Health After 50*, Feb 2008.
242. "Treatment for early prostate cancer not better than 'wait and see,'" *HealthFacts*, March 2009.
243. "Clues to prostate cancer," B Liebman, *Nutrition Action*, March 1996.
244. "Hormone-blockers hailed for prostate cancer," *New York Post*, 9 Dec 1999. (*JAMA*, Edward Messing MD)
245. *HealthFacts*, March 2009.
246. "State of the heart therapy for prostate cancer," *Harvard Heart Letter*, April 2008.
247. "Blocking a key gene could reduce prostate cancer's deadliness," *HealthNews*, March 2005.
248. *HealthNews*, Aug 2006. (*British Journal of Urology International*)
249. "Exploring a prostate therapy called PC-SPES," *Cedars-Sinai Medical Center*. (www.wholehealthmd.com, 2001.)
250. *Urology*, 57:122, 2001.
251. "Prostate cancer," *The* Integrative Medicine *Consult*, May 2000.
• Info on PC-SPES: www.pcspes.com (1-800-CEDARS-1)
252. Press release from Dendreon Corp. (the developer), 15 April 2009.
253. "Prostate cancer 'vaccine'," *Mayo Clinic Health Letter*, Dec 2009.
254. "Can fasting blunt chemotherapy's debilitating side effects?" *Science*, 321: 1146-7, 29 Aug 2008.
255. "Medications for enlarged prostate do not increase hip fracture risk," *JAMA*, 8 October 2008. (*UCLA Healthcare*, Dec 2008)
256. *European Urology*, vol 54:924, 2009.
257. "Prostate cancer treatment recommendations biased according to specialty," *HealthFacts*, July 2000. (quote: Tim Wilt MD)
258. *New England J. of Medicine*, 12 May 2005. (*Science News*, 14 May 2005)

259. "Facing incontinence after prostate surgery," *JHML*, June 2008. (*Archives of Internal Medicine*)
260. "Prostate paradox," *The New Yorker*, 29 May 2000. (quote: Dr. Talcott)
261. *Archives of Internal Medicine*, 8 Oct 2007. (*HealthNews*, Jan 2008)
262. "Prostate surgery OK for elders," *Duke Med.*, March 2007. (*Urology*)
263. "Treating prostate cancer," *HealthNews*, 5 Aug. 1997.
264. "Sex after prostatectomy?," *Health After 50*, July 2009.
265. "Keeping dry after prostate surgery," *HealthNews*, March 2000. (*JAMA*, 19 Jan 2000)
266. "After prostate surgery," *JHML*, June 2008.
267. "Treating prostate cancer," *HealthNews*, 5 Aug 1997.
268. "The prostate predicament," *B* Carey,*Health*, May/June 1994.
269. "After prostate surgery," *JHML*, June 2008.
270. *Ibid.*
271. *Lancet*, 8 Jan 2000.
• Continence audio tape/ training manual: 1-800-BLADDER.
272. "The prostate predicament," B Carey, *Health*, May/June 1994.
273. "Prostate surgery OK for elders," *Duke Med.*, March 2007. (*Urology*)
274. "Rising PSA after prostate surgery may guide subsequent treatment," *HealthNews*, July 2001. (*JAMA*, 5 May, 2001)
275. "Ultrasound's new focus," *Science News*, 29 April 2006.
276. *Tufts Health & Nutrition Newletter*, Dec 2004.
277. "Treating prostate cancer," *HealthNews*, 5 Aug 1997.
278. *Tufts Health & Nutrition Newletter*, Dec 2004. (report from NCI)
279. *Lancet*, 23 Jan 2001.
280. *Ibid.*
281. "Radiation reaction,"*Saturday Evening Post*, July 2007.
282. *Tufts Health & Nutrition Newletter*, Dec 2004.
283. "The prostate predicament," B Carey, *Health*, May/June 1994.
284. *Ibid.*
285. "Intensity modulated radiation therapy safe, effective for prostate cancer," *HealthNews*, Jan 2007. (*J. of Urology*)
286. "Proton beam therapy/prostate cancer," *Health Afer 50*, April 2009.
287. "New weapons against prostate cancer," Richard Saltus, *Popular Science*, Aug 2000.
288. *Journal of Urology*, vol. 181:1665. (*Health After 50*, Nov 2009.)
289. *HealthNews*, April 2005.
290. "Cryosurgery for recurrent prostate cancer following radiation therapy," *US Dept. of Health and Human Services*, June 1999.
291. "Treating prostate cancer," *HealthNews*, 5 Aug 1997.
292. *Hit Below the Belt*, F. Ralph Berberich, Celestial Arts, 2000.

Saw Palmetto

293. *NEJM*, August 1996.
294. *Dr. Duke's Essential Herbs*, page 219.
295. *Endocrine*, 9(1):65-59, Aug. 1998.
296. *The Botanical Pharmacy*, Heather Boon, Quarry Press, 1999. (Includes 39 references to scientific studies on saw palmetto.)
297. "Extract of *Serenoa repens* in the treatment of BPH: A multicentre study," J Braeckman, *Current Therapy Research*, 55(7):776-85, 1994.
298. WJ Vahlensieck et al., "BPH – treatment with sabal fruit extract, a study of 1,334 patients," *Fortschritte der Medizin*, 111:323-326, 1993.
299. *Dr. Duke's Essential Herbs*, page 219.
300. *Ibid.*, page 224.
301. *Ibid.*
302. "Palmetto and the prostate," *Nutrition Action Healthletter*, Sept 2000.
303. vitanetonline.com/forums/1/thread/1534
304. "Comparison of phytotherapy with finasteride in the treatment of BPH: A randomized international study of 1,098 patients," JC Carraro et al., *Prostate*, 29:231-40, 1996.(*Nut. Action Healthletter*, Sept 2000)
305. *Dr. Duke's Essential Herbs*, page 224.
306. *Ibid.*
307. "Natural relief for prostate problems," Denise Webb, *Natural Foods Merchandiser*, Sept 2006.
308. *Dr. Duke's Essential Herbs*, page 219.

Dear reader, dear friends,

I loathe and despise footnotes.

The sun is shining, the flowers are blooming, the baby goats are romping, and I am sitting here stuck at the computer making the f-ing footnotes as clear, comprehensive, and complete as possible.

Yes, yes, I know how important they are. I know you want them; I understand they are necessary, needed. (But I'd rather be out in the woods.)

"Show your work!" my favorite math teacher always admonished me. And the footnotes show my work. (Or at least a part of it. For every reference cited, I read four or five that I didn't cite.)

This section is a tad less polished than I (and my editor Betsy) would like. Some holes here and there. (How could I have misplaced the source for that quote!!!) But, sweet goddess, fourty-four pages of footnotes; more than 1200 references, plus lots of yummy resources. It's a lovely offering, even if it isn't perfect. Let's just call it a work in progress. My website – susunwed.com – and the wise woman web stand ready to help you.

Green blessings.

Susun

Grandmother Growth and Grandfather Growth hold hands as they turn and walk into the woods, lope across the savannah, dive off the cliff into the ocean, disappear into the mist, glow so brightly you have to shut your eyes, sink into the earth, call out to you: "Listen, listen, listen."

Is it words or is it music? Is it a sense or is it a feeling? Somehow you know you have not seen the last of this old couple.

In your dreams, in your meditations, in your visions, in your waking fantasies, they will arise and speak the truth of your own being to you. Listen. Listen. . . .

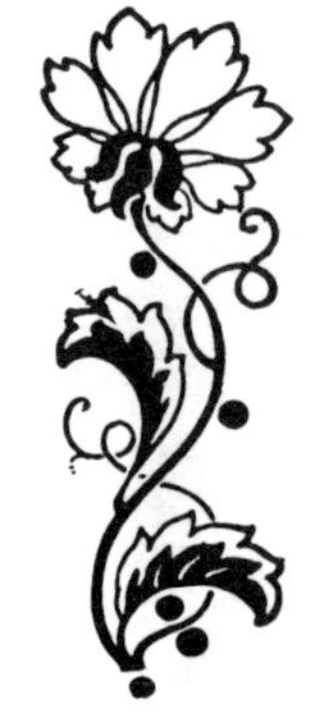

Other books you will want to read from

Ash Tree Publishing

Women's Health, Women's Spirituality

Wise Woman Herbal Series

best-sellers by

Susun S Weed

Wise Woman Herbal for the Childbearing Year $11.95
Healing Wise, Everyone's Herbal $17.95
New Menopausal Years, the Wise Woman Way $16.95
Breast Cancer? Breast Health! The Wise Woman Way . . $21.95
Down There: Sexual and Reproductive Health $29.95

Herbals of Our Foremothers Series

classics by

Juliette de Bairacli Levy

Nature's Children $15.95
Common Herbs for Natural Health $15.95
Traveler's Joy $11.95
Spanish Mountain Life $16.95
Summer in Galilee $24.95
Gypsy in New York $21.95

and, by **Maida Silverman**

A City Herbal $13.95

To order:

- *Visit* **www.wisewomanbookshop.com**
- *Write to* PO Box 64, Woodstock, NY 12498

Prices subject to change.